Saunders' Pocket Essentials of

Clinical
Medicine

SAUNDERS' POCKET ESSENTIALS

Series Editors
Parveen Kumar and Michael Clark
Medical College of St Bartholomew's Hospital
London

Titles in this series:

Basant Puri, Psychiatry

Saunders' Pocket Essentials of

Clinical Medicine

**Anne Ballinger and
Stephen Patchett**
*Department of Gastroenterology
St Bartholomew's Hospital
London, UK*

Series editors
Parveen Kumar and Michael Clark

W.B. Saunders Company Limited
London   Philadelphia   Toronto   Sydney   Tokyo

W.B. Saunders Company Ltd 24–28 Oval Road
London NW1 7DX, UK

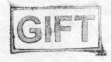

The Curtis Center
Independence Square West
Philadelphia, PA 19106–3399
USA

Harcourt Brace & Company
55 Horner Avenue, Toronto,
Ontario, M8Z 4X6, Canada

Harcourt Brace & Company,
Australia
30–52 Smidmore Street
Marrackville, NSW 2204
Australia

Harcourt Brace & Company,
Japan Inc.
Ichibancho Central Building
22–1 Ichibancho
Chiyoda-ku, Tokyo 102, Japan

A catalogue record is available from the British Library

ISBN 0–7020–1921–6

Typeset by Columns Design and Production Services Ltd,
Reading and printed in Great Britain by
Mackays of Chatham PLC, Chatham, Kent

Contents

Series Preface

Medical students and doctors in training are expected to travel to different hospitals and community health centres as part of their education. Many books are too large to carry on a regular basis but are still necessary for the basic understanding of disease processes. This series of books is designed to provide portable, pocket-sized companions to larger texts such as *Clinical Medicine*. They all contain core material for quick revision, easy reference and practical management. The modern format makes them easy to read providing an indispensable 'pocket essential'.

PARVEEN KUMAR AND MICHAEL CLARK
Series Editors

Preface

Medical students are confronted with the daunting task of assimilating a vast quantity of information for their final examinations. This compact textbook of clinical medicine aims to facilitate this process by providing a concise yet comprehensive account of general medical topics. Certain restrictions become necessary in a 'compact' textbook, with topics such as childhood diseases, psychiatry and most basic physiology being deliberately omitted. The section on tropical medicine includes only those conditions that a medical student is likely to encounter in the UK.

The design of this book facilitates cross-referencing to its larger companion *Clinical Medicine* (cross-references appear in the form of [CM p. ...]). The inclusion of sample examination questions at the end of each chapter will not only allow the student to test his knowledge on the subject but also to focus his attention on areas most commonly addressed in the final medical examination. A dictionary of terms has been provided in most chapters as a convenient source of definitions and explanations of specialised investigations.

We would particularly like to thank Mike Clark and Parveen Kumar for their support and assistance in the writing of this book. We are also indebted to all the contributors of the parent text *Clinical Medicine* on which this book is based.

ANNE BALLINGER AND STEPHEN PATCHETT

Abbreviations

ACE	angiotensin converting enzyme
ACTH	adrenocorticotrophic hormone
ADH	antidiuretic hormone
AF	atrial fibrillation
AIDS	acquired immunodeficiency syndrome
ANA	antinuclear antibodies
ANCA	antineutrophil cytoplasmic antibodies
ANF	antinuclear factor
ARDS	adult respiratory distress syndrome
AST	aspartate aminotransferase
AV	atrioventricular
AXR	abdominal X-ray
BCG	bacille Calmette-Guérin
BNF	*British National Formulary*
BP	blood pressure
CAL	chronic airflow limitation
CAPD	continuous ambulatory peritoneal dialysis
CCF	congestive cardiac failure
CCU	coronary care unit
CLL	chronic lymphatic leukaemia
CM	*Clinical Medicine* (Baillière Tindall 1994)
CML	chronic myeloid leukaemia
CNS	central nervous system
CRP	C-reactive protein
CSF	cerebrospinal fluid
CT	computerized tomography
CVP	central venous pressure
CXR	chest X-ray
DIC	disseminated intravascular coagulation
DNA	deoxyribonucleic acid
DVT	deep venous thrombosis
ECG	electrocardiogram
EEG	electroencephalogram
ERCP	endoscopic retrograde cholangiopancreatography
ESR	erythrocyte sedimentation rate
FBC	full blood count
GABA	γ–aminobutyric acid
γGT	γ-glutamyltranspeptidase
GFR	glomerular filtration rate
Hb	haemoglobin
5HIAA	5-hydroxyindoleacetic acid
HIV	human immunodeficiency virus

HLA	human leucocyte antigen
Ig	immunoglobulin (e.g. IgM = immunoglobulin of the M class)
INR	international normalized ratio
iu/IU	international unit
iv	intravenous
IVP	intravenous pyelogram
JVP	jugular venous pressure
LP	lumbar puncture
LVF	left ventricular failure
MCV	mean corpuscular volume
ME	myalgic encephalomyelitis
MRI	magnetic resonance imaging
MRSA	methicillin-resistant *staphylococcus aureus*
MSU	mid-stream urine
NSAIDs	non-steroidal anti-inflammatory drugs
P_aCO_2	partial pressure of carbon dioxide in arterial blood
P_aO_2	partial pressure of oxygen in arterial blood
PCV	packed cell volume
PR	per rectum (rectal instillation)
PT	prothrombin time
PTC	percutaneous transhepatic cholangiography
PTCA	percutaneous transluminal coronary angioplasty
PTTK	partial thromboplastin time with kaolin
RCC	red cell count
RNA	ribonucleic acid
SLE	systemic lupus erythematosis
STD	sexually transmitted disease
SVC	superior vena cava
SVT	supraventricular tachycardia
TIA	transient ischaemic attack
TPN	total parenteral nutrition
TRH	thyroid releasing hormone
TSH	thyroid stimulating hormone
VDRL	Venereal Disease Research Laboratory (test for syphilis)
VF	ventricular fibrillation
VIP	vasoactive intestinal polypeptide
VT	ventricular tachycardia
WBC	white blood (cell) count
WCC	white cell count

Normal Values

Haemotology

Haemoglobin
   Male   14.0–17.7 g/dl
   Female   12.0–16.0 g/dl

Haemoglobin	
Male	14.0–17.7 g/dl
Female	12.0–16.0 g/dl
Mean corpuscular volume (MCV)	80–96 fl
White cell count	$4–11 \times 10^9$/litre
Platelet count	$150–400 \times 10^9$/litre
Serum B_{12}	160–925 ng/litre (150–675 pmol/litre)
Serum folate	4–18 µg/litre (5–63 nmol/litre)
Erythrocyte sedimentation rate (ESR)	<20 mm in 1 hour

Coagulation

Partial thromboplastin time (PTTK)	35–50 s
Prothrombin time	12–16 s

Serum Biochemistry

Alanine aminotransferase (ALT)	5–40 U/litre
Albumin	34–48 g/litre
Alkaline phosphatase	25–115 U/litre
Amylase	<220 U/litre
Aspartate aminotransferase (AST)	10–40 U/litre
Bicarbonate	22–30 mmol/litre
Bilirubin	<17 µmol/litre (0.3–1.5 mg/dl)
Calcium	2.20–2.67 mmol/litre (8.5–10.5 mg/dl)
Chloride	95–106 mmol/litre
Creatinine	0.06–0.12 mmol/litre (0.6–1.5 mg/dl)
Ferritin	5.8–144 nmol/litre (15–300 µg/litre)
Glucose	4.5–5.6 mmol/litre (70–110 mg/dl)
Potassium	3.5–5.0 mmol/litre
Sodium	135–146 mmol/litre
Urea	2.5–6.7 mmol/litre (8–25 mg/dl)

CHAPTER 1

Infectious Diseases and Tropical Medicine

Infectious diseases are the most common diseases of humans and a major source of morbidity and mortality in both developed and developing countries. Upper respiratory tract infections and gastroenteritis are commonly seen in the community and do not often need admission to hospital. With increasing travel abroad more tropical diseases are now seen in the UK and, with the emergence of AIDS, opportunistic infections are seen more commonly. In the UK some infectious diseases must be notified to the local Medical Officer for Environmental Health; these are indicated by **ND** where appropriate.

Table 1.1 Causes of pyrexia of unknown origin

Infection (40%)
Pyogenic abscess: liver, pelvic, subphrenic
Biliary infection
Urinary infection
Tuberculosis
Subacute infective endocarditis
Viruses, e.g. Epstein–Barr, cytomegalovirus, HIV-related
Brucellosis

Cancer (30%)
Lymphoma
Leukaemia
Solid tumours, e.g. renal carcinoma, hepatocellular carcinoma, pancreatic cancer

Immunogenic (20%)
Drugs
Connective tissue diseases
Rheumatoid arthritis
Sarcoidosis
Polymyalgia rheumatica/cranial arteritis

Factitious (1–5%)
Switching thermometers
Injection of pyogenic material

Remains unknown (5–9%)

Pyrexia of unknown origin

Pyrexia of unknown origin (PUO) is defined as a documented fever (>38°C) lasting more than 2 weeks in which a clinical history, thorough physical examination and routine investigations have failed to reveal a cause. Occult infection remains the most common cause in adults. Connective tissue diseases, drug hypersensitivity and malignancy are other causes (Table 1.1).

Investigations

FIRST-LINE INVESTIGATIONS should be repeated as results may have changed since the tests were first performed:

- Full blood count including a differential white cell count (WCC) and blood film
- Erythrocyte sedimentation rate (ESR)
- Urea and electrolytes, serum liver biochemistry and blood glucose
- Blood cultures: several sets from different sites at different times
- Microscopy and culture of urine, sputum and faeces
- Baseline serum for virology
- Chest radiograph

SECOND-LINE INVESTIGATIONS are performed in patients who remain undiagnosed and repeat physical examination is unhelpful.

- Abdominal ultrasonography and CT + ? MRI to detect occult abscesses and malignancy
- Echocardiography for infective endocarditis
- Serum rheumatoid factor and antinuclear antibody
- Needle biopsy of the liver
- Bone marrow examination
- ?? Exploratory laparotomy in patients who remain undiagnosed (very rarely needed)

Management

The treatment is of the underlying cause.

Septicaemia

The term *bacteraemia* refers to the transient presence of organisms in the blood (generally without causing symptoms) as a result of local infection or penetrating injury. The term *septicaemia*, on the other hand, is usually reserved for when bacteria or fungi are actually multiplying in the blood, usually with the production of severe systemic symptoms such as fever and hypotension. Septicaemia has a high mortality, without treatment, and demands immediate attention. The pathogenesis and management of septic shock is discussed on pages 364, 365 and 367.

Aetiology

Overall, about 40% of cases are the result of Gram-positive organisms and 60% of Gram-negative ones. Fungi are much less common but should be considered, particularly in the immunocompromised. In the previously healthy adult, septicaemia may occur from a source of infection in the chest (e.g. with pneumonia), urinary tract (often Gram-negative rods) or biliary tree (commonly *Enterococcus faecalis*, *Escherichia coli*). Intravenous drug abusers frequently suffer septicaemia caused by *Staphylococcus aureus* and *Pseudomonas* sp. Hospitalized patients are susceptible to infection from wounds, indwelling urinary catheters and intravenous cannulae.

Clinical features

Fever, rigors and hypotension are the cardinal features of severe septicaemia. Lethargy, headache and a minor change in conscious level may be preceding features. In elderly and immunocompromised patients, clinical features may be quite subtle and a high index of suspicion is needed.

Certain bacteria are associated with a particularly fulminating course:

- Staphylococci that produce an exotoxin called toxic shock syndrome toxin-1. The toxic shock syndrome is characterized by an abrupt onset of fever, rash, diarrhoea and shock. It is associated with the use of infected tampons in women but may occur in anyone including children.
- ND Meningococci that produce the Waterhouse–Friderichsen syndrome. This is a rapidly fatal illness (without treatment) with purpuric skin rash and shock. Adrenal haemorrhage (and hypoadrenalism) may or may not be present.

Investigations

In addition to blood count, serum electrolytes and liver biochemistry:

- BLOOD CULTURES
- CULTURES FROM POSSIBLE SOURCE: urine, abscess aspirate, sputum
- IN SOME CASES: chest radiography, abdominal ultrasonography and C T scan.

Management

Antibiotic therapy should be started immediately the diagnosis is suspected. The probable site of origin of sepsis will often be apparent and knowledge of the likely microbial flora can be used to choose appropriate treatment. In cases where 'blind antibiotic' treatment is started, a reasonable combination would be intravenous gentamicin and cefuroxime with flucloxacillin if staphylococcal infection is a possibility. Therapy may subsequently be altered on the basis of culture and sensitivity results.

COMMON VIRAL INFECTIONS

Measles ND

Measles is caused by infection with an RNA paramyxovirus which is spread by droplets. With the introduction of immunization policies in the West (live attenuated vaccine), the incidence has fallen but it remains a common infection in developing countries where it is associated with a high morbidity and mortality. One attack confers lifelong immunity.

Clinical features

The incubation period is 8–14 days. Two distinct phases of the disease can be recognized.

THE INFECTIOUS PRE-ERUPTIVE AND CATARRHAL STAGE
There is fever, cough, rhinorrhoea, conjunctivitis and Koplik's spots in the mouth (small, grey, irregular lesions on an erythematous base, commonly on the inside of the cheek).

THE NON-INFECTIOUS ERUPTIVE OR EXANTHEMATOUS STAGE
Characterized by the presence of a maculopapular rash which starts on the face and spreads to involve the whole body. The rash becomes confluent and blotchy.

COMPLICATIONS (UNCOMMON IN THE HEALTHY CHILD)
Gastroenteritis, pneumonia, otitis media, encephalitis, myocarditis, subacute sclerosing panencephalitis (rare).

Management

The diagnosis is usually clinical and treatment is symptomatic. Measles vaccine is given to children between 12 and 18 months of age in combination with mumps and rubella vaccine (MMR).

Mumps ND

Mumps is also caused by infection with a paramyxovirus, spread by droplets. The incubation period averages 18 days.

Clinical features

Mumps is predominantly an infection of school-aged children and young adults. There is fever, headache and malaise, followed by the development of parotid gland swelling. Less common features are orchitis, meningitis, pancreatitis, oophoritis, myocarditis and hepatitis.

Management

Diagnosis is usually clinical. In doubtful cases demonstration of a rise in serum antibody titres is necessary for diagnosis. Treatment is symptomatic. The disease is prevented by administration of a live attenuated mumps virus vaccine.

Rubella ND

Rubella is caused by an RNA virus and has a peak age of incidence of 15 years. The incubation period is 14–21 days.

During the prodrome the patient complains of malaise, fever and lymphadenopathy (suboccipital, postauricular, posterior cervical nodes). A pinkish macular rash appears on the face and trunk after about 7 days and lasts for up to 3 days.

Diagnosis
Diagnosis is made by demonstrating a rising serum antibody titre in paired samples taken 2 weeks apart or by the detection of rubella-specific IgM.

Management
Treatment is symptomatic. Complications are uncommon but include arthralgia, encephalitis and thrombocytopenia.

Congenital rubella syndrome
Maternal infection during pregnancy may affect the fetus, particularly if infection is acquired in the first trimester. Congenital rubella syndrome is characterized by the presence of congenital cardiac defects, eye lesions particularly cataracts, microcephaly, mental handicap and deafness. There may also be persistent viral infection of the liver, lungs and heart, with hepatomegaly, pneumonitis and myocarditis. The teratogenic effects of rubella underly the importance of preventing maternal infection with immunization.

Herpes viruses

Herpes simplex virus (HSV) infection
HSV-1 causes:

- Herpetic stomatitis with buccal ulceration, fever and local lymphadenopathy
- Herpetic whitlow: damage to the skin over a finger allows access of the virus with development of irritating vesicles
- Keratoconjunctivitis
- Encephalitis
- Systemic infection in immunocompromised patients

HSV-2 is transmitted sexually and causes genital herpes with painful genital ulceration, fever and lymphadenopathy. There may be systemic infection in the immunocompromised host. These divisions are not rigid, because HSV-1 can give rise to genital herpes.

Recurrent HSV infection occurs when the virus lies dormant in ganglion cells and is reactivated by trauma, febrile illnesses and ultraviolet irradiation. This leads to recurrent labialis ('cold sores') or recurrent genital herpes.

Investigations
The diagnosis is often clinical but the virus may be cultured from lesions. Herpes simplex encephalitis is discussed on page 487.

Management
Acyclovir cream is used topically for HSV-1 infection. Oral acyclovir tablets are given for genital herpes.

Herpes zoster
VARICELLA (CHICKENPOX)
Primary infection with this virus causes chickenpox which may produce a mild childhood illness, although this can be severe in adults and immunocompromised patients.

Clinical features
After an incubation period of 14–21 days there is a brief prodromal period of fever, headache and malaise. The rash, predominantly on the face, scalp and trunk, begins as macules and develops into papules and vesicles which heal with crusting. Complications include pneumonia and central nervous system involvement.

Investigations
The diagnosis is usually clinical. Electron microscopy of vesicle fluid may reveal the virus.

Management
Healthy children require no treatment. Immunocompromised patients are treated with intravenous acyclovir and varicella-zoster immunoglobulin (VZIg).

HERPES ZOSTER (SHINGLES)
After the primary infection herpes zoster remains dormant in dorsal root ganglia and reactivation causes shingles.

Clinical features
Pain and tingling in a dermatomal distribution precede the rash by a few days. The rash consists of papules and vesicles in the same dermatome. The most common sites are the lower thoracic dermatomes and the ophthalmic division of the trigeminal nerve (pages 454 and 455).

Management
Treatment is with oral acyclovir given as early as possible. The main complication is postherpetic neuralgia which can be severe and last for years. Treatment is with carbamazepine or phenytoin.

Infectious mononucleosis
Infectious mononucleosis is caused by the Epstein–Barr virus (EBV) and predominantly affects young adults. EBV is probably transmitted in saliva and by aerosol.

Clinical features
Many infections are asymptomatic. In symptomatic patients the main features are fever, headache, sore throat and a transient macular rash. There may be palatal petechiae, cervical lymphadenopathy, splenomegaly and mild hepatitis.

Rare complications include splenic rupture, myocarditis and meningitis.

Investigations

Atypical lymphocytes on a peripheral blood film strongly suggest infection. The diagnosis is confirmed by a positive Paul–Bunnell reaction (agglutination of sheep red cells by heterophile antibodies) and IgM antibodies to EBV.

Management

Most cases require no treatment. Corticosteroids are given if there are systemic complications. Infection with *Toxoplasma gondii* or cytomegalovirus may produce a similar clinical picture in immunocompetent adults.

TROPICAL MEDICINE

Malaria ND

Malaria is a protozoan parasite widespread in the tropics and subtropics (Figure 1.1). Each year 270 million people are affected with a mortality rate of 1%.

Aetiology

Travellers abroad are infected following the bite of an infected female mosquito of the genus *Anopheles*. Rarely the parasite is transmitted by importation of infected mosquitoes by air (airport malaria).

Four malaria parasites may infect humans; by far the most hazardous is *Plasmodium falciparum* the symptoms of which can rapidly progress from an acute fever with rigors to severe multiorgan failure, coma and death. Once successfully treated this form does not relapse. The other malaria parasites *P. vivax, P. ovale* and *P. malariae* cause a more benign illness which may relapse.

Pathogenesis

The infective form of the parasite (*sporozoites*) pass through the skin and via the blood stream to the liver. After a variable number of days they invade red blood cells and pass through further stages of development which terminates with the rupture of the red cell. Rupture of red blood cells contributes to anaemia and releases pyrogens causing fever. Red blood cells infected with *P. falciparum* adhere to the endothelium of small vessels and the consequent vascular occlusion causes severe organ damage, chiefly in the kidney, liver and brain. All the different forms, except *P. falciparum*, may remain latent in the liver and this is believed to be responsible for the relapses which may occur.

Clinical features

The incubation period varies:

- 10–14 days in *P. vivax, P. ovale* and *P. falciparum* infection.
- 18 days to 6 weeks in *P. malariae* infection.

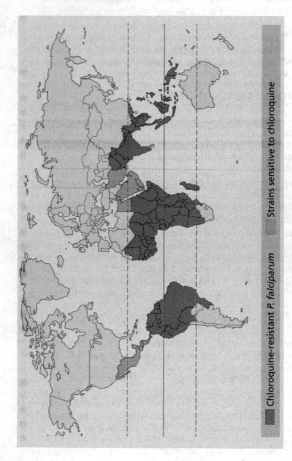

Figure 1.1 Malaria – geographical distribution

Chloroquine-resistant *P. falciparum*   Strains sensitive to chloroquine

The onset of symptoms may be delayed in the partially immune or after prophylaxis.

There is an abrupt onset of fever (>40°C), tachycardia and rigors, followed by profuse sweating some hours later. This may be accompanied by anaemia and hepatosplenomegaly.

P. falciparum should be considered a medical emergency because patients may deteriorate rapidly. The following clinical forms are recognized and are more likely to occur when more than 2% of the red blood cells are parasitized.

CEREBRAL MALARIA is characterized by high fever, convulsions, coma and eventually death. Hypoglycaemia, a complication of severe malaria, may present in a similar way and must be excluded.

BLACKWATER FEVER, so called because of the production of dark brown–black urine (haemoglobinuria) resulting from severe intravascular haemolysis.

Table 1.2 Possible features of falciparum malaria

Central nervous system
Cerebral malaria

Renal
Haemoglobinuria (Blackwater fever)
Oliguria
Uraemia (acute tubular necrosis)

Blood
Severe anaemia
Disseminated intravascular coagulation

Respiratory
Adult respiratory distress syndrome

Metabolic
Hypoglycaemia
Metabolic acidosis

Gastrointestinal
Diarrhoea
Jaundice
Splenic rupture

Other
Shock
Hyperpyrexia

Investigations
The diagnosis is made by finding malaria parasites on thick and thin blood smears stained with Giemsa, Wright or Leishman stains. The four species of malaria are distinguishable from each other on examination of peripheral

smears. Other investigations include full blood count, serum urea and electrolytes, and blood glucose.

Management

The acute treatment and eradication therapy of malaria is summarized in Table 1.3. Chloroquine is not used in treatment if it has been used as prophylaxis.

Table 1.3 Treatment of an acute attack of malaria

Treatment	
Uncomplicated malaria in a chloroquine-sensitive area	Oral chloroquine 600 mg of base, 300 mg 6 h later, then 300 mg/ 24 h for 3 days*
Uncomplicated malaria in a chloroquine-resistant area	Oral quinine sulphate 650 mg three times daily + sulphadiazine 500 mg twice daily for 5 days + pyrimethamine 25 mg twice daily for 3 days Other treatments: mefloquine halofantrine
Complicated *P. falciparum* malaria	Intravenous quinine until tablets tolerated
ERADICATION	
For *P. vivax, P. malariae, P. ovale*	Oral primaquine 7.5 mg daily for 14 days

* The active component of many drugs, whether acid or base, is relatively insoluble and this presents a problem in formulation. This is overcome by using a soluble salt e.g. adding a base to an acid and vice versa. Hence, the base chloroquine is available as chloroquine sulphate or chloroquine phosphate. Chloroquine base 150 mg = chloroquine sulphate 200 mg = chloroquine phosphate 250 mg. The amount of drug prescribed is given as the active component, i.e. the base, to avoid confusion as to how much chloroquine is actually to be given.

Prevention and control

As a result of changing patterns of resistance, advice about chemoprophylaxis should be sought before leaving for a malaria-endemic area. Prophylaxis does not afford full protection. Drug regimens should be started at least 1 week before departure and continued without interruption for 6 weeks after return. The rationale for this advice is to ensure therapeutic drug levels before travelling and to enable unwanted effects to be dealt with before departure. The continued use of drugs after returning home will deal with infection contracted on the last day of exposure.

CHLOROQUINE

In low-risk areas chloroquine 300 mg weekly is
recommended. In areas of limited chloroquine resistance this
is combined with proguanil 200 mg daily. This regimen has
few side effects and is safe in pregnancy.

MEFLOQUINE

Mefloquine 250 mg weekly is used in areas where falciparum
malaria is highly resistant to chloroquine (east and central
Africa).

MALOPRIM + CHLOROQUINE

Maloprim + chloroquine are administered weekly to
travellers to the Pacific Islands.

Individual measures to control insect bites include mosquito
repellents, impregnated bed nets and protective clothing.

Enteric fever

Typhoid fever and paratyphoid fever are caused by
Salmonella typhi and *Salmonella paratyphi* (types A, B and
C) respectively.

Typhoid fever ND

Humans are the only known reservoir of infection and the
spread is faecal–oral.

Clinical features

After an incubation period of 10–14 days there is an insidious
onset of headache, dry cough and constipation, and a rising
fever with relative bradycardia. In the second week of the
illness an erythematous maculopapular rash that blanches on
pressure and is referred to as 'rose spots' appears, chiefly on
the upper abdomen and thorax, and lasts for only 2–3 days.
There is splenomegaly (75%), cervical lymphadenopathy and
hepatomegaly (30%). Diarrhoea may develop.

Complications, usually occurring in the third week, are
pneumonia, meningitis, acute cholecystitis, osteomyelitis,
intestinal perforation and haemorrhage. Recovery occurs in
the fourth week.

Investigations

CULTURE OF THE ORGANISM FROM:

- Blood in the first 2 weeks
- Urine in the second week
- Stool cultures in weeks 2–4

BLOOD COUNT shows leukopenia.

SEROLOGY (Widal test) may show a sequential rise in
antibody titre.

Management

Chloramphenicol for 2 weeks is the treatment of choice.
Alternatives are co-trimoxazole and ampicillin.

Infection is cleared when consecutive cultures of urine and faeces are negative. Some patients become chronic carriers with the focus of infection in the gallbladder. Treatment is with ampicillin and probenecid for 6 weeks, but cholecystectomy may be needed. A live oral vaccine and a parenteral vaccine are available which both give protection for about 3 years.

Paratyphoid fever ND

Paratyphoid results in a milder illness that is otherwise clinically indistinguishable from typhoid fever. Treatment is with co-trimoxazole for 2 weeks.

Enterocolitis ND

Other *Salmonella* species (*S. choleraesuis* and *S. enteritidis*) cause a self-limiting infection presenting with diarrhoea and vomiting.

Amoebiasis ND

Amoebiasis is caused by infection of the human gastrointestinal tract with the protozoal organism *Entamoeba histolytica*. Infection occurs worldwide although much higher incidence rates are found in the tropics and subtropics. The modes of transmission are:

- Ingestion of cysts in contaminated food and water
- Person-to-person spread
- Sexual transmission among homosexual men

Clinical features
INTESTINAL AMOEBIASIS (AMOEBIC DYSENTERY)
Invasion of the colonic epithelium by *E. histolytica* leads to tissue necrosis and ulceration. Ulceration may deepen and progress under the mucosa to form typical 'flask-like ulcers'. The presentation of amoebic colitis varies from mild bloody diarrhoea to fulminating colitis with the risk of toxic dilatation, perforation and peritonitis. In 10% of cases an amoeboma (inflammatory fibrotic mass) develops, commonly in the caecum or rectosigmoid region, which may bleed, cause obstruction or intussusception, or be mistaken for a carcinoma.
AMOEBIC LIVER ABSCESS
An amoebic liver abscess develops when organisms invade through the bowel serosa, enter the portal vein and pass into the liver. The abscess is usually single and in the right lobe of the liver. There is tender hepatomegaly, high swinging fever and profound malaise.

Investigations
SEROLOGY
Amoebic fluorescent antibody test (FAT) is positive in 90% of patients with liver abscess and in 75% of patients with active colitis.

COLONIC DISEASE

The most important diagnostic investigation in amoebic dysentery is sigmoidoscopy and immediate microscopic examination of a rectal smear. This shows the motile trophozoites which contain red blood cells. A fresh stool sample shows the same features but is less sensitive.

LIVER DISEASE

Liver abscesses should be suspected when the serum alkaline phosphatase is elevated. Liver ultrasonography or CT scan will confirm the presence of an abscess.

Differential diagnosis

Amoebic colitis must be differentiated from the other causes of bloody diarrhoea: inflammatory bowel disease, bacillary dysentery, *E. coli*, *Campylobacter* sp., salmonellae, and, rarely, pseudomembranous colitis. Amoebic liver abscess must be differentiated from a pyogenic abscess and/or a hydatid cyst.

Management

Metronidazole for 5 days is given in amoebic colitis and a more prolonged course for 10–14 days in liver abscess. A large tense abscess may require percutaneous drainage under ultrasonic control.

Control and prevention

Improved standards of personal hygiene and water supply are important. Travellers are advised to drink bottled water. Individual chemoprophylaxis is not advised because the risk of acquiring infection is low. There is no effective vaccine.

Shigellosis (bacillary dysentery) ND

Shigellosis is an acute, self-limiting, intestinal infection which occurs worldwide but is more common in tropical countries and in areas of poor hygiene. Transmission is by the faecal–oral route. The four *Shigella* species (*S. dysenteriae*, *S. flexneri*, *S. boydii* and *S. sonnei*) produce colonic inflammation with liberation of a cytotoxin (predominantly *S. dysenteriae*) which results in diarrhoea.

Clinical features

After an incubation period of about 2 days there is an abrupt onset of fever, malaise, abdominal pain and watery diarrhoea, which may progress to bloody diarrhoea with mucus and tenesmus.

Investigations

The diagnosis is made on the basis of the stool culture.

Differential diagnosis

This is from other causes of bloody diarrhoea (see above). Sigmoidoscopic appearances may be the same as those in inflammatory bowel disease.

Management

Treatment is symptomatic with antidiarrhoeals, e.g. loperamide, and rehydration. In severe cases treatment is with trimethoprim 200 mg twice daily or ciprofloxacillin 500 mg twice daily.

Cholera ND

Cholera is caused by the Gram-negative bacillus *Vibrio cholera*. Infection is common in tropical and subtropical countries in areas of poor hygiene. Infection is by the faecal–oral route, and spread is predominantly by ingestion of water contaminated with faeces of infected humans. There is no identified animal reservoir.

Clinical features

Infection is confined to the small bowel where a powerful enterotoxin is formed. The B subunit of the toxin attaches to receptors on the enterocyte; this allows migration of the A subunit into the cell to stimulate adenylate cyclase activity and increase cAMP levels. This produces massive secretion of isotonic fluid into the intestinal lumen.

Clinical features

The incubation period varies from a few hours to 6 days. The illness varies from mild diarrhoea to profuse watery diarrhoea ('rice water stools') resulting in dehydration, hypotension and death.

Investigations

The diagnosis is largely clinical. Fresh stool microscopy may show the motile vibrios.

Management

Management is aimed at effective rehydration which is mainly oral, but in severe cases intravenous fluids are given. Oral rehydration solutions (ORS) depend on the fact that there is a glucose-dependent sodium absorption mechanism not related to cAMP and thus unaffected by cholera toxin. The traditional World Health Organization ORS contains sodium (90 mmol/l) and glucose (111 mmol/l) along with potassium, chloride and citrate. New ORS solutions based on rice water may be more effective and are being evaluated.

Tetracycline for 3 days helps to eradicate the infection, decrease stool output and shorten the duration of the illness.

Prevention and control

Good hygiene and sanitation are the most effective measures for the reduction of infection. Oral cholera vaccines are under development.

Giardiasis

Giardia lamblia is a flagellated protozoan that is found worldwide but is more common in tropical areas. It is a cause of traveller's diarrhoea (see later).

Clinical features
The clinical features are the result of damage to the small intestine with subtotal villous atrophy in severe cases. There is diarrhoea, nausea, abdominal pain and distension, with malabsorption and steatorrhoea in some cases. Chronic giardiasis can result in growth retardation in children.

Investigations
The diagnosis is made by finding cysts on stool examination or parasites in duodenal aspirates.

Management
Metronidazole 2 g daily for 3 days will cure most infections; some patients need two or three courses.

Hydatid disease

Hydatid disease is not a tropical disease but occurs worldwide, particularly in sheep-rearing areas. The disease is caused by ingestion and infection with the dog tapeworm, *Echinococcus granulosus* or *E. multilocularis*. Sheep perpetuate the lifecycle of these parasites.

Clinical features
Parasites enter the body via the duodenum where they form cysts in many organs, particularly the lungs and liver. Clinical features include haemoptysis, dyspnoea, hepatomegaly, jaundice or pyrexia of unknown origin. Occasional rupture into the peritoneal cavity may cause anaphylaxis.

Investigations
Blood count shows eosinophilia. The cysts may be seen on ultrasonography or CT scan, when characteristic daughter cysts are seen. Diagnosis is made on a positive hydatid complement fixation test. Needle aspiration of cysts is not usually performed because of the risk of dissemination or fatal anaphylaxis.

Management
The treatment is surgical removal of the cyst in combination with albendazole.

ACUTE INFECTIOUS DIARRHOEA

Three clinical syndromes are recognized:
- Acute food poisoning **ND**
- Watery diarrhoea
- Bloody diarrhoea

Gastroenteritis and food poisoning

Most cases of food poisoning are caused by either *Salmonella* (page 12) or *Campylobacter* spp. The clinical features associated with the causative organisms are summarized in Table 1.4. Listeriosis (infection with *Listeria monocytogenes*) is associated with contaminated coleslaw, non-pasteurized soft cheeses and other packaged chilled foods. The main

Table 1:4 Bacterial causes and clinical features of food poisoning. ND

Organism	Source	Incubation period (h)	Symptoms	Diagnosis	Recovery
Salmonellae	Bowels of animals, especially fowl	12–24	Abrupt diarrhoea, fever and vomiting	Culture organism in the stool	Usually 2–5 days but may be up to 2 weeks
Campylobacter jejuni	Bowels of animals, especially fowl; also milk	48–96	Diarrhoea + blood, fever, malaise and abdominal pain	Culture organism in the stool	3–5 days
Staphylococcus aureus	Contaminated food, usually by humans	2–6	Vomiting, diarrhoea and dehydration	Culture organism in remaining food	Rapid (few hours)
Bacillus cereus	Spores in food survive boiling	1–6	Vomiting, diarrhoea and dehydration	Culture organism in faeces or food	Rapid
Clostridium perfringens	Spores in food survive boiling	8–22	Watery diarrhoea and abdominal pain	Culture organism in faeces or food	2–3 days
Clostridium botulinum	Spores survive cooking, but germinate in anaerobic conditions, e.g. canned or bottled food	18–36	Brief diarrhoea and paralysis caused by neuromuscular blockade	Demonstrate toxin in food or faeces	10–14 days
Vibrio parahaemolyticus (rare in UK)	Shellfish	6–36	Diarrhoea and vomiting	Culture of faeces	3 days

The main clinical features are those that are underlined.

feature of listeria infection is meningitis occurring perinatally and in immunocompromised adults (page 485).

Watery diarrhoea

Some serotypes of *E. coli* produce diarrhoea by one of several mechanisms:

- Enterotoxigenic *E. coli* (ETEC) produces a toxin that stimulates water and electrolyte secretion by activation of intracellular messengers (such as cholera toxin). It accounts for 40–75% of cases of traveller's diarrhoea (see below).
- Enteropathogenic *E. coli* attaches to and damages the intestine and produces diarrhoea in children.
- Enterohaemorrhagic and enteroinvasive *E.coli* tend to produce an illness with bloody diarrhoea.

Other infectious causes of watery diarrhoea are *V. cholera* (see above), *Salmonella* sp., *Giardia lamblia* and viruses (Rotavirus and Norwalk family of viruses). *Clostridium difficile*, the causative organism of pseudomembranous colitis, produces diarrhoea by production of a toxin. Rarely there is bloody diarrhoea. It usually occurs a few days after institution of antibiotic therapy. Diagnosis is by demonstration of the toxin in stool and by typical sigmoidoscopic appearances (pseudomembranes on an erythematous background). Culture of the organism alone in faeces is insufficient because 5% of healthy adults carry *C. difficile*. Treatment is with oral metronidazole or vancomycin.

Bloody diarrhoea

Organisms causing bloody diarrhoea include *Salmonella* sp., *Shigella* sp., *Campylobacter jejuni* and some strains of *E. coli*.

Traveller's diarrhoea

Traveller's diarrhoea commonly occurs in travellers to foreign countries. Symptoms may start during the visit or soon after the return home. The causes are listed in Table 1.5.

Table 1.5 Causes of traveller's diarrhoea

Pathogen	Proportion of cases (%)
Enterotoxigenic *E. coli*	40–75
Shigella sp.	0–15
Salmonella sp.	0–10
Rotavirus, Norwalk family of viruses	0–10
Giardia lamblia, Entamoeba histolytica	0–3
Unknown	22–25

SEXUALLY TRANSMITTED DISEASES

Sexually transmitted diseases (STDs) remain endemic in all societies and the range of diseases spread by sexual activity continues to increase. The three common presenting symptoms are:

- Urethral discharge (see below)
- Genital ulcers (see below)
- Vaginal discharge caused by *Candida albicans, Trichomonas vaginalis, Neisseria gonorrhoeae, Chlamydia trachomatis,* herpes simplex, cervical polyps, neoplasia, retained tampon, chemical irritants.

STDs predominantly seen in the tropics are chancroid, granuloma inguinale and lymphogranuloma venereum. They may present with genital ulceration and inguinal lymphadenopathy.

The important aspects of management of all the STDs are:

- Accurate diagnosis and effective treatment
- Screening for other STDs (multiple STDs may coexist)
- Patient education
- Contact tracing; the patient's sexual partners must be traced so that they can be treated, thus preventing the disease from spreading further
- Follow-up to ensure that infection is adequately treated

Urethritis

Urethritis in men presents with urethral discharge and dysuria. It is often asymptomatic in women.

Gonorrhoea

The causative organism, *Neisseria gonorrhoeae* (gonococcus), is a Gram-negative intracellular diplococcus which infects epithelium particularly of the urogenital tract, rectum, pharynx and conjunctivae.

Clinical features

The incubation period ranges from 2 to 14 days. In men the symptoms are purulent urethral discharge and dysuria. In homosexual men proctitis may produce anal pain, discharge and itch. Women are often asymptomatic but may complain of vaginal discharge, dysuria and intermenstrual bleeding. Complications include salpingitis and Bartholin's abscess in women, epididymitis and prostatitis in men, and systemic spread with a rash and arthritis (page 172). Infants born to infected mothers may develop ophthalmia neonatorum.

Diagnosis

Gram stain and culture of swab taken from the urethra in men and the endocervix in women.

Management

- Single-dose amoxycillin (3 g) plus probenecid (1 g)
- Ciprofloxacillin in patients allergic to penicillin
- Longer course of treatment in complicated infection

Non-gonococcal urethritis (NGU)

The most common cause is infection with *Chlamydia*

trachomatis which presents in men with urethral discharge and dysuria. In women infection may be asymptomatic and only found during investigations for infertility (secondary to salpingitis). The diagnosis is made on cell culture or direct antigen detection (available in some centres) of swabs taken from the urethra or endocervix. Treatment is with oxytetracycline or erythromycin (in pregnancy). Other causes of NGU are *Ureaplasma urealyticum*, *Bacteroides* sp. and *Mycoplasma* sp.

Genital ulcers

The infective causes of genital ulceration in the UK include syphilis, herpes simplex and herpes zoster (page 6). Non-infective causes are Behçet's syndrome, Steven–Johnson syndrome (page 518), carcinoma and trauma.

Syphilis

The causative organism, *Treponema pallidum*, is a motile spirochaete which enters via a skin abrasion during close sexual contact. The organism may also pass transplacentally from mother to fetus.

PRIMARY INFECTION

After an incubation period of 10–90 days a papule develops at the site of infection. This ulcerates to become a painless, firm chancre which heals spontaneously within 2–3 weeks.

SECONDARY INFECTION

This occurs 4–10 weeks after the appearance of the primary lesion. There may be one or more of the following features: fever, sore throat, arthralgia, generalized lymphadenopathy, widespread skin rash (except the face), superficial ulcers in the mouth (snail-track ulcers) and condylomata lata (warty perianal lesions). In most patients symptoms subside within one year.

TERTIARY SYPHILIS

Occurs after a latent period of 2 years or more. The characteristic lesion is a *gumma* (granulomatous lesion) occurring in the skin, bones, liver and testes. Cardiovascular syphilis is mentioned on pages 301 and 315 and neurosyphilis is described on page 488.

CONGENITAL SYPHILIS

This usually becomes apparent between the second and sixth week after birth, early signs being nasal discharge, skin and mucous membrane lesions, and failure to thrive. Signs of late syphilis appear after 2 years of age when there are also characteristic bone and teeth abnormalities from earlier damage.

Diagnosis

Dark ground microscopy of fluid taken from lesions shows organisms in primary and secondary disease. Serological tests may be negative in primary disease.

SEROLOGY

The VDRL (Venereal Disease Research Laboratory) test is detectable within 3–4 weeks of infection; it becomes negative in treated patients and in some untreated patients with late tertiary syphilis. Other diseases, e.g. autoimmune disease and malignancy, may give false positive results.

T. pallidum haemagglutination assay (TPHA) and fluorescent treponemal antibody test are positive in most patients in primary disease and remain positive in spite of treatment. They do not distinguish between syphilis and other treponemes, e.g. yaws.

Management

Intramuscular procaine penicillin for 10 days is given for primary and secondary syphilis. For tertiary syphilis treatment is continued for 4 weeks. The Jarisch–Herxheimer reaction occurs most commonly in secondary syphilis and is the result of release of endotoxin when organisms are killed by antibiotics. The symptoms of malaise, fever and headache may be ameliorated by giving prednisolone for 24 hours before penicillin.

HIV AND AIDS

Human immunodeficiency virus (HIV) infection was identified as the causative organism of acquired immunodeficiency syndrome (AIDS) in 1983. Current WHO estimates are of 13 million adults infected worldwide of whom 2.5 million have died.

Epidemiology

Transmission is by:

- Sexual intercourse: in Europe, the USA and Australia sexual spread is predominantly among homosexual men. In central and sub-Saharan Africa spread is predominantly through heterosexual intercourse with equal numbers of men and women affected.
- Mother to child: transmission can occur *in utero*, during childbirth and via breast milk.
- Contaminated blood, blood products and organ donations: the risk is now minimal in developed countries since the introduction of screening blood products in 1985.
- Contaminated needles: intravenous drug addicts, needlestick injuries in healthcare workers.

HIV infection is not spread by ordinary social or household contact.

Viral structure

The virus (p. 24) consists of an outer envelope and an inner core. The core contains RNA and the enzyme reverse transcriptase which allows viral RNA to be transcribed into DNA and then incorporated into the host cell genome.

HIV binds to CD4 receptors on T-helper cells (CD4 cells).

Other cells of the immune system bearing the CD4 receptor are also affected. There is a progressive and severe depletion of CD4 lymphocytes and it is this that leads to the clinical manifestations of AIDS.

Clinical features

The spectrum of illness associated with HIV infection is broad. Several classification systems exist, the most widely used being the Centers for Disease Control (CDC) classification.

GROUP I: ACUTE SEROCONVERSION ILLNESS
A self-limiting non-specific illness occurs 4–8 weeks after exposure in some patients. Symptoms include fever, myalgia, oral ulceration, generalized lymphadenopathy and a maculopapular rash. An 'aseptic-meningitis' picture is common.

GROUP II: ASYMPTOMATIC INFECTION
The number of HIV-infected lymphocytes gradually increases and although the patients remain well, they remain infectious. This stage may last up to 10 years.

GROUP III: PERSISTENT GENERALIZED LYMPHADENOPATHY
Defined as nodes more than 1 cm in diameter at two or more extrainguinal sites for more than 3 months in the absence of causes other than HIV infection.

GROUP IV: SYMPTOMATIC HIV INFECTION
Divided into subgroups A–E:

- A – constitutional symptoms of fever, weight loss and diarrhoea
- B – neurological disease: dementia, peripheral neuropathy, myelopathy
- C – opportunistic infections (see below)
- D – secondary cancers (see below)
- E – other conditions: lymphoid interstitial pneumonia, thrombocytopenia

---

Opportunistic infections

As immunosuppression increases patients are susceptible to a wide range of infections. The organisms requiring an intact cell-mediated immunity for their control are most likely to cause clinical problems. High-grade pathogens, e.g. *Mycobacterium tuberculosis*, *Candida* sp. and herpes virus are relatively common in the early stages of infection. Susceptibility to infections such as that caused by *Pneumocystis carinii* occur at late stages of immuno-suppression (usually when the CD4 cell count is less than $200/mm^3$). With severe immunosuppression there is infection with atypical mycobacteria and cryptosporidia. Numerous organisms cause infection in AIDS patients The more common opportunistic infections are:

- PULMONARY: *Pneumocystis carinii* pneumonia causes dyspnoea, cough and fever. The chest radiograph may be normal or show bilateral midzone shadowing. Diagnosis is by microscopy of bronchial washings or biopsies taken at bronchoscopy. Treatment is with co-trimoxazole or intravenous pentamidine for 3 weeks. Corticosteroids reduce the mortality in severe cases. Recurrence is largely prevented (secondary prophylaxis) by the use of low-dose co-trimoxazole (960 mg three times weekly) or nebulized pentamidine (300 mg monthly). Prophylaxis is also offered (primary prophylaxis) to those at high risk of infection (CD4 cell count < 200/mm^3).

- CNS: The fungus, *Cryptococcus* sp., usually causes meningitis and presents with headache, fever and impaired conscious level. Diagnosis is made by CSF microscopy (India ink staining shows the organisms directly) and treatment is with intravenous amphotericin B or fluconazole (continued long term to suppress infection). *Toxoplasma gondii* commonly causes encephalitis and cerebral abscesses in AIDS patients. Presentation is with headache and focal neurological signs. Multiple ring-enhancing lesions are seen on a CT scan; if there is doubt about the diagnosis a brain biopsy is sometimes performed. Treatment is with pyrimethamine and sulphonamide continued lifelong to prevent relapse. Cytomegalovirus (CMV) causes a retinitis with visual field defects, deteriorating vision and blindness. Diagnosis is made on funduscopy and treatment is with intravenous ganciclovir or foscarnet (continued long term, via an indwelling venous catheter, to prevent relapse).

- GUT: the protozoan, *Cryptosporidium parvum*, causes a mild self-limiting diarrhoea in an immunocompetent individual but may cause severe watery diarrhoea in AIDS patients. Diagnosis is made by stool microscopy and treatment is largely supportive. Other causes of diarrhoea in AIDS patients are AIDS enteropathy, *Mycobacterium avium-intracellulare*, *microsporidia*, *Isospora belli* and CMV colitis. Most of these will be identified on several stool cultures and a rectal biopsy.

Candida infection of the oesophagus may cause dysphagia; treatment is with fluconazole or ketoconazole.

Tumours

- Kaposi's sarcoma is caused by proliferation of vascular endothelial cells. It presents with purple papules on the skin, and in the lung and gut. Spread is to the lymph nodes. Localized disease is treated with radiotherapy; systemic disease is treated with chemotherapy.

- Non-Hodgkin's lymphoma occurs in the CNS, gut and lung.

Diagnosis

- VIRAL P24 ANTIGEN (p24 Ag) is detected in the serum usually for 8–10 weeks after exposure, and is a useful marker of infection in patients who have not yet developed antibodies.
- IgG ANTIBODIES in the serum may not appear for up to 3 months after infection. They are the most commonly used marker of HIV infection.

Table 1.6 AIDS-defining diagnoses (1993 classification, Europe*)

The following can be used as indicator diseases for AIDS providing other causes of immunodeficiency have been excluded (congenital immune deficiency, lymphoma, leukaemia, recent use of steroids or other immunosuppressive drugs).

Bacterial chest infection (recurrent in 12 month period)

Candidiasis, trachea, bronchi or lungs

Cervical carcinoma, invasive

Coccidioidomycosis, disseminated or extrapulmonary

Cryptococcus, extrapulmonary

Cryptosporidiosis, with diarrhoea for > 1 month

Cytomegalovirus disease (onset after age 1 month) not in liver, spleen or nodes

Encephalopathy (dementia) due to HIV

Herpes simplex ulcers for 1 month or bronchitis, pneumonitis or oesophagitis (onset in infants > 1 month old)

Histoplasmosis, disseminated or extrapulmonary

Isosporiasis, with diarrhoea for > 1 month

Kaposi's sarcoma

Lymphoid interstitial pneumonitis and/or pulmonary lymphoid hyperplasia in a child aged < 13 years

Mycobacteriosis (including extrapulmonary tuberculosis), disseminated

Mycobacteriosis, pulmonary tuberculosis

Pneumocystis carinii pneumonia

Progressive multifocal leucoencephalopathy

Salmonella (non-typhoid) septicaemia, recurrent

Toxoplasmosis of brain, onset after 1 month age

Wasting syndrome caused by HIV (weight loss > 10% baseline, with no other cause identified)

* USA definition also includes those with a CD4 count <200/mm^3.

The diagnosis of AIDS is made when an HIV-positive patient develops one or more of a defined list of opportunistic infections, malignancies or HIV-associated illness in the absence of other causes of immunosuppression, e.g. leukaemia, immunosuppressive drugs. In the USA, AIDS is also diagnosed on the basis of the the CD4 count ($<200/mm^3$) (Table 1.6).

Management
Zidovudine inhibits reverse transcriptase. It reduces mortality and opportunistic infections in patients with symptomatic HIV infection (CDC group IV) but offers no survival advantage if given at an earlier stage. Side effects include headache, nausea, bone marrow suppression and myopathy.

Prevention and control
- Screening of blood products
- Use of condoms reduces sexual transmission of HIV
- Advise drug addicts not to share needles; some areas provide free sterile needles

FINAL MEDICINE EXAMINATION: INFECTIOUS DISEASES

1. Discuss the management of an otherwise healthy 32-year-old man who has just been found to be HIV positive.

2. What are the early symptoms and signs of rubella? Write short notes on its prevention.

3. How would you investigate and treat a young male patient presenting with urethral discharge?

4. Write short notes on diarrhoea one week after return from the Far East.

5. Describe briefly the intestinal infections produced by:
   (a) *Campylobacter* sp.
   (b) *Yersinia* sp.
   (c) *Clostridium difficile* sp.

6. A one-year-old boy has been unwell for 6 hours, temperature 40.5°C with eight petechial spots on the trunk and legs. He is drowsy with systolic blood pressure of 45 mmHg.
   (a) What is the probable diagnosis ?
   (b) What immediate treatment would you give?
   (c) What treatment would you give the rest of the family?
   (d) Can the disease be prevented in this age group?
   (e) What complications would you examine for at an outpatient visit 6 weeks later?

ANSWERS

1. Most patients are found to be positive on antibody testing. Before any patient is tested for evidence of HIV infection they must be counselled by a trained counsellor (often a nurse) and a full explanation is given of what a positive test means. Some patients will require this information to be discussed again when they are subsequently found to have a positive test. They must be told that the result is confidential and will only be known by those staff involved with the care. A risk history must be established (e.g. intravenous drug abuse, sexual history) and advice given about avoiding transmission to others (i.e. non-penetrative sex, no sharing of needles). This patient is said to be healthy but a full physical examination must be carried out to look for evidence of AIDS. A full list of those diseases which indicate AIDS in an HIV-positive patient is given in Table 1.6.

   The natural history of the disease must be discussed (in asymptomatic people the average is 10 years between infection and AIDS). Baseline investigations include FBC, CD4 count (used to monitor disease progression, prophylaxis against some infections, e.g. pneumocystis, is instituted at low CD4 counts).

2. The clinical features of rubella are dicussed on page 4. Prevention is *active* (live attenuated rubella vaccine given with mumps and measles as a single dose at 1–2 years of age) or *passive* (human immunoglobulin reduces symptoms but does not reduce teratogenic effects).

3. This is discussed on pages 18–19.

4. This is traveller's diarrhoea and the causes are listed in Table 1.5. This question does not say if this is bloody diarrhoea but the presence of blood narrows the differential diagnosis. Most cases are self-limiting but antibiotics may be necessary for severe infections. Ciprofloxacillin covers most of these organisms. Metronidazole is given for amoebiasis or giardiasis.

5. (a) The only campylobacter producing intestinal infection is *Campylobacter jejuni*, which belongs to the genus Vibrio (other members are *Vibrio cholerae* and *Vibrio parahaemolyticus*). *Campylobacter* and *Salmonella* species account for most cases of food poisoning (poultry is the main source of infection in both). *Campylobacter* infection produces a prodromal febrile infection lasting 1–4 days followed by a diarrhoeal phase

which may last 1–2 weeks. Severe abdominal pains often accompany the diarrhoea which may be blood-stained. Septicaemia may occur, but rarely death. Sigmoidoscopy may show an acute colitis resembling ulcerative colitis. Diagnosis is made by microscopy (seen as motile rods) and culture of faeces. Infection is usually self-limiting, antibiotic treatment with erythromycin is given to those with systemic symptoms. Complications include cholecystitis, pancreatitis and reactive arthritis.

(b) There are three main *Yersinia* species in humans, all of which are uncommon in Britain. *Y. pseudo-tuberculosis* and *Y. enterocolitic* cause diarrhoea, terminal ileitis and mesenteric adenitis (may be confused with appendicitis). Diagnosis is usually by serology, demonstrating a rise in antibody titre on paired samples. The illness is usually self-limiting but tetracycline may be helpful for treating a severe infection. The third yersinia species, *Y. pestis*, causes plague.

(c) *Clostridium difficile* produces pseudomembranous colitis which is an uncommon complication of antibiotic therapy. *C. difficile* is present in the colon of some healthy individuals and colitis has been attributed to the selection of drug-resistant *C. difficile* that proliferates in the colon and pro-duces a necrotizing toxin. The diagnosis and management is discussed on page 17.

6. The temperature and hypotension indicate septicaemic shock. The petechial spots suggest this is caused by infection with *N. meningitidis* (not all of these infections produce meningitis).

(a) Fulminant meningococcaemia is a severe life-threatening illness with a rapidly progressive downhill course.

(b) The initial treatment is intravenous benzylpenicillin which must be started **immediately** the diagnosis is clinically suspected. In addition, shock should be treated urgently (page 2).

(c) Family contacts should receive prophylaxis with rifampicin 600 mg twice daily for 2 days.

(d) A vaccine is available, but is generally only given when travelling to high-risk places, e.g. Africa, Asia, South America and the Middle East.

(e) A small number of patients develop chronic complications, e.g. arthritis, vasculitis and pericarditis, which may be due to immune complex disease.

CHAPTER 2

Gastroenterology

Symptoms of gastrointestinal disease

DYSPHAGIA
Dysphagia is difficulty in swallowing. The causes are listed on page 30.

HEARTBURN
Heartburn is a retrosternal burning discomfort which spreads up towards the throat and is a common symptom of acid reflux (page 32). The pain can sometimes be difficult to distinguish from the pain of ischaemic heart disease, although a careful history will usually differentiate between the two (page 262).

DYSPEPSIA
Dyspepsia is a general term often used to describe a range of symptoms referable to the upper gastrointestinal tract, e.g. nausea, heartburn, acidity, pain or distension.

FLATULENCE
Flatulence is a term used to describe excessive wind, presenting as belching, abdominal distension and the passage of flatus per rectum. It is rarely indicative of serious underlying disease.

VOMITING
Vomiting occurs as a result of stimulation of the vomiting centres in the lateral reticular formation of the medulla. This may result from stimulation of the chemoreceptor trigger zones in the floor of the fourth ventricle or from vagal afferents from the gut. It is associated with many gastrointestinal conditions, but nausea and vomiting without pain are frequently non-gastrointestinal in origin.

CONSTIPATION
Constipation is difficult to define because there is considerable individual variation, but it is usually taken to mean infrequent passage of stool or the difficult passage of hard stool.

DIARRHOEA
Diarrhoea implies the passage of increased amounts of loose stool (>300 g per 24 hours). This must be differentiated from the frequent passage of small amounts of stool (which patients often refer to as diarrhoea), which is commonly seen in functional bowel disease.

STEATORRHOEA
Steatorrhoea is the passage of pale bulky stools that contain fat. The stools often float because of increased air content and are difficult to flush away.

THE MOUTH

Problems in the mouth are common and often trivial although they can cause severe symptoms.

Mouth ulcers

NON-INFECTIVE

- Recurrent aphthous ulceration is the most common cause of mouth ulcers and affects at least 20% of the population; in most cases the aetiology is unknown. The history is of recurrent self-limiting episodes of painful oral ulcers (rarely on the palate). Topical corticosteroids are used for symptomatic relief but they have no effect on the natural history. In a few cases aphthous ulcers are associated with trauma or gastrointestinal and systemic diseases, e.g. anaemia, inflammatory bowel disease, coeliac disease, Behçet's syndrome, Reiter's disease and systemic lupus erythematosus.

- Squamous cell carcinoma presents as an indolent ulcer, usually on the tongue or floor of the mouth. Aetiological factors include tobacco (smoking and chewing) and alcohol. Treatment is with surgery and radiotherapy.

INFECTIVE

- Herpes simplex virus type 1
- Coxsackie A virus
- Herpes zoster virus

Oral white patches

Oral white patches are caused by smoking, candida infection, lichen planus, trauma and syphilis. *Leukoplakia* is the term used to describe oral white patches or plaques that cannot be diagnosed clinically or pathologically as any other disease (i.e. a diagnosis of exclusion). Leukoplakia is a premalignant lesion and thus oral white patches must be biopsied to exclude malignancy. *Hairy leukoplakia* is a white patch on the side of the tongue seen in patients with AIDS; it is not premalignant.

Atrophic glossitis

A smooth sore tongue with loss of filliform papillae may occur in patients with iron, vitamin B_{12} or folate deficiency.

Geographical tongue

This affects up to 10% of the population and describes discrete areas of depapillation on the dorsum of the tongue. This may be asymptomatic or produce a sore tongue. The aetiology is unknown and there is no specific treatment.

Gum disorders

Gum bleeding is most commonly caused by gingivitis, an inflammatory condition of the gums, associated with dental plaque. Bleeding may also be associated with generalized conditions such as bleeding disorders and leukaemia. Acute ulcerative gingivitis (Vincent's infection) is characterized by the development of crater-like ulcers, with bleeding, involving the interdental papillae, followed by lateral spread along the gingival margins. It is thought to be the result of infection occurring in the malnourished and immuno-compromised. Treatment is with oral metronidazole and good oral hygiene.

Salivary gland disorders

XEROSTOMIA (mouth dryness) may be caused by anxiety, drugs, Sjögren's syndrome and dehydration.

INFECTION (parotitis) may be viral, i.e. mumps virus, or bacterial (staphylococci or streptococci).

SARCOIDOSIS produces enlargement of parotid glands and, if combined with lacrimal gland enlargement, it is known as Mikulicz's syndrome.

CALCULUS formation usually involves the duct of the submandibular gland, and causes painful swelling of the gland after eating.

TUMOURS most commonly affect the parotid gland and are usually mixed cell (pleomorphic adenoma) in type. Treatment is with surgical resection.

THE OESOPHAGUS

The main oesophageal symptoms are dysphagia, heartburn and painful swallowing.

- DYSPHAGIA (difficulty in swallowing) is usually investigated with a barium swallow followed by endoscopy where appropriate. The causes are listed in Table 2.1. Typically, mechanical narrowing of the oesophagus, e.g. by carcinoma or benign peptic strictures, produce progressive dysphagia initially for solids and eventually for liquids. Motor disorders, e.g. achalasia and scleroderma, produce dysphagia for both solids and liquids.

- HEARTBURN is a retrosternal or epigastric burning sensation produced by reflux of gastric acid into the oesophagus. The pain may radiate up to the throat and be confused with chest pain of cardiac origin. It is often aggravated by bending or lying down.

- PAINFUL SWALLOWING occurs with infections of the oesophagus or in gastro-oesophageal reflux disease particularly with alcohol and hot liquids (see later).

Table 2.1 Causes of dysphagia

Neuromuscular disorders
Bulbar palsy
Pharyngeal disorders
Myasthenia gravis

Motility disorders
Achalasia
Scleroderma
Diffuse oesophageal spasm
Presbyoesophagus (oesophagus of old age)
Diabetes
Chagas' disease

Extrinsic pressure
Goitre
Mediastinal glands
Enlarged left atrium in mitral valve disease

Intrinsic lesion
Foreign body
Benign stricture
Malignant stricture
Oesophageal ring or web
Pharyngeal pouch

Achalasia

Achalasia is a disease of unknown aetiology, characterized by
aperistalsis in the body of the oesophagus, and the failure of
relaxation of the lower oesophageal sphincter (LOS) on
initiation of swallowing.

Pathology
There is a decrease in ganglionic cells in the nerve plexus of
the oesophageal wall and degeneration in the vagus nerve.

Clinical features
The disease can present at any age but is rare in childhood.
There is usually a long history of dysphagia for both liquids
and solids, which may be associated with regurgitation.
Severe retrosternal chest pain may occur, particularly in
younger patients.

Investigations
BARIUM SWALLOW will show dilatation of the oesophagus,
lack of peristalsis, a gradually tapering lower end (beak
deformity) and synchronous contractions of the oesophagus.

OESOPHAGOSCOPY may be necessary to exclude a carcinoma.

MANOMETRY demonstrates aperistalsis and failure of LOS
relaxation.

CHEST RADIOGRAPHS may show a dilated oesophagus with a fluid level behind the heart. The fundal gas shadow is not present.

Management
Endoscopic pneumatic dilatation of the LOS, under radiographic screening, is currently the procedure of choice and is successful in 80% of cases. Surgical division of the sphincter (Heller's cardiomyotomy) is used in resistant cases and is now being performed by laparoscopy. Reflux oesophagitis is a complication of both procedures.

Complications
There is an increased incidence of 5–10% of carcinoma of the oesophagus regardless of treatment.

Systemic sclerosis

There is oesophageal involvement in over 90% of patients with systemic sclerosis. The smooth muscle layer is replaced by fibrous tissue. The LOS pressure is reduced permitting reflux. Patients may be asymptomatic or complain of reflux and dysphagia. Dysphagia is caused by stricture formation complicating reflux. Treatment is as for reflux and stricture formation.

Diffuse oesophageal spasm

This is a severe form of abnormal oesophageal motility which can produce chest pain and dysphagia. A 'corkscrew' appearance may be seen on barium swallow. 'Nutcracker oesophagus' is a variant characterized by high amplitude peristaltic waves in the oesophagus. Treatment of these disorders is difficult but calcium channel blockers may be helpful.

Hiatus hernia

On its own, a hiatus hernia is not responsible for symptoms unless there is associated reflux. There are two main forms:

● Sliding: the gastro-oesophageal junction slides through the hiatus and lies above the diaphragm.

● Paraoesophageal: a part of the stomach rolls up through the hiatus alongside the oesophagus, the sphincter remaining below the diaphragm

Gastro-oesophageal reflux disease

Reflux of gastric contents into the oesophagus occurs as a normal event and clinical symptoms occur only when there is prolonged contact of gastric contents with the oesophageal mucosa.

Pathophysiology
There is low oesophageal sphincter tone, with reduced mucosal resistance to acid and reduced oesophageal

clearance of acid. Delayed gastric emptying and prolonged postprandial and nocturnal reflux also contribute.

Clinical features

Heartburn is the major symptom of reflux oesophagitis. The burning is aggravated by bending, stooping and lying down and may be relieved by antacids. There may be pain on drinking hot drinks. Cough and nocturnal asthma can occur from aspiration of gastric contents into the lungs. Symptoms do not correlate well with the severity of oesophagitis.

Investigations

BARIUM SWALLOW. This may show an ulcerated lower oesophagus and/or reflux of barium at the time of the examination.

OESOPHAGOSCOPY shows the presence of oesophagitis. The mucosa can be normal in gastro-oesophageal reflux disease.

24-HOUR INTRALUMINAL pH MONITORING AND A BERNSTEIN TEST. These are not routine investigations and are used in difficult diagnostic cases or where there is a poor response to treatment [CM p. 186].

Management

Conservative measures with simple antacids, raising the head of the bed, losing weight, reduction in alcohol intake and cessation of smoking are often sufficient for mild symptoms.

ALGINATES prevent reflux by forming a 'foam raft' on gastric contents.

H_2-RECEPTOR ANTAGONISTS (e.g. ranitidine) improve symptoms of heartburn.

PROKINETIC AGENTS, such as metoclopramide and cisapride, enhance peristalsis and may be of value particularly as maintenance treatment.

PROTON PUMP INHIBITORS (e.g. omeprazole and lansoprazole) inhibit hydrogen–potassium ATPase and block luminal secretion of gastric acid. They are potent acid blockers and the drugs of choice for all but mild cases.

Surgery is necessary for the few patients who continue to have symptoms in spite of full medical therapy. The fundus of the stomach is sutured around the lower oesophagus to produce an antireflux valve (*Nissen fundoplication*). In some centres the operation is done via the laparoscope (*lap-wrap*) rather than by open surgery.

Complications

Oesophageal stricture formation is the major complication of reflux and presents with intermittent dysphagia. It is treated with endoscopic dilatation. Long-standing acid reflux causes columnization of the lower oesophageal mucosa (Barrett's oesophagus) which is premalignant.

Malignant oesophageal tumours

Pathology

- Squamous cell, usually of the middle third of oesophagus
- Adenocarcinoma
- Kaposi's sarcoma is seen in patients with AIDS but is rarely symptomatic

Epidemiology

SQUAMOUS CARCINOMA. The incidence is 5–10 per 100 000 in the UK though the incidence varies greatly throughout the world, being particularly high in China and parts of Africa and Iran. It is most common in the 60–70 year age group. It is associated with heavy alcohol intake, heavy smoking and a high intake of salted fish and pickled vegetables. Other predisposing factors include the Plummer-Vinson syndrome (iron deficiency anaemia and oesophageal web causing dysphagia), tylosis (autosomal dominant condition with hyperkeratosis of palms and soles), achalasia, and coeliac disease.

ADENOCARCINOMA. This arises from the columnar lined epithelium of the lower oesophagus which results from long-standing reflux (Barrett's oesophagus).

Clinical features

Symptoms include progressive dysphagia, initially for solids and later for liquids, weight loss, and chest pain which may be due to bolus food impaction or local infiltration. Physical signs are usually absent.

Investigations

BARIUM SWALLOW OR ENDOSCOPY are the initial investigations.

CT, MRI, AND ENDOSCOPIC ULTRASONOGRAPHY may be helpful in staging the lesion for surgery.

Management

In many patients only symptomatic treatment to relieve dysphagia is possible. This is usually done via the endoscope:

- Dilatation and insertion of a tube to keep the oesophagus open
- Laser to photocoagulate the tumour
- Alcohol injections to slough the tumour

Surgical resection may be done in the few patients with localized disease (25% 5-year survival). Radiation and chemotherapy have provided limited success with squamous cell carcinoma.

Prognosis

The prognosis overall is poor (2% 5-year survival) as most patients can only be treated palliatively.

Benign oesophageal tumours

Leiomyomas are the most common benign tumours. They are usually discovered incidentally and do not often produce symptoms.

THE STOMACH AND DUODENUM

Acute gastritis, acute ulceration and erosions

There is no universally accepted classification for these conditions, partly because there is a poor correlation among clinical, pathological and endoscopic findings.

Aetiology

The most common cause is aspirin or other non-steroidal anti-inflammatory drugs (NSAIDs), resulting, in part, from depletion of mucosal prostaglandins. Other causes include infections, e.g. cytomegalovirus and herpes simplex virus, and alcohol in high concentrations. Acute ulcers may be seen after severe stress (stress ulcer), burns (Curling's ulcer), and in renal and liver disease.

Pathology

There is an acute inflammatory cell infiltrate in the superficial gastric mucosa, predominantly with neutrophils. Multiple erosions (small superficial mucosal breaks) are described as acute erosive gastritis. Acute gastric ulceration occurs in the same setting as erosions but are larger.

Clinical features

Common symptoms include indigestion, vomiting and haemorrhage although these correlate poorly with endoscopic and pathological findings.

Investigations

Symptoms often settle spontaneously although endoscopy and biopsy are sometimes required to clarify the diagnosis.

Management

Treatment is symptomatic with removal of the offending cause if possible.

Chronic gastritis

Aetiology

The most common cause of chronic gastritis is *Helicobacter pylori* infection (see below). Other causes are autoimmune gastritis (the cause of pernicious anaemia associated with antibodies to gastric parietal cells and intrinsic factor) and biliary reflux.

Pathology

There is infiltration of the lamina propria with lymphocytes and plasma cells, which over a long period may lead to gastritis with atrophy and subsequent metaplasia.

Clinical features
Chronic gastritis is usually asymptomatic and discovered incidentally.

Management
No specific treatment is required.

Helicobacter pylori and the upper gastrointestinal tract

Helicobacter pylori is a Gram-negative, urease-producing, spiral-shaped bacterium found predominantly in the gastric antrum and in areas of gastric metaplasia in the duodenum. It is closely associated with chronic active gastritis, peptic ulcer disease and, possibly, gastric cancer and lymphoma.

Epidemiology
The incidence of *H. pylori* infection increases with age (60% at 60 years) and is associated with lower socioeconomic status. The exact mode of transmission is unclear, but epidemiological studies and recent culture of the organism in faeces suggests person-to-person spread.

Clinical features
Initially *H. pylori* infection produces an acute gastritis which rapidly becomes chronic active gastritis and, in some, peptic ulcer disease may develop. Long-standing chronic active gastritis leads to atrophy, intestinal metaplasia and an increased risk of gastric carcinoma.

Investigations
INVASIVE TESTS *(endoscopic antral biopsy)*

- Rapid urease test (*H. pylori* added to a urea-containing solution breaks down urea and produces a colour change in the indicator present)
- Gram stain and culture
- Histology with direct visualization of the organism

NON-INVASIVE TESTS

- Urea breath test ^{13}C(or ^{14}C) labelled urea is given by mouth; the detection of ^{13}C in expired air indicates infection with urease-producing *H. pylori*)
- Serum antibodies

Management
Eradication of *H. pylori* is indicated for all patients with proven peptic disease. Recurrence is substantially reduced in those in whom the infection is successfully eradicated. Treatment regimens are evolving but two that are commonly used are:

- Bismuth chelate one tablet four times daily for 1 week
  Metronidazole 400 mg three times daily for 1 week
  Tetracycline 500 mg three times daily for 1 week
- Omeprazole 20 mg twice daily and amoxycillin 1 g twice daily or clarithromycin 500 mg three times daily for 2 weeks

Peptic ulcer disease

A peptic ulcer is an ulcer of the mucosa in or adjacent to an acid-bearing area. Most occur in the stomach or proximal duodenum.

Epidemiology

Duodenal ulcers are three to four times more common than gastric ulcers and occur in 15% of the population at some time. They are more common in men than in women (4 : 1) and both are more common in elderly people. There is a significant geographical variation.

Aetiology

There is an imbalance between acid and pepsin and mucosal defences (mucus, bicarbonate and prostaglandins). *H. pylori* plays a central role although the mechanisms are unclear (Table 2.2). Genetic factors may have a role to play. NSAIDs are an important cause of gastric ulceration though probably not duodenal ulcers. Peptic ulceration is also seen in hyperparathyroidism and the Zollinger–Ellison syndrome.

Table 2.2 Pathogenic mechanisms of *H. pylori*

Increased fasting and meal stimulated serum gastrin
Decreased somatostatin (D) cells in the antrum
Increased parietal cell mass
Increased pepsinogen 1
Disruption of mucous protective layer
Cytotoxin release

Clinical features

Epigastric pain is the most common presenting symptom. This is typically relieved by antacids but has a variable relationship to food. Duodenal ulcer pain, however, often occurs when the subject is hungry and classically occurs at night. Other symptoms such as nausea, heartburn and flatulence may occur. Occasionally ulcers may present with the complications of perforation or painless upper gastrointestinal haemorrhage.

Investigations

Many young patients can be treated symptomatically without investigation. A gastroscopy is the investigation of choice. A barium meal is useful if gastric outlet obstruction is suspected.

Management

H. PYLORI ERADICATION

Treatment regimens that successfully eradicate *H. pylori* from the gastric antrum result in healing rates of over 90% and prevent recurrence unless reinfection occurs which is unusual. This approach to treatment is indicated in ulcers that recur or those that present with a complication such as haemorrhage or perforation.

ACID SUPPRESSION THERAPY

- H_2-receptor antagonists (ranitidine, cimetidine) will heal over 80% of ulcers with a 2-month course of treatment. The choice of drug is often based on cost. However, at least 60% will recur within one year and thus most patients are usually treated by eradication of *H. pylori*.

- Proton pump inhibitors (omeprazole, lansoprazole) inhibit hydrogen–potassium ATPase ($H^+/K^+ATPase$), producing 80–90% inhibition of 24-hour intragastric acidity and almost 100% healing rates after 4 weeks of treatment

- Antacids are now usually only prescribed for symptomatic relief of mild episodes of indigestion

SURGERY

With the introduction of modern drugs, surgery is rarely performed for peptic ulceration but reserved for the treatment of complications, namely recurrent haemorrhage, perforation and outflow obstruction.

Complications

PERFORATION

This is becoming less common partly as a result of the introduction of H_2-receptor antagonists. Duodenal ulcers perforate more commonly than gastric ulcers, usually into the peritoneal cavity. Management is initially surgical with closure of the perforation and drainage of the abdomen. *H. pylori* should subsequently be eradicated. Conservative treatment with fluids and antibiotics may be indicated in elderly or very ill patients.

GASTRIC OUTLET OBSTRUCTION

Outflow obstruction occurs because of surrounding oedema or scarring following healing. Copious projectile vomiting is the main symptom and a succussion splash may be detectable clinically. Metabolic alkalosis may develop as a result of loss of acid. Management is initially with nasogastric suction and replacement of fluids and electrolytes. In some cases oedema may settle with conservative management but treatment with surgery or balloon dilatation is often required.

HAEMORRHAGE – see below.

Malignant gastric tumours

Epidemiology

Gastric cancer is the sixth most common fatal cancer in the UK. The incidence increases with age and is more common in men. The frequency varies throughout the world being more common in Japan and Chile, and relatively less common in the USA. The incidence overall is decreasing worldwide.

Aetiology

This is unknown although the association with long-standing *H. pylori* infection is thought to be a factor. Dietary factors, such as alcohol, spiced, salted or pickled foods, and nitrate ingestion may also have a role. Smoking and achlorhydria (e.g. pernicious anaemia) are also significantly associated with gastric cancer.

Pathology

Tumours most commonly occur in the antrum and are almost always adenocarcinomas. They may be localized ulcerated lesions with rolled edges (*intestinal type*) or more diffuse with extensive submucosal spread giving the picture of linitus plastica (*diffuse type*).

Clinical features

Pain similar to peptic ulcer pain is the most common symptom. With advanced disease, nausea, anorexia and weight loss are common. Vomiting with outflow obstruction occurs if the tumour is near the pylorus, or dysphagia can occur with lesions in the cardia. Almost 50% have a palpable epigastric mass, and a lymph node is sometimes felt in the supraclavicular fossa (Virchow's node). In patients with advanced disease, there may be evidence of metastatic spread to the peritoneum and liver with ascites and hepatomegaly. Skin manifestations of malignancy, such as dermatomyositis and acanthosis nigricans, are occasionally associated.

Investigations

Barium meal or gastroscopy and biopsy are the investigations of choice, biopsy providing histological confirmation. CT, MRI and endoscopic ultrasonography may be useful in staging the tumour and guiding operability.

Management

Surgery is the best form of treatment if the tumour is operable. Chemotherapy has made little impact and is not justifiable outside clinical trials.

Prognosis

The overall survival is poor (10% 5-year survival). Those patients undergoing curative operations, however, have a 5-year survival of 50%. In Japan, where there is an active screening programme, earlier diagnosis and an aggressive surgical approach have resulted in a 5-year survival of 90%.

Benign gastric tumours

The most common is a leiomyoma which is usually asymptomatic although it can ulcerate and bleed. Gastric polyps are uncommon and usually regenerative. Adenomatous polyps can occur but are rare.

GASTROINTESTINAL BLEEDING

Acute upper gastrointestinal bleeding

Haematemesis is the vomiting of blood. Melaena is the passage of black tarry stools which are the result of altered blood from the upper intestine (50 ml or more is required to produce this).

Aetiology

Chronic peptic ulceration is still the most common cause of upper gastrointestinal bleeding (Figure 2.1). Relative incidences vary according to patient population. Aspirin and NSAIDs may be responsible for bleeding from both duodenal and gastric ulcers, particularly in elderly people.

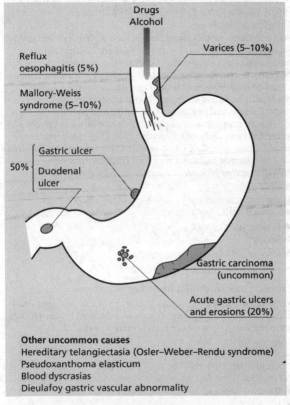

Figure 2.1 Causes of acute upper gastrointestinal haemorrhage.

Corticosteroids have been implicated, but in the usual therapeutic dosage they probably have no relationship to gastrointestinal bleeding.

Management

RESUSCITATE

In many patients no specific treatment is required, bleeding stops spontaneously and the patient remains well compensated. In patients with large bleeds or clinical signs of shock, urgent transfusion, ideally with whole blood, is required (page 366). Monitoring pulse rate and venous pressure will guide transfusion requirements.

DETERMINE SITE OF BLEEDING

This may be evident from the history but endoscopy should be performed as soon as possible. Endoscopy can detect the site of haemorrhage in 80% or more of cases.

Specific management

At endoscopy varices should be treated with sclerotherapy (injection of a sclerosant, e.g. ethanolamine, directly into or next to the varix) or banding. Ulcers that are actively bleeding or demonstrate stigmata of recent bleeding (visible vessel or overlying clot) should be treated by injection of dilute adrenaline or coagulated with the heater probe or laser. There is little evidence that drug therapy with H_2-receptor antagonists or proton pump inhibitors improve immediate mortality or rebleeding rates, but these agents are usually given to induce ulcer healing. Surgery may be required for persistent or recurrent bleeding from ulcers. Further management of bleeding varices is described on page 82.

Prognosis

The overall mortality rate is 5–10%. The following are associated with a poor prognosis:

- Old age (>65 years)
- Shock
- Continued bleeding or rebleeding
- Presence of chronic liver disease

Lower gastrointestinal bleeding

Massive bleeding is rare and usually the result of diverticular disease or ischaemic colitis. Minor bleeds from haemorrhoids are common. Other causes are listed in Figure 2.2

Management

With large bleeds resuscitation with intravenous fluids / whole blood may be required. The site of bleeding must then be determined using the following investigations as appropriate:

- Rectal examination, e.g. carcinoma
- Proctoscopy, e.g. haemorrhoids
- Sigmoidoscopy, e.g. inflammatory bowel disease

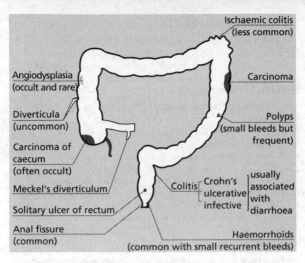

Figure 2.2 Causes of lower gastrointestinal bleeding.

- Barium enema, – any mucosal lesion
- Colonoscopy – diagnosis and removal of polyps
- Angiography – vascular abnormality, e.g. angiodysplasia

Specific management
Lesions should be treated as appropriate.

Chronic gastrointestinal bleeding

Chronic gastrointestinal bleeding usually presents with iron deficiency anaemia and chronic blood loss. Blood loss producing anaemia in all men and in women after the menopause is always the result of bleeding from the gastrointestinal tract. The causes of chronic blood loss are those that cause acute bleeding (see Figures 2.1 and 2.2). However, oesophageal varices, duodenal ulcers and diverticular disease very rarely bleed chronically.

Investigations
Initial investigations are a 'top' and 'tail' performed at the same endoscopic session, i.e. gastroscopy and colonoscopy.

Further investigations are reserved for difficult cases where the above tests have not identified a source of bleeding.

- Small bowel follow-through
- Angiography
- Technetium-labelled red cell scan
- Small bowel enteroscopy

THE SMALL INTESTINE

The small intestine has a number of functions, many of which are concerned with digestion and absorption of nutrients. Nutrients are absorbed throughout the small intestine with the exception of vitamin B_{12} and bile salts which have specific receptors in the terminal ileum. [CM pp. 200–207]

The presenting features of small-bowel disease are diarrhoea, steatorrhoea (pale, bulky stools that contain fat), abdominal pain or discomfort, and weight loss which is the result of accompanying anorexia. The two most common causes of small-bowel disease in developed countries are coeliac disease and Crohn's disease. In many small-bowel diseases, malabsorption of specific substances occurs, but these deficiencies do not dominate the clinical picture. An example is Crohn's disease in which malabsorption of vitamin B_{12} can be demonstrated, but this is not usually a clinical problem. The major disorders of the small intestine that cause malabsorption are shown in Table 2.3.

Table 2.3 Disorders of the small intestine causing malabsorption

Coeliac disease
Dermatitis herpetiformis
Tropical sprue
Bacterial overgrowth
Intestinal resection
Whipple's disease
Radiation enteritis
Parasite infection, e.g. *Giardia lamblia*

Coeliac disease (gluten-sensitive enteropathy)

Coeliac disease is a condition in which there is an abnormal jejunal mucosa that improves morphologically when the patient is treated with a gluten-free diet and relapses when gluten is reintroduced. Gluten is contained in wheat, rye, barley and possibly oats.

Epidemiology

Worldwide distribution but it is rare in the African people and more common in Ireland (incidence 1 in 300; 1 in 2000 in UK).

Aetiology

The toxic portion of gluten is the peptide gliadin. The exact mechanism by which gluten causes damage to the intestinal mucosa is not known. The strong association with the haplotypes HLA-A1, -B8, -DR3, -DR7 and -DQW2 suggests a possible immunological origin.

Pathology

There are absent villi with elongation of crypts (*subtotal villous atrophy*). There is a chronic inflammatory cell infiltrate in the lamina propria with an increase in intraepithelial cell lymphocytes. [CM p. 209]

Clinical features

Coeliac disease can present at any age but there are two peaks in incidence: in infancy after weaning onto gluten-containing foods and in adults at 30–40 years. It often presents with non-specific symptoms of tiredness and malaise or symptoms of small intestinal disease (see above).

Physical signs are usually few and non-specific, and related to anaemia and nutritional deficiency. There is an increased incidence of atopy and autoimmune disease.

Investigations

JEJUNAL MUCOSAL BIOPSY is obtained via the endoscope or Crosby–Kugler capsule. The capsule is swallowed on the end of a tube and guided into the jejunum by radiographic screening; a biopsy is then obtained by suction on the tubing. The biopsy shows the histological features described above. Other causes (Table 2.4) of a flat mucosa are rare in adults.

SERUM ANTIBODIES: antigliadin and antiendomysial antibodies are present in most cases.

BLOOD COUNT: a mild anaemia is present in 50% of cases. There is almost always folate deficiency, commonly iron deficiency and, rarely, vitamin B_{12} deficiency.

RADIOLOGY: small bowel follow-through shows a dilated bowel with thickened folds.

Table 2.4 Causes of villous atrophy

Giardiasis
Malnutrition
Ischaemia
Lymphoma
Whipple's disease
Tropical sprue
Coeliac disease

Management

Treatment is with a gluten-free diet. A repeat biopsy after treatment shows morphological improvement in the mucosa and confirms the diagnosis.

Complications

There is an increased incidence of malignancy, particularly intestinal lymphoma, small bowel cancer and oesophageal cancer.

Dermatitis herpetiformis

Dermatitis herpetiformis is an itchy, symmetrical eruption of vesicles and crusts over the extensor surfaces of the body. Most patients also have a gluten-sensitive enteropathy which is usually asymptomatic. The skin condition responds to dapsone but both the gut and the skin will improve on a gluten-free diet.

Tropical sprue

Tropical sprue is a chronic, progressive, small intestinal disorder presenting with malabsorption which occurs in residents or visitors to a tropical area where the disease is endemic (Asia, some Caribbean islands, Puerto Rico, parts of South America).

Aetiology

The aetiology is unknown but the disease occurs in epidemics and responds to antibiotics, suggesting an infectious aetiology.

Clinical features

The disease may present many years after being in the tropics. There is diarrhoea, anorexia and abdominal distension. Nutritional deficiencies develop over a variable period of time.

Investigations

Malabsorption should be demonstrated, particularly of fat and vitamin B_{12}. The jejunal mucosa shows villous atrophy affecting the whole small bowel. It is necessary to exclude infective causes of diarrhoea, particularly *Giardia lamblia*.

Management

Treatment is with a combination of folic acid and tetracycline which may be required for up to 6 months. In addition, nutritional deficiencies must be corrected.

Bacterial overgrowth

The upper small intestine is almost sterile. Bacterial overgrowth may occur when there is stasis of intestinal contents as a result of abnormal motility, eg. systemic sclerosis or a structural abnormality, e.g. diverticulum.

Clinical features

There may be diarrhoea and/or steatorrhoea caused by deconjugation of bile salts by bacteria. Vitamin B_{12} deficiency, resulting from its metabolism by bacteria, can also occur.

Diagnosis

BREATH TESTS

The hydrogen or ^{14}C breath tests are the investigations of choice. These depend on the ability of the organisms to metabolize either glucose or labelled bile salts, given by mouth, with the production of either hydrogen (from glucose) or $^{14}CO_2$ (from bile salts) which are then absorbed and can be measured in the exhaled air.

PROXIMAL SMALL INTESTINAL ASPIRATES

Proximal small intestinal aspirates (obtained via the endoscope or by a peroral tube) will reveal high numbers of coliforms and *Bacteroides* sp.

Management

If possible the underlying cause should be corrected. This may not be possible and rotating courses of antibiotics are necessary such as tetracycline and metronidazole.

Whipple's disease

Whipple's disease is a rare systemic disease which almost always involves the small intestine. Common clinical features include steatorrhoea, abdominal pain, fever, lymphadeno-pathy, arthritis and neurological involvement. Intestinal biopsy shows PAS positive macrophages. On electron microscopy, the macrophages are seen to contain bacteria now called *Tropheryma whippei*. Treatment of the disease is with antibiotics.

Intestinal resection

The effects of small intestinal resection depend on the extent and the area involved. Resection of the terminal ileum leads to malabsorption of:

- Vitamin B_{12} leading to megaloblastic anaemia.
- Bile salts which overflow into the colon and interfere with salt and water absorption producing diarrhoea. Bile salts in the colon also increase oxalate absorption which may result in renal oxalate stones (page 234).

If there is extensive resection, increased hepatic bile salt synthesis cannot compensate for faecal loss and there is steatorrhoea secondary to bile salt deficiency. After massive intestinal resection there is severe loss of water and electrolytes with malnutrition.

Miscellaneous intestinal conditions [CM pp. 212–213]

Tuberculosis

This results from reactivation of primary disease caused by *M. tuberculosis* (page 343) and is most commonly seen in Asian immigrants. The ileocaecal valve is the most common site affected.

Clinical features

There is abdominal pain, diarrhoea, anorexia, weight loss and fever. A mass may be palpable. The symptoms, signs and radiology (see below) can be similar to those of Crohn's disease and TB must always be considered in the differential diagnosis of Asians presenting with apparent Crohn's disease.

Diagnosis

RADIOLOGY

The chest radiograph will show evidence of pulmonary

tuberculosis in 50% of cases. The small bowel follow-through may show features similar to those of Crohn's disease (pages 47–52). Abdominal ultrasonography shows mesenteric thickening and lymphadenopathy.

ENDOSCOPY

Colonoscopy with terminal ileal biopsies is usually performed. It is not always possible to obtain bacteriological confirmation on tissue culture and treatment is started if there is a high degree of suspicion.

SURGERY

Laparotomy is rarely needed for diagnosis.

Management

Treatment is similar to pulmonary tuberculosis, i.e. isoniazid, rifampicin and pyrazinamide, although 1 year's treatment is required.

Protein-losing enteropathy

This involves increased protein loss across an abnormal intestinal mucosa. If there is inadequate hepatic synthesis of albumin to compensate for the intestinal loss, patients develop hypoalbuminaemia and oedema. Causes include Crohn's disease, Ménétrièr's disease (thickening and enlargement of gastric folds), coeliac disease and lymphatic disorders, e.g. lymphangiectasia.

Meckel's diverticulum

This is a congenital abnormality affecting 2–3% of the population. A diverticulum projects from the wall of the ileum approximately 60 cm from the ileocaecal valve. About half will contain gastric mucosa which secretes acid, and peptic ulceration may occur with complications of bleeding or perforation. They may also become inflamed and present similar to appendicitis. Treatment is surgical removal.

Chronic intestinal ischaemia

This is rare and results from atheromatous occlusion of mesenteric vessels in elderly people. The characteristic symptom is abdominal pain occurring after food. Diagnosis is made using angiography.

Malignant small intestinal tumours

These are rare and present with abdominal pain, diarrhoea, anorexia and anaemia. Carcinoid tumours have additional clinical features described below.

Carcinoid tumours

Pathology

These originate from argentaffin cells (serotonin-producing) of the intestine. The most common sites are the appendix, terminal ileum and rectum. Carcinoid tumours produce serotonin (5-hydroxytryptamine or 5-HT), kinins, histamine and a variety of other hormones that are metabolized by the liver.

Clinical features
In the presence of liver metastases tumour products are able to drain directly into the hepatic vein (without being metabolized) and then into the systemic circulation where they produce a variety of effects resulting in the carcinoid syndrome: flushing, wheezing, diarrhoea and abdominal pain, and right-sided cardiac valvular fibrosis causing stenosis and regurgitation.

Investigations
A high level of 5-hydroxyindole acetic acid (5-HIAA), the breakdown product of serotonin, is found in the urine and this is useful in diagnosing carcinoid syndrome. Ultrasonography examination of the liver confirms the presence of secondary deposits.

Management
Treatment is symptomatic and aimed at:

- Reducing tumour mass through surgical resection, hepatic artery embolization or chemotherapy
- Inhibition of tumour products with 5-HT antagonists, e.g. cyproheptadine, or octreotide (a long-acting somatostatin analogue)

Adenocarcinoma

Adenocarcinoma accounts for 50% of malignant small bowel tumours; there is an increased incidence in coeliac disease and Crohn's disease.

Lymphoma

Non-Hodgkin's lymphoma constitutes 15% of malignant small bowel tumours and may be B cell or T cell in origin. The latter occur with increased frequency in coeliac disease.

Benign small bowel tumours

- The Peutz–Jegher syndrome is an autosomal dominant condition with mucocutaneous pigmentation (circumoral, hands and feet) and hamartomatous gastrointestinal polyps. Polyps may occur anywhere in the gastrointestinal tract but are most common in the small bowel. They may bleed or cause intussusception and virtually never become malignant.
- Adenomas, leiomyomas and lipomas are rare. They are usually asymptomatic and discovered incidentally.
- Familial adenomatous polyposis (page 54).

INFLAMMATORY BOWEL DISEASE

Two main forms are recognized: Crohn's disease which affects any part of the gastrointestinal tract and ulcerative colitis which affects the large bowel only.

Epidemiology

Inflammatory bowel disease is more common in the Western World occurring at any age but most commonly between the ages of 20 and 40 years. Both sexes are affected but ulcerative colitis is more common in women. There is a familial tendency and an increased incidence of HLA-B27 in inflammatory bowel disease with ankylosing spondylitis. Crohn's disease is more common in smokers and ulcerative colitis less common in smokers.

Aetiology

This is unknown but possible factors include:

● Infective agents – mycobacteria, measles, other viruses

● Immunological factors – autoimmunity, altered macrophage function

● Multifocal gastrointestinal infarction

Pathology

Ulcerative colitis and Crohn's disease have important differences macroscopically and microscopically (Table 2.5).

Table 2.5 Histological differences between Crohn's disease and ulcerative colitis

	Crohn's disease	Ulcerative colitis
Macroscopic	Affects any part of the gut from mouth to anus	Affects only the colon Begins in the rectum and extends proximally in varying degrees
	Discontinuous involvement ('skip lesions')	Continuous involvement
	Deep ulcers and fissures in the mucosa – "cobblestone appearance"	Red mucosa which bleeds easily Ulcers and pseudopolyps (regenerating mucosa) in severe disease
Microscopic	Transmural inflammation	Mucosal inflammation
	Granulomata ++	No granulomata but goblet cell depletion and crypt abscesses

Clinical features

CROHN'S DISEASE is a progressive chronic disease with symptomatology depending on the region of involved bowel. It presents insidiously with abdominal pain, diarrhoea and weight loss. Less commonly it presents as an acute abdomen with right iliac fossa pain mimicking appendicitis. In perianal disease there are anal tags, fissures, fistulae and abscess formation.

ULCERATIVE COLITIS presents with diarrhoea containing blood and mucus. The clinical course may be one of persistent diarrhoea, relapses and remissions or severe fulminating colitis (Table 2.6).

Table 2.6 Definition of a severe attack of ulcerative colitis

Bloody diarrhoea	> 6/day
Fever	> 37.5°C
Tachycardia	> 90/min
ESR	> 30 mm/hour
Anaemia	Hb < 10 g/dl
Albumin	< 30 g/l

Patients with inflammatory bowel disease, particularly Crohn's disease, may have one or more extraintestinal manifestations and these are listed in Table 2.7.

Table 2.7 Extra-gastrointestinal manifestations of inflammatory bowel disease

Eyes
Uveitis
Episcleritis
Conjunctivitis

Joints
Monoarticular arthritis (knees and ankles)
Ankylosing spondylitis*
Sacroiliitis

Skin
Erythema nodosum
Pyoderma gangrenosum (necrotizing ulceration of the skin)
Vasculitis (rare)

Liver* †
Fatty change
Pericholangitis
Sclerosing cholangitis
Chronic active hepatitis
Cirrhosis

Calculi*
Increased incidence of kidney and gallbladder stones in Crohn's disease

* These manifestations are not related to disease activity.
† Biochemical abnormalities are common, clinically overt disease is uncommon.

Investigations
BLOOD COUNT: anaemia is common and usually the normochromic/normocytic anaemia of chronic disease,

although iron deficiency may occur. The white cell count, ESR and C-reactive protein are often raised and the albumin may be low in severe disease. '

RADIOLOGY: in Crohn's disease, a small-bowel follow-through shows an asymmetrical alteration in the mucosal pattern, with deep ulceration and areas of narrowing (string sign) largely confined to the ileum. Skip lesions may be seen. A barium enema may demonstrate aphthous ulceration or deeper ulceration in the colon. Ultrasonography and CT scanning are particularly helpful in delineating abscesses, and will show thickened bowel in involved areas.

In ulcerative colitis a barium enema shows the extent of disease and in long-standing disease the colon is shortened and narrowed. A plain radiograph should be performed during a severe attack to look for toxic dilatation of the colon.

COLONOSCOPY: this is useful for delineating the exact extent of disease and for obtaining biopsies for histological examination to differentiate between Crohn's disease and ulcerative colitis.

Differential diagnosis
Crohn's disease must be differentiated from other causes of chronic diarrhoea, malabsorption and malnutrition. In children it is a cause of short stature. Other causes of terminal ileitis are TB and *Yersinia enterocolitica* infection (causing an acute illness). Inflammatory bowel disease affecting the colon must be differentiated from other causes of colitis: infection (page 15), ischaemia and microscopic colitis (macroscopically normal mucosa but inflammation detected histologically).

Management
MEDICAL

- Oral sulphasalazine (5-aminosalicylic acid + sulphapyridine carrier) or other 5-acetylsalicylic acid preparations (mesalazine, olsalazine) will induce a remission in mild attacks of ulcerative colitis and colonic Crohn's disease. In a lower dose it is useful as a maintenance treatment to reduce the number of relapses. 5-Acetylsalicylic acid preparations can also be administered as an enema or suppository to treat proctosigmoiditis (i.e. inflammation of the rectum and sigmoid colon).

- Corticosteroids: oral steroids are used to treat acute attacks and the dose tailed off as symptoms improve. In severe attacks intravenous steroids are necessary (Table 2.8). Proctosigmoiditis can be treated locally with steroid enemas and suppositories.

- Azathioprine is used in some patients to maintain a steroid-induced remission.

- Elemental diet (liquid preparation of amino acids, carbohydrate and fat) will induce a remission in a relapse of small-bowel Crohn's disease. The exact mode of action is not known. These diets are unpalatable and often have to be given via a nasogastric tube.

- Metronidazole is useful in severe perianal Crohn's disease resulting from its antibacterial action.

- Cyclosporin is occasionally used in the treatment of refractory ulcerative colitis.

Table 2.8 Management of acute severe colitis

Admit to hospital

Investigations
  Full blood count, ESR
  Serum albumin
  Urea and electrolytes
  Blood cultures (Gram-negative sepsis is common)
  Plain abdominal radiograph ?toxic dilatation (diameter, colon >5 cm), perforation

Intravenous steroids
  Hydrocortisone 100 mg 6-hourly

Correct electrolyte and fluid imbalance

Surgical treatment (colectomy) may be necessary

SURGERY is indicated for:
- Failure of medical therapy
- Complications (Table 2.9)
- Failure to grow in children

In Crohn's disease resections are kept to a minimum as recurrence is almost inevitable in the remaining bowel. The surgical options in ulcerative colitis are panproctocolectomy with ileostomy (the whole colon and rectum are removed and the ileum brought out onto the abdominal wall as a stoma) or colectomy with an ileorectal (diseased rectum left *in situ* and diarrhoea may still occur) or ileoanal anastamosis (the terminal ileum is used to form a reservoir and the patient is continent with a few bowel motions per day).

Table 2.9 Complications of inflammatory bowel disease

Toxic dilatation + perforation
Stricture formation
Abscess formation (Crohn's disease)
Fistulae and fissures (Crohn's)
Cancer:
    In ulcerative colitis the risk of colon cancer increases with extent and
    duration of disease (30% after 30 years in total colitis)
    Slightly increased risk in Crohn's disease.

Prognosis

Both diseases are characterized by relapses and remissions.
Almost all patients with Crohn's disease have a significant
relapse over a 20-year period. The mortality rate is twice as
high as that of the general population. The prognosis of
ulcerative colitis is variable. Only 10% of patients with
proctitis develop more extensive disease, but with severe
fulminant disease the mortality rate is 15–25%.

THE COLON AND RECTUM

Diverticular disease

Pouches of mucosa extrude through the muscular wall through
weakened areas near blood vessels to form diverticula. The
term *diverticulosis* indicates the presence of diverticula.
Diverticulitis implies inflammation which occurs when faeces
obstruct the neck of the diverticulum. Diverticula are common,
affecting 50% of the population over 50 years of age.

Aetiology

The precise cause of diverticular disease is unknown,
although it appears to be related to the low-fibre diet eaten in
Western populations.

Clinical features

It is asymptomatic in 90% and usually discovered incidentally
when a barium enema or colonoscopy is performed for other
reasons. Symptoms are usually the result of bleeding or acute
diverticulitis (left iliac fossa pain, fever, nausea, vomiting).
Complications include abscess formation, perforation, fistula
formation and intestinal obstruction.

Management

Acute attacks are treated with bowel rest, intravenous fluids
and antibiotics. Surgery is indicated rarely for complications
and for attacks that occur frequently in spite of medical therapy.

Constipation

This is a very common problem in the general population
which often requires no more than dietary advice and
reassurance. It is particularly common in elderly people in
whom it is often associated with immobility and poor diet,

and in young women in whom it may be associated with slow colonic transit or postpartum pelvic floor abnormalities. Most have simple constipation associated with low fibre intake. Colorectal cancer should always be excluded in middle-aged and elderly people.

Table 2.10. Causes of constipation

Simple
Obstruction
Painful anal conditions
Drugs, e.g. opiates, aluminium antacids
Hypothyroidism
Depression
Immobility
Hirschsprung's disease

Management
A high-fibre diet and bulking agents should be the first line of treatment. Laxatives should only be used as a short-term treatment.

Miscellaneous conditions

Megacolon

This term describes a number of conditions in which the colon is dilated. The most common cause is chronic constipation. Other causes are Chagas' and Hirschsprung's disease (congenital aganglionic segment in the rectum). Treatment is similar to that for simple constipation, although Hirschsprung's disease responds to surgical resection.

Ischaemic colitis

This usually presents in the older age group with abdominal pain and rectal bleeding, and occasionally shock. Sigmoidoscopy is often normal apart from blood. Treatment is symptomatic although surgery may be required for gangrene, perforation or stricture formation.

Colon polyps and the polyposis syndromes

A polyp is an elevation above the mucosal surface. They may be single or multiple, are usually asymptomatic and are almost always adenomas (70–80%). In the polyposis syndromes, hundreds of polyps may be present.

Hamartomatous polyps

Hamartomas are benign tumours composed of an overgrowth of mature cells and tissues that normally occur in the affected part, in this case the colon. They may be one of two types:

JUVENILE POLYPS
These are dominantly inherited polyps which occur in

children and teenagers, and present early with diarrhoea, bleeding or intussusception.

PEUTZ–JEGHERS POLYPS

Peutz–Jeghers polyps may be single but are usually multiple. The Peutz–Jeghers syndrome consists of mucocutaneous pigmentation, multiple polyps in the large and small bowel, and a dominant inheritance.

Adenomatous polyps

Adenomatous polyps are tumours of benign neoplastic epithelium. They are common, occurring in about 10% of the population. The aetiology is unknown although genetic and environmental factors have been implicated. They rarely produce symptoms although large polyps can bleed or cause anaemia, and villous adenomas can occasionally present with diarrhoea and hypokalaemia. Adenomatous polyps carry a malignant risk which increases with polyp size. Treatment is by endoscopic removal.

FAMILIAL ADENOMATOUS POLYPOSIS

This is an autosomal dominantly inherited condition characterized by the presence of multiple adenomatous polyps throughout the gastrointestinal tract and resulting inevitably in colon cancer unless the large bowel is removed. As a result a prophylactic colectomy is usually performed in young adulthood. These patients remain at risk of small bowel cancer particularly of the duodenum. The gene responsible has been localized to the long arm of chromosome 5. Many of these patients have congenital hypertrophy of the retinal pigment epithelium (CHRPE) and this, along with genetic analysis, facilitates screening of young patients. Gardener's syndrome is a variant of this condition which includes multiple bone and soft tissue tumours in addition to adenomas.

Colorectal cancer

Epidemiology

This is the second most common tumour in the UK and the incidence increases with age. It is rare in Africa and Asia largely through environmental differences. A diet high in meat and animal fat and low in fibre is thought to be an important aetiological factor. Ulcerative colitis and familial adenomatous polyposis are predisposing factors. First degree relatives of a patient are at increased risk.

Inheritance

Multiple molecular genetic abnormalities are now thought to be involved in the development of sporadic colon cancer. These include the activation of tumour-promoting genes or oncogenes (*c-Ki-ras*, *c-myc*) and the inactivation of tumour suppressor genes (*MCC*, *DCC*, *p53*). The risk of a tumour developing increases with increasing number of genetic abnormalities. [CM p. 225]

Pathology
Two-thirds of the tumours are in the rectosigmoid area. Spread
is by direct invasion through the bowel wall with later invasion
of blood vessels and lymphatics and spread to the liver. The
mortality of colorectal cancer is directly related to the stage at
presentation, and the stage is most commonly classified
according to the modified Dukes' classification (Table 2.11).
Synchronous tumours are present in 2% of cases.

Table 2.11 Dukes' grading of colon cancer

Dukes' A	Tumour confined to the bowel wall
Dukes' B	Tumour extending through the bowel wall
Dukes' C	Regional lymph nodes involved
Dukes' D	Distant metastases

Clinical features
Alteration in bowel habit, abdominal pain, rectal bleeding
and anaemia are common presenting features of colon
cancer. Clinical examination is usually unhelpful although a
mass may be palpable transabdominally or in the rectum.
Hepatomegaly may be present with liver metastases.

Investigation
Examination of the colon is performed with a double-
contrast barium enema or colonoscopy. A full blood count
may show anaemia and abnormal serum liver biochemistry
suggests the presence of liver secondaries. Feacal occult
blood tests have been used for mass screening but are not of
value in hospital practice.

Management
Treatment is surgical with tumour resection and end-to-end
anastomosis of bowel if possible. Adjuvant chemotherapy
with 5-fluorouracil and levamisole increases survival in
Dukes' grade C cases.

Prognosis
Overall 5-year survival rate is 40%, but is over 95% in
tumours confined to the bowel wall (Dukes' grade A).

Cancer families
Hereditary non-polyposis colon cancer (HNPCC) accounts
for 5–10% of colon cancers. These patients have an increased
risk of developing tumours at an early age, and more often
develop right-sided tumours. Many of these patients have a
high rate of endometrial and other non-gastrointestinal
cancers. Recently the genetic abnormality associated with
HNPCC has been localized to chromosome 2.

DIARRHOEA

True diarrhoea is defined as an increase in stool weight to
more than 300 g in 24 hours. This must be differentiated from

frequent passage of small amounts of stool (usually functional).

There are four main mechanisms: osmotic, secretory, inflammatory and related to motility.

Osmotic diarrhoea

This occurs when there are large quantities of non-absorbed hypertonic substances in the bowel lumen. The diarrhoea stops when the patient stops eating or the malabsorptive substance is discontinued. Causes of osmotic diarrhoea are the following:

- Ingestion of non-absorbable substance, e.g. magnesium sulphate
- Generalized malabsorption
- Specific malabsorptive defect, e.g. disaccharidase deficiency.

Secretory diarrhoea

Secretory diarrhoea results from net secretion of fluid and electrolytes into the bowel lumen and continues when the patient fasts. The causes are:

- Enterotoxins, e.g. from *E. coli*, cholera toxin
- Hormone-secreting tumours, e.g. VIPoma (page 101)
- Bile salts (in the colon) following ileal resection
- Fatty acids (in the colon) following ileal resection
- Some laxatives

Inflammatory diarrhoea

Mucosal damage with infection, e.g. shigella dysentery, or inflammation, e.g. ulcerative colitis, leads to fluid and blood loss.

Motility related

Abnormal motility often produces frequency rather than true diarrhoea. Causes are thyrotoxicosis, diabetic autonomic neuropathy and post vagotomy.

Investigation

Acute diarrhoea lasting a few days is the result of dietary indiscretion or an infection. Investigation is not needed and treatment is symptomatic to maintain hydration. Chronic diarrhoea always requires investigation. Figure 2.3 outlines an approach to the investigation of a patient with chronic diarrhoea. Laxative abuse, usually seen in young females, must be excluded as a cause of chronic diarrhoea. Patients taking anthraquinone purgatives, e.g. Senokot, develop pigmentation of the colonic mucosa which may be seen at sigmoidoscopy. Other laxatives may be detected in the stool or urine.

Diarrhoea is a common problem in patients with AIDS resulting either from a specific AIDS enteropathy or from an

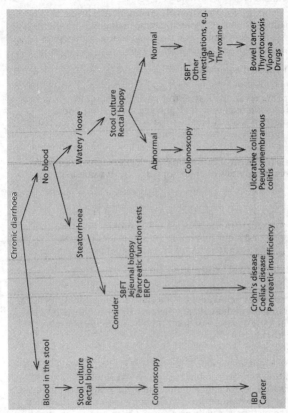

Figure 2.3 An approach to the investigation of chronic diarrhoea. SFBT, small bowel follow-through; ERCP, endoscopic retrograde cholangiopancreatography; VIP, vasoactive intestinal polypeptide; IBD, inflammatory bowel disease.

Chronic diarrhoea

Blood in the stool

No blood

Stool culture
Rectal biopsy

→

Colonoscopy

→

IBD
Cancer

Steatorrhoea

Consider
SBFT
Jejeunal biopsy
Pancreatic function tests
ERCP

→

Crohn's disease
Coeliac disease
Pancreatic insufficiency

Watery / loose

Stool culture
Rectal biopsy

Abnormal

→

Colonoscopy

→

Ulcerative colitis
Pseudomembranous
colitis

Normal

→

SBFT
Other
investigations, e.g.
VIP
Thyroxine

→

Bowel cancer
Thyrotoxicosis
Vipoma
Drugs

infection (cryptosporidia, microsporidia, cytomegalovirus infection).

FUNCTIONAL BOWEL DISEASE

This is a general term used to embrace two syndromes:

- Non-ulcer dyspepsia
- Irritable bowel syndrome

These conditions are extremely common worldwide accounting for 60–70% of patients seen in the gastroenterology clinic. The two conditions overlap, with some symptoms being common to both.

Non-ulcer dyspepsia

Clinical features

There are a variety of symptoms which are usually stress related. Common symptoms include indigestion, wind, nausea, early satiety and heartburn. Symptoms are sometimes very similar to peptic ulceration.

Investigation

This is frequently unnecessary, particularly in young people, but barium studies or endoscopy may be of value to exclude peptic disease.

Management

This is mainly by reassurance. Antacids and H_2-receptor antagonists are rarely of benefit. The prokinetic agents cisapride and metaclopramide are sometimes helpful, particularly in those with fullness and bloating.

Irritable bowel syndrome

Aetiology

The aetiology is unknown. Abnormalities in gut motility have been found but these do not always correlate with symptoms. Psychological factors are important and symptoms are often exacerbated by stress.

Clinical features

Crampy abdominal pain relieved by defaecation or passage of wind, altered bowel habit, a sensation of incomplete evacuation, abdominal bloating and distension are common symptoms. Symptoms are more common in women than men and the history is usually prolonged. Characteristically the patients look healthy. Examination is usually normal, although sigmoidoscopy and air insufflation may reproduce the pain. If frequency of defaecation is a feature, a rectal biopsy should be performed to exclude inflammatory bowel disease.

Investigation

This depends on the individual patient. Young patients with classic symptoms do not require investigation. New symptoms in an elderly patient should prompt a search for underlying disease.

Management

Reassurance with discussion of lifestyle and diet is valuable. A high-fibre diet and antispasmodics, e.g. mebeverine, are useful in some patients. Other treatments such as antidepressants, biofeedback and hypnotherapy may be tried.

THE ACUTE ABDOMEN

This section deals with acute abdominal conditions that cause patients to be hospitalized within a few hours of the onset of their pain. Most patients are admitted under the care of the surgical team and some patients will need a laparotomy. Medical conditions that may present as an acute abdomen include diabetic ketoacidosis, myocardial infarction and pneumonia. The irritable bowel syndrome may also present with acute severe abdominal pain.

History

A detailed history will often point to the cause of the pain. In addition a full medical, surgical and gynaecological history must be taken.

- Acute abdominal pain may be *intermittent* or *continuous*. Intermittent (colicky) pain describes pain that occurs for a short period (usually a few minutes) and is interspersed with pain-free periods lasting a few minutes or up to half an hour. This is characteristic of *mechanical obstruction* of a hollow viscus, e.g. ureteric calculus or bowel obstruction (Table 2.12). Additional symptoms of bowel obstruction, which may or may not be present, are abdominal distension, vomiting and absolute constipation (i.e. failure to pass flatus or stool). Biliary pain (previously called biliary colic) resulting from obstruction of the gallbladder or bile duct (page 96) is not colicky but usually a constant upper abdominal pain.

  Continuous pain is constant with no periods of complete relief. It occurs in many abdominal conditions.

- The *onset* of pain may be sudden or gradual. Sudden onset of pain suggests perforation of a viscus (e.g. duodenal ulcer), rupture of an organ (e.g. aortic aneurysm) or torsion (e.g. ovarian cyst). The pain of acute pancreatitis often begins suddenly.

- The *site* of the pain must be noted. In general, upper abdominal pain is produced by pathology of either the upper abdominal viscera, e.g. acute cholecystitis, acute pancreatitis, or the stomach and duodenum. The pain of small bowel obstruction is often in the centre of the abdomen. A common cause of acute right iliac fossa pain is acute appendicitis.

- *Radiation* of pain to the back suggests acute pancreatitis, rupture of an aortic aneurysm or renal tract disease.

Examination

A general physical examination should be made and the following points noted:

- The presence of shock (pale cool peripheries, tachycardia, hypotension) suggests rupture of an organ, e.g aortic aneurysm, ruptured ectopic pregnancy. It may also occur in the later stages of generalized peritonitis resulting from bowel perforation (see below).
- Fever is common in acute inflammatory conditions.
- Peritonitis and bowel obstruction produce specific signs on abdominal examination.

The signs of *peritonitis* are tenderness, guarding, and rigidity on palpation. Guarding describes an involuntary contraction of the abdominal muscles when the abdomen is palpated. Peritonitis may be localized or generalized (see below). Bowel sounds are absent with generalized peritonitis.

Mechanical bowel obstruction produces distension and active 'tinkling' bowel sounds. A strangulated hernia may produce obstruction and the hernial orifices must always be examined.

A complete examination must include a rectal and pelvic examination.

Investigations

BLOOD TESTS. The white cell count may be raised in inflammatory conditions. The serum amylase may be raised in any acute abdomen but levels greater than five times normal indicate acute pancreatitis.

RADIOLOGY. An erect chest radiograph may show air under the diaphragm with a perforated viscus. A plain abdominal radiograph shows dilated loops of bowel and fluid levels in obstruction. Ultrasonography examination is useful in the diagnosis of acute cholangitis, appendicitis and gynae-cological conditions.

SURGERY. Laparoscopy or laparotomy may occasionally be required.

Acute appendicitis

Acute appendicitis occurs when the lumen of the appendix becomes obstructed by a faecolith.

Epidemiology
It affects all age groups but is rare in the very young and very old.

Clinical features
The typical clinical presentation is onset of central abdominal pain which then becomes localized to the right iliac fossa (RIF), accompanied by anorexia and sometimes vomiting and diarrhoea. The patient is pyrexial with tenderness and guarding in the RIF.

Investigations
There is a raised white cell count and ultrasonography may show an inflamed appendix. In most cases the diagnosis is clinical.

Management
The treatment is surgical with removal of the appendix. This is now often performed via the laparoscope.

Complications
These arise from gangrene and perforation leading to localized abscess formation or generalized peritonitis.

Acute peritonitis

LOCALIZED PERITONITIS occurs with all acute inflammatory conditions of the gastrointestinal tract and management depends on the underlying condition, e.g. acute appendicitis, acute cholecystitis.

GENERALIZED PERITONITIS occurs as a result of rupture of an abdominal viscus, e.g. perforated duodenal ulcer, perforated appendix. There is a sudden onset of abdominal pain which rapidly becomes generalized. The patient is shocked and lies still as movement exacerbates the pain. A plain abdominal radiograph shows air under the diaphragm; serum amylase must be checked to exclude acute pancreatitis.

Intestinal obstruction

Intestinal obstruction is either mechanical or functional.
MECHANICAL (Table 2.12)
The bowel above the level of the obstruction is dilated, with increased secretion of fluid into the lumen. The patient complains of colicky abdominal pain associated with vomiting and absolute constipation. On examination there is distension and 'tinkling' bowel sounds. Small bowel obstruction may settle with conservative management (i.e. nasogastric suction and intravenous fluids to maintain hydration). Large-bowel obstruction is treated surgically.

Table 2.12 Causes of mechanical intestinal obstruction

Constriction from the outside	Bowel entrapped in a hernia
	Adhesions
	Volvulus particularly of sigmoid
Disease of the bowel wall	Crohn's disease
	Carcinoma
	Diverticular disease
Intraluminal obstruction	Foreign body
	Gallstones

FUNCTIONAL

This occurs with a paralytic ileus which is often seen in the postoperative stage of peritonitis or of major abdominal surgery. It also occurs when the nerves or muscles of the intestine are damaged causing intestinal pseudo-obstruction. Unlike mechanical obstruction, pain is often not present and bowel sounds may be decreased. Gas is seen throughout the bowel on a plain abdominal radiograph. Management is conservative.

The peritoneum

The peritoneal cavity is a closed sac lined by mesothelium. It contains a little fluid to allow the abdominal contents to move freely. Conditions which affect the peritoneum are listed below.

- Infective *(peritonitis)*   Secondary to gut disease, e.g. appendicitis, perforation
  Chronic peritoneal dialysis
  Spontaneous (associated with ascites)
  Tuberculous
- Neoplasia   Secondary deposits, e.g. from ovary
  Primary mesothelioma
- Vasculitis   Connective tissue disease

FINAL MEDICINE EXAMINATION: GASTROENTEROLOGY

1. State the causes of bloody diarrhoea. What are the most common infectious causes and what specific antibacterial therapy is available to treat these?
2. Write short notes on the management of massive haematemesis.
3. A 30-year-old man presents with a 10-week history of

discomfort in the right iliac fossa. He has also noticed some weight loss. The ESR is raised (50 mm/h). What are the likely causes? What imaging tests might be appropriate?

4. A 23-year-old beautician, who is otherwise well, gives a 5-year history of alternating morning diarrhoea, constipation, flatulence and left lower quadrant abdominal pain. What is the most likely diagnosis and how would you manage the problem?

5. A man of 30 presents with a 3-month history of difficulty in swallowing. What features of the history and clinical examination would help in making a diagnosis?

6. How would you investigate and manage a 44-year-old patient found to have a lesser curve gastric ulcer on a barium meal examination?

7. Give five common causes of malabsorption. List the clinical features.

ANSWERS

1. Bloody diarrhoea strongly suggests colonic disease. The common causes are inflammatory bowel disease and infections, although colon cancer (usually blood mixed in with the stools, not frank diarrhoea) and acute intestinal ischaemia should be borne in mind. The infectious causes of bloody diarrhoea are *Campylobacter jejuni*, *Shigella* sp. (bacillary dysentery), *Entamoeba histolytica* (amoebic dysentery, occurring in the tropics), some types of *Escherichia coli* and rarely *Salmonella* sp. and *Clostridium difficile*. Ciprofloxacillin will cover the common organisms except *Entamoeba histolytica* which is treated with metronidazole.

2. Massive haematemesis is usually the result of bleeding from varices or large gastric ulcers. Patients are usually shocked on presentation and must be aggressively resuscitated, initially with plasma expanders (page 366) and subsequently with whole blood. After adequate resuscitation the source of bleeding is localized at gastroscopy; further management depends on the cause (page 39).

3. In a young person right iliac fossa discomfort associated with weight loss and a raised ESR strongly suggests Crohn's disease (page 48). An appendix mass must be considered, although the history is long. In immigrants, ileocaecal tuberculosis should be considered (page 45). Amoebiasis may sometimes cause right iliac fossa pain,

usually with the formation of an 'amoeboma', and this should be considered in travellers from the tropics. Imaging is with abdominal ultrasonography and small-bowel follow-through.

4. These features, particularly in a young, otherwise healthy female, are very suggestive of irritable bowel syndrome. The approach to management is outlined on page 59.

5. The causes of dysphagia are listed on page 30. Progressive dysphagia associated with weight loss is suggestive of malignancy although this would be unusual in a young man. A preceding history of heartburn suggests reflux with a complicating peptic stricture. Chest pain, regurgitation and dysphagia for liquids points to a motility disorder such as achalasia. Oesophageal candidiasis or cytomegalovirus infection may cause dysphagia in patients with AIDS.

6. The investigation and management of gastric ulceration is described on pages 36–37. Benign gastric ulcers may appear radiologically similar to gastric cancer and therefore endoscopy with multiple biopsies is usually recommended. Treatment is initially with H_2-receptor antagonists for 6 weeks. Gastric ulcers must be followed up (by endoscopy) to ensure healing. An ulcer that is resistant to treatment raises the question of malignancy (initial biopsies may be negative because of sampling error) and repeat biopsies must be taken. *H. pylori* eradication treatment (page 36) is considered for benign ulcers which relapse after healing. Remember that NSAIDs are an important cause of gastric ulceration, so these should be withdrawn if possible.

7. This question is discussed on page 42.

CHAPTER 3

Liver, Biliary Tract and Pancreatic Diseases

Symptoms of liver disease

ACUTE LIVER DISEASE, e.g. viral hepatitis, may be asymptomatic or present with generalized symptoms of lethargy, anorexia and malaise in the early stages, with jaundice developing later (page 66).

CHRONIC LIVER DISEASE may also be asymptomatic and discovered from an incidental finding of abnormal liver biochemistry. Some patients with chronic liver disease may present at a late stage with complications of cirrhosis causing:

- Ascites with abdominal swelling and discomfort (page 83).
- Haematemesis and melaena from (often massive) gastrointestinal bleeding (page 82).
- Confusion and drowsiness (page 85).

Patients presenting in this way are often extremely unwell and a detailed history may not be obtained. However, physical examination will often reveal the signs of chronic liver disease (page 79) and thus point to liver disease as the cause of the presenting illness.

Pruritus (itching) occurs in cholestatic jaundice from any cause (page 68) but is particularly common in primary biliary cirrhosis when it may be the only symptom at presentation. Pruritus may occur in association with other systemic diseases (e.g. hyperthyroidism, polycythaemia, renal failure, malignant disease) and skin diseases (e.g scabies, eczema), but in these cases there are usually additional symptoms or signs that suggest the diagnosis.

Interpreting liver biochemistry and liver function tests

A routine blood sample sent to the laboratory for *liver biochemistry* will be processed by an automated multichannel analyser to produce serum levels of bilirubin, aminotransferases, alkaline phosphatase, γ-glutamyl transpeptidase and serum proteins. *Liver synthetic function* is determined by measuring the serum albumin and the prothrombin time (clotting factors of the intrinsic pathway are synthesized in the liver). A prolonged prothrombin time may also occur as a result of vitamin K deficiency in biliary obstruction (low concentration of intestinal bile salts results in poor absorption of vitamin K); however, unlike liver disease, clotting is corrected by giving intravenous vitamin K.

- BILIRUBIN (normal range <17 μmol/l). A small or moderate rise in the serum bilirubin without other abnormalities of liver enzymes is usually the result of Gilbert's syndrome, haemolysis or ineffective erythropoiesis. Hyperbilirubinaemia caused by hepatobiliary disease is almost always accompanied by other abnormalities of liver biochemistry; very high levels occur most frequently in biliary tract obstruction. Serial measurements are useful in following the progress of some diseases, e.g. primary biliary cirrhosis, or the response to treatment, e.g. after placement of a stent in cancer of the head of the pancreas.

- AMINOTRANSFERASES. These enzymes are present in hepatocytes and leak into the blood with liver cell damage. Very high levels may occur with acute hepatitis (20–50 times normal). *Aspartate aminotransferase* (AST) (normal range 10–40 U/l) is also present in heart and skeletal muscle and raised serum concentrations are seen with myocardial infarction and skeletal muscle damage. *Alanine aminotransferase* (ALT) (normal range 5–40 U/l) is more specific to the liver than AST.

- ALKALINE PHOSPHATASE (normal range 25–115 U/l) is situated in the canalicular and sinusoidal membranes of the liver. Raised serum alkaline phosphatase concentrations are seen in cholestasis from any cause, whether intra- or extrahepatic disease. Circulating alkaline phosphatase is also derived from bone, and raised serum levels occur in Paget's disease, osteomalacia, growing children, metastases and hyperthyroidism. In these cases differentiation from cholestasis is made by absence of a rise in serum γ-glutamyl transferase (γGT) (see below). The placenta secretes its own isoenzyme and its level is raised in pregnancy.

- γ-GLUTAMYL TRANSPEPTIDASE (normal range, male <50 U/l, female <32 U/l) is a liver microsomal enzyme which may be induced by alcohol and enzyme-inducing drugs, e.g. phenytoin. A raised serum concentration is a useful screen of alcohol abuse. In cholestasis the γGT rises in parallel with the serum alkaline phosphatase because it has a similar pathway of excretion.

JAUNDICE

Jaundice (icterus) is a yellow discoloration of the sclerae and skin as a result of a raised serum bilirubin and is usually detectable when the bilirubin is greater than 30–60 μmol/l (normal range < 17 μmol/l).

Bilirubin is derived predominantly from breakdown of haemoglobin in the spleen and is carried in the blood bound

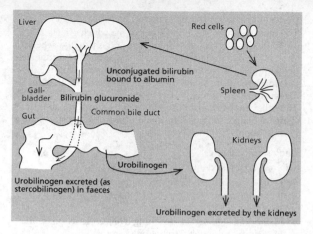

Figure 3.1 Pathways in bilirubin metabolism.

to albumin. Unconjugated bilirubin is conjugated in the liver by glucuronyl transferase to bilirubin glucuronide, and this is excreted into the small intestine in bile. In the terminal ileum conjugated bilirubin is converted to urobilinogen and excreted in the faeces (as stercobilinogen) or reabsorbed and excreted by the kidneys (Figure 3.1).

The usual division of jaundice into prehepatic, hepatocellular and obstructive jaundice is an oversimplification, because in hepatocellular jaundice there is invariably cholestasis and the clinical problem is whether the cholestasis is intrahepatic or extrahepatic. Jaundice is therefore considered under the following headings:

- Haemolytic jaundice
- Congenital hyperbilirubinaemias
- Cholestatic jaundice

Haemolytic jaundice

Increased breakdown of red cells leads to increased production of bilirubin which may result in mild jaundice. The unconjugated bilirubin is not water soluble and therefore does not pass into the urine, unlike the conjugated hyperbilirubinaemia of cholestatic jaundice. The urinary urobilinogen is increased. The causes are those of haemolytic anaemia (page 115), with the clinical features dependent on the cause. Investigations show features of haemolysis (page 116), with raised serum unconjugated bilirubin and normal alkaline phosphatase and transaminases.

Congenital hyperbilirubinaemia

The most common is Gilbert's syndrome which affects 2–5% of the population. It is asymptomatic and is usually picked up as an incidental finding of a slightly raised serum bilirubin (up to 80 μmol/l). There are no signs of liver disease and the liver enzymes are normal. The cause is multifactorial with many defects in bilirubin metabolism having been demonstrated. The other congenital abnormalities of bilirubin metabolism (Crigler–Najjar, Dubin–Johnson, and Rotor syndromes) are rare. [CM p 247]

Cholestatic jaundice

This can be divided into the following (Table 3.1):

● *Intrahepatic cholestasis* caused by hepatocellular swelling in parenchymal liver disease or to abnormalities at a cellular level of bile excretion.

● *Extrahepatic cholestasis* resulting from obstruction of bile flow at any point distal to the bile canaliculi.

Table 3.1 Causes of cholestatic jaundice

Intrahepatic
Viral hepatitis
Drugs
Alcoholic hepatitis
Cirrhosis
Pregnancy
Extrahepatic
Common bile duct stone
Carcinoma
Head of pancreas
Ampulla
Bile duct
Biliary stricture
Pancreatitis
Sclerosing cholangitis

Investigation

An outline of the approach to investigation of jaundice is shown in Figure 3.2.

SERUM LIVER BIOCHEMISTRY will confirm the jaundice. The AST tends to be high early in the course of hepatitis, with a smaller rise in alkaline phosphatase. Conversely, in extrahepatic obstruction, the alkaline phosphatase is elevated with a smaller rise in the AST.

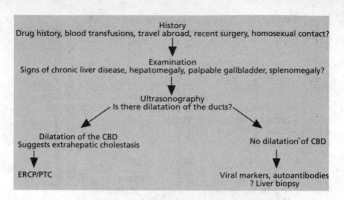

Figure 3.2 An approach to the investigation of cholestatic jaundice. PTC, percutaneous transhepatic cholangiography; ERCP, endoscopic retrograde cholangiopancreatography; CBD, common bile duct.

ULTRASONOGRAPHY examination will show dilated bile ducts in extrahepatic cholestasis and identify the level of obstruction. Mass lesions may also be identified.

SERUM VIRAL MARKERS for hepatitis A and hepatitis B may be present. Antibodies to hepatitis C virus develop late in the course of acute infection.

OTHER TESTS. The prothrombin time is often prolonged in long-standing liver disease and the serum albumin is low. Serum autoantibodies are present in autoimmune liver disease (see later).

HEPATITIS

The pathological features of hepatitis are liver cell necrosis and inflammatory cell infiltration. Clinically the liver may be enlarged and tender with or without jaundice, and laboratory evidence of hepatocellular damage is invariably found in the form of elevated serum transferase levels. Hepatitis is divided into *acute* and *chronic* types (Table 3.2) on the basis of clinical and pathological criteria. Acute hepatitis is most commonly caused by one of the hepatitis viruses. Usually there is complete resolution of the liver cell damage with return to normal structure and function. Occasionally there is progression to massive liver cell necrosis which may result in death. Chronic hepatitis is defined as sustained inflammatory disease of the liver lasting for more than 6 months.

Table 3.2 The causes of acute and chronic hepatitis

ACUTE	CHRONIC
Viruses	Viruses
Hepatitis A, B, C, D and E	Hepatitis B, C and D
Epstein–Barr virus	
Cytomegalovirus	
Non-viral infections	Autoimmune hepatitis
Leptospira icterohaemorrhagiae	
Toxoplasma gondii	
Coxiella burnetii (Q fever)	
Alcohol (superimposed on cirrhosis)	Alcohol
Drugs	Drugs
Anti-TB, e.g. isoniazid	Methyldopa
Halothane	Nitrofurantoin
Paracetamol poisoning	
Others	Metabolic disorders
Pregnancy	Wilson's disease
Poisons, e.g. carbon tetrachloride	α_1-Antitrypsin deficiency
Wilson's disease	

Viral hepatitis ND

The most important causes of viral hepatitis are the well-characterized hepatotrophic viruses named hepatitis A, B and C. Hepatitis D and E are infrequent causes in the UK. Important features of these viruses are summarized in Table 3.3. All cases of viral hepatitis must be notified to the appropriate public health authority. This allows contacts to be traced and provides data on disease incidence.

Hepatitis A ND

Epidemiology
Hepatitis A is the most common type of viral hepatitis, responsible for 20–40% of clinically apparent acute hepatitis. It occurs worldwide and affects particularly children and young adults. Spread is mainly faecal–oral and arises from the ingestion of contaminated food (e.g. shellfish, clams) or water. The virus is excreted in the faeces of infected individuals for about 2 weeks before, and 7 days after, the onset of the illness. It is most infectious just before the onset of the jaundice.

Clinical features
A pre-icteric phase lasting about 2 weeks is characterized by nausea, vomiting, diarrhoea, malaise, abdominal discomfort and mild fever. This is followed by the development of jaundice with dark urine and pale stools, at which stage the

Table 3.3 Some features of the hepatitis viruses

			HEPATITIS		
FEATURE	A	B	C	D	E
Virus	RNA	DNA	RNA	RNA	RNA
Transmission	Faecal–oral	Parenteral Sexual Vertical	Parenteral	Parenteral	Faecal–oral
Incubation	Short (2–3 weeks)	Long (1–5 months)	Long	Intermediate	Short
Chronicity	No	Yes	Yes	Yes	No
Mortality rate (%) (acute)	<0.5	<1	<1	(Only with B)	1–2 (10% in pregnancy)

patient often begins to feel better. There is moderate hepatomegaly and the spleen is enlarged in 10% of cases. Occasionally lymphadenopathy and a skin rash are present. The illness is self-limiting and usually over in 3–6 weeks. Rarely the disease is very severe with fulminant hepatitis (page 77), liver coma and death.

Investigations

LIVER BIOCHEMISTRY shows a raised serum AST and raised bilirubin when jaundice develops.

THE BLOOD COUNT shows a leucopenia with relative lymphocytosis and a high ESR.

SERUM ANTIBODIES to hepatitis A virus (HAV) are present with anti-HAV IgM indicating an acute infection.

ULTRASONOGRAPHY is performed in the older patient to exclude bile duct obstruction as a cause of jaundice.

Management

No specific treatment is required.

Prophylaxis

Active immunization with an inactivated HAV vaccine is now available and recommended for people travelling frequently to areas of high hepatitis A prevalence (Africa, Asia, South America, eastern Europe and the Middle East). Passive immunization with human normal immunoglobulin gives protection for 2–3 months and is given to people making a brief single visit to a high-risk area or to close contacts of a case who present within 2 weeks of exposure to hepatitis A.

Control of hepatitis also depends on good hygiene. Travellers to high-risk areas should drink only boiled or bottled water and avoid risky foods.

Hepatitis B ND

Epidemiology

Hepatitis B virus (HBV) is present worldwide but is particularly prevalent in parts of Africa, the Middle and the Far East. It is spread through the intravenous route (infected blood products, contaminated needles of intravenous drug abusers and tattooists) and through sexual intercourse, particularly in male homosexuals. Vertical transmission from mother to child during parturition is the most important means of transmission worldwide.

Viral structure

The whole virus is the Dane particle (Figure 3.3) which consists of an inner core and an outer surface coat, the hepatitis B surface antigen (HBsAg). The inner core contains double-stranded DNA, DNA polymerase, the core antigen

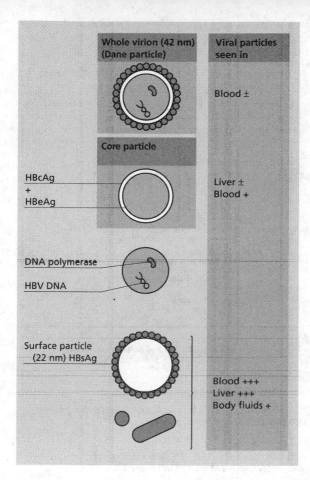

Whole virion (42 nm) (Dane particle) — Viral particles seen in: Blood ±

Core particle

HBcAg + HBeAg — Liver ± / Blood +

DNA polymerase

HBV DNA

Surface particle (22 nm) HBsAg — Blood +++ / Liver +++ / Body fluids +

Figure 3.3 Hepatitis B virus – the antigenic components.

(HBcAg) and e antigen (HBeAg). HBeAg is produced in excess during active viral replication and its detection in the serum indicates a high degree of infectivity.

Acute infection

Acute infection with HBV may be asymptomatic or produce symptoms and signs similar to those seen in hepatitis A. Occasionally it is associated with a rash or polyarthritis

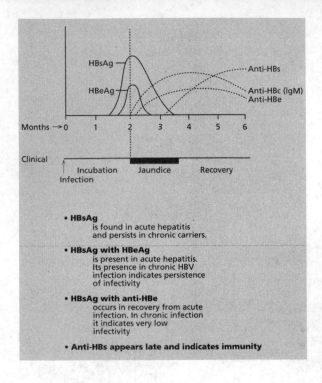

Figure 3.4 Time course of the events and serological changes seen following infection with hepatitis B virus.

affecting the small joints. The sequence of events following acute infection are depicted in Figure 3.4.

Investigation is generally the same as for hepatitis A. The viral markers for HBV are shown in Figure 3.4. If HBsAg is present, a full viral profile is then performed. There is no specific therapy for acute HBV infection and management is supportive.

Most patients recover completely. This is marked by disappearance of HBsAg from the serum, development of antibodies to surface antigen (anti-HBsAg) and immunity to subsequent infection (Figure 3.4). One per cent of patients with acute hepatitis develop fulminant liver failure.

A minority of patients do not clear HBsAg from the serum and become chronic carriers (5–10%).

Chronic carriers

The persistence of HBsAg in the serum for more than 6 months after acute infection defines the carrier status. Carriers who, in addition, have HBeAg or viral DNA in the serum (i.e. have active viral replication) are highly infectious and are at greatest risk of developing chronic hepatitis (see below) and cirrhosis, with the attendant increased risk of hepatocellular carcinoma. Patients with only HBsAg are usually asymptomatic with normal liver biochemistry and are of relatively low infective risk.

Chronic hepatitis

Approximately 3% of patients with acute viral hepatitis B progress to chronic active hepatitis. The condition may be asymptomatic or present with established liver disease and the signs of chronic liver disease on physical examination (Figure 3.5). Serum liver biochemistry, particularly the transferases, is usually abnormal. Liver biopsy and histological examination will show the severity of the disease varying from mild inflammatory changes to established cirrhosis.

Treatment of chronic hepatitis B

Treatment is with interferon alpha (interferon-α) administered subcutaneously (by the patient) three times weekly for 4–6 months. The aim of treatment is to clear HBeAg and HBV DNA from the serum, and this is accomplished in about 50% of treated patients.

Prophylaxis

Avoidance of high-risk factors (needle sharing, prostitutes and multiple male homosexual partners) and counselling patients who are potentially infective are important aspects of prevention. Active immunization is available with a recombinant yeast vaccine and is recommended for those at increased risk, e.g. healthcare workers, homosexuals, intravenous drug abusers and haemodialysis patients.

Combined prophylaxis (i.e. active immunization and passive immunization with specific antihepatitis B immunoglobulin) is given to non-immune individuals after high-risk exposure, e.g. a needle-stick injury from a carrier, newborn babies of HBsAg-positive mothers and HBV-negative sexual partners of HBsAg-positive patients.

Hepatitis D (delta or δ agent) ND

Hepatitis D virus is an incomplete RNA virus enclosed in a shell of HBsAg. It is unable to replicate on its own but is activated by the presence of HBV. It can affect all risk groups for HBV infection, but is seen particularly in intravenous drug abusers. HDV infection can occur as a *co-infection* with HBV or as a *superinfection* in an HBsAg-positive patient, and thus presents as an illness indistinguishable from acute HBV infection or as a flare-up of previously quiescent chronic HBV infection. Diagnosis is by finding IgM anti-δ in the serum.

Hepatitis C ND

Epidemiology
Hepatitis C virus (HCV) is an RNA virus that was discovered in 1988 and found to be responsible for most of the post-transfusion hepatitides before screening for HCV in donated blood. It is present worldwide but is more common in southern Europe and Japan. It is transmitted by blood products and perhaps also by sexual intercourse. In some cases the exact mode of transmission is unknown (community acquired).

Clinical features
Acute infection is usually mild with jaundice developing in less than 20% of cases. At least 50% of patients go on to develop chronic liver disease and many patients present for the first time with the complications of chronic liver disease.

Diagnosis
SERUM ANTIBODIES to HCV are found with both past and present infection. Negative serology excludes HCV infection and is thus the initial screening test in a patient with chronic liver disease of undetermined cause. However, antibodies may take 3 months to appear after acute infection and thus a negative result does not exclude acute HCV infection.

Patients with antibodies to hepatitis C should undergo further tests to look for the presence of HCV RNA (detected by the polymerase chain reaction) in the serum. A positive result indicates ongoing infection and a liver biopsy is usually then performed to detect the presence or absence of chronic hepatitis and cirrhosis.

Management
It is unclear which patients will progress to chronic liver disease and cirrhosis, and therefore who should be treated in an attempt to prevent progression. Currently interferon-α is used in most patients with *active* chronic liver disease. In 50% of treated patients liver biochemistry improves, but, of these, 50% relapse with discontinuation of treatment so that repeated courses are necessary.

Hepatitis E ND

This is an RNA virus which causes enteral (epidemic or

waterborne) hepatitis, particularly in developing countries. There is no chronic carrier state, and it does not progress to chronic liver disease, but the mortality rate from fulminant hepatic failure is about 1–2% rising to 20% in pregnant women.

Fulminant hepatic failure

Fulminant hepatic failure is an infrequent complication of acute hepatitis (from any cause) and occurs as a result of massive liver cell necrosis. In the UK, viral hepatitis and paracetamol overdose are the most common causes. Presentation is with hepatic encephalopathy of varying severity (Table 3.4), accompanied by severe jaundice and a marked coagulopathy. The complications include cerebral oedema, hypoglycaemia, hypotension and renal failure (hepatorenal syndrome). Fulminant hepatic failure is managed with supportive treatment in a specialist liver unit. Emergency liver transplantation has become a useful treatment for the very severe cases (grade IV encephalopathy), of which 80% may otherwise die.

Table 3.4 Grading of hepatic encephalopathy

Grade I	Daytime somnolence, asterixis (flapping tremor of outstretched hands)
Grade II	Confusion, disorientation, agitation and impaired coordination
Grade III	Increasing drowsiness, stupor, no communication possible
Grade IV	Coma, increased rigidity, extensor plantar response

Autoimmune hepatitis

Autoimmune hepatitis is a chronic, usually progressive liver disease which is often associated with other autoimmune diseases. It is most common in young and middle-aged females but can occur in any age in either sex.

Aetiology
The aetiology is unknown but there are many immunological abnormalities present. These include hypergamma-globulinaemia, circulating antibodies such as nuclear, smooth muscle and liver kidney microsomal antibodies, and an increased helper/suppressor T-cell ratio.

Clinical features
The onset is often insidious with anorexia, malaise, nausea and fatigue. Twenty-five per cent present as an acute hepatitis with rapidly progressive liver disease. The signs of chronic liver disease are often present with palmar erythema, spider

naevae, hepatosplenomegaly and jaundice. Features of other autoimmune diseases may be present.

Investigations
Circulating autoantibodies (antinuclear and antismooth muscle antibodies) are the hallmarks of the disease. There is hypergammaglobulinaemia, and the serum bilirubin and aminotransferases are elevated. Liver biopsy will show the changes of chronic active hepatitis with piecemeal necrosis.

Treatment
Prednisolone 30 mg daily is given for 2–3 weeks. Subsequent reduction of dose depends on clinical response but maintenance doses of 10–15 mg are usually required. Azathioprine may be used as a steroid-sparing agent.

Prognosis
In treated patients the 5-year survival rate is 90%.

CIRRHOSIS

Cirrhosis is a histological diagnosis. It is a diffuse process that results from necrosis of liver cells followed by fibrosis and nodule formation. The end result is impairment of liver cell function and gross distortion of liver architecture leading to portal hypertension.

Aetiology
The causes of cirrhosis are shown in Table 3.5. Alcohol is the most common cause in the Western World, but hepatitis B is the most common cause worldwide.

Table 3.5 Causes of cirrhosis

Common
Alcohol
Chronic active hepatitis caused by:
   Hepatitis B
   Hepatitis C
   ? Other hepatitis viruses

Others
Biliary cirrhosis: primary and secondary
Autoimmune chronic active hepatitis
Haemochromatosis
Cystic fibrosis
Budd–Chiari syndrome
Wilson's disease
Drugs, e.g. methotrexate
α_1-Antitrypsin
Idiopathic
Rare causes

Pathology

Histologically two types have been described: micronodular and macronodular cirrhosis.

- MICRONODULAR CIRRHOSIS, characterized by uniform, small nodules up to 3 mm in diameter. This type is often caused by alcohol damage.
- MACRONODULAR CIRRHOSIS, in which large nodules up to several centimetres in diameter are present. This type is often seen following hepatitis B infection.
- MIXED PICTURE with both small and large nodules.

Clinical features

These are secondary to portal hypertension and liver cell failure (Figure 3.5). Cirrhosis with the complications of encephalopathy, ascites or variceal haemorrhage is designated *decompensated cirrhosis*. Cirrhosis without any of these complications is termed *compensated cirrhosis*.

Investigations

These are performed to identify the aetiology and assess the severity of liver disease.

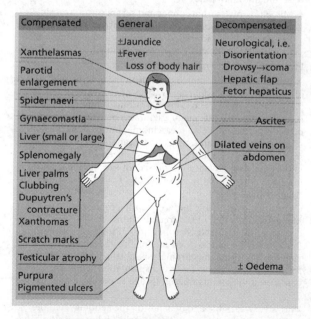

Figure 3.5 Physical signs in chronic liver disease.

- Liver biochemistry may be normal. In most cases there is at least a slight elevation of the serum alkaline phosphatase and amino transferase. A low serum albumin reflects reduced hepatic synthetic function and is the best guide to the severity of liver disease.

- Serum electrolytes: a low sodium indicates severe liver disease secondary to either impaired free water clearance or excess diuretic therapy.

- Haematology: the prothrombin time is prolonged as a result of decreased hepatic synthesis of clotting factors.

- Serum α-fetoprotein (AFP). This is usually undetectable after fetal life but raised levels may be found in chronic liver disease. Very high levels (greater than 500 U/ml) suggest the complication of hepatocellular carcinoma.

AETIOLOGY

This is determined by the following:

- Hepatitis B and C serology
- Serum autoantibodies
- Miscellaneous: serum copper and serum α_1-antitrypsin should always be measured in young cirrhotic individuals. Serum iron, total iron-binding capacity and ferritin should be measured to exclude haemochromatosis.

FURTHER INVESTIGATIONS

A liver biopsy is performed to confirm the severity and type of liver disease. Oesophageal varices are sought with a barium swallow or endoscopy. Ultrasonography examination is often performed, its major usefulness being in the early detection of hepatocellular carcinoma. Intravenous injection of technetium-99m and subsequent scanning (^{99m}Tc colloid scan) shows uptake in the bones and spleen, but poor uptake in the liver with advanced cirrhosis. This technique is used less frequently since the introduction of ultrasonography.

Management

Cirrhosis is irreversible and frequently progresses. Management is that of the complications seen in decompensated cirrhosis as they arise. Progression of liver disease may be halted by correcting the underlying cause, e.g. venesection for haemochromatosis, abstinence from alcohol for alcoholic cirrhosis. Liver transplantation should be considered in patients with end-stage cirrhosis.

Prognosis

This is very variable and depends on the aetiology and the presence of complications. The severity and prognosis of liver disease can be graded according to five variables:

encephalopathy, ascites, prothrombin time, serum bilirubin and albumin (Child's grading or modifications thereof).

Complications

The complications of cirrhosis are shown in Table 3.6.

Table 3.6 Complications and effects of cirrhosis

Portal hypertension and gastrointestinal haemorrhage
Ascites
Portosystemic encephalopathy
Renal failure
Primary liver cell carcinoma (hepatoma)

Portal hypertension

The portal vein carries blood from the gut and spleen to the liver and accounts for 85% of hepatic vascular inflow (15% is via the hepatic artery). The inflow of portal blood to the liver can be partially or completely obstructed at a number of sites, leading to high pressure proximal to the obstruction and diversion of blood into portosystemic collaterals. The most important site for collateral formation is at the gastro-oesophageal junction (varices), where they are superficial and liable to rupture causing massive gastrointestinal haemorrhage.

The main sites of obstruction are:

- Prehepatic caused by blockage of the portal vein before the liver
- Intrahepatic resulting from distortion of the liver architecture
- Posthepatic as a result of obstruction of the hepatic veins

Aetiology

The causes of portal hypertension are outlined in Table 3.7. In the UK 90% of cases are caused by cirrhosis.

Table 3.7 Causes of portal hypertension

Prehepatic
Portal vein thrombosis

Intrahepatic
Cirrhosis
Alcoholic hepatitis
Schistosomiasis
Granulomata

Posthepatic
Budd–Chiari syndrome
Veno-occlusive disease
Right heart failure – rare
Constrictive pericarditis

Clinical features

The characteristic clinical manifestations of portal hypertension are:

- Gastrointestinal bleeding from oesophageal or gastric varices
- Ascites
- Hepatic encephalopathy

Variceal haemorrhage

Only 30% of patients with varices ever have bleeds from them and this is most common in those with large varices. Bleeding is often massive and may be fatal.

Management

ACUTE BLEEDING. Patients should be resuscitated (see page 366) and undergo urgent gastroscopy to confirm the diagnosis and exclude bleeding from other sites.

- Endoscopic therapy: injection sclerotherapy or banding of varices is the treatment of choice. Bleeding stops in 80% of cases.
- Pharmacological treatment is used as a holding measure if sclerotherapy or banding is not available. The alternatives are an intravenous infusion of octreotide (a long-acting somatostatin analogue) or vasopressin which both restrict portal inflow by splanchnic arterial constriction.
- Balloon tamponade with a Sengstaken–Blakemore tube is used if bleeding continues (Figure 3.6). It has serious complications such as aspiration pneumonia, oesophageal rupture and mucosal ulceration; to reduce complications, the tube is only left *in situ* for up to 24 hours.
- Surgery (oesophageal transection and ligation of varices) is occasionally necessary if bleeding continues in spite of all the above measures. A less invasive approach is TIPSS (transjugular intrahepatic portosystemic shunting) but this is only available in specialist centres. A metal stent is passed over a guidewire in the jugular vein. The stent is then pushed into the liver substance, under ultrasonic guidance, to form a shunt between the portal and hepatic veins, thus lowering portal pressure.

PROPHYLAXIS. Following an episode of variceal bleeding there is a high risk of recurrence (60–80% over a 2-year period) and therefore treatment is given to prevent further bleeds (*secondary prophylaxis*). The main options are:

- Injection sclerotherapy until the varices are obliterated.
- Oral propranolol, which reduces portal pressure and is as effective as sclerotherapy. This is also given to patients with varices who have never bled (*primary prophylaxis*).

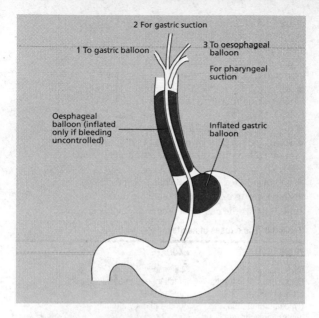

Figure 3.6 Diagram of a Sengstaken–Blakemore tube *in situ*.

● Portosystemic shunts (portal vein to vena cava – or splenorenal) are rarely performed. They carry a very low risk of rebleeding but there is a high operative mortality in patients with severe liver disease, and encephalopathy in those surviving the operation. Liver transplantation should always be considered.

Ascites

This is the presence of fluid in the peritoneal cavity and is a common complication of cirrhosis of the liver.

Aetiology

In cirrhosis, peripheral arterial vasodilatation (?mediated by nitric oxide) leads to a reduction in effective blood volume with activation of the sympathetic nervous system and renin–angiotensin system, thus promoting salt and water retention. Formation of oedema is encouraged by hypoalbuminaemia and mainly localized to the peritoneal cavity as a result of the portal hypertension.

Clinical features

There is fullness in the flanks with shifting dullness. Tense ascites is uncomfortable and may produce respiratory distress. A pleural effusion (usually right-sided) and peripheral oedema may be present.

Investigations

A diagnostic paracentesis of 10–20 ml of fluid should be carried out in all patients and the following performed:

- A CELL COUNT: a neutrophil count > 250 cells/mm^3 indicates underlying peritonitis (usually spontaneous bacterial peritonitis)
- GRAM STAIN and culture for bacteria and acid-fast bacilli
- PROTEIN: an ascitic protein of 11 g/l or more below the serum albumin level suggests a transudate (exudate > 11 g/l)
- CYTOLOGY for malignant cells
- AMYLASE to exclude pancreatic ascites

Table 3.8 lists the causes of ascites, including cirrhosis.

Table 3.8 The causes of ascites

TRANSUDATE	EXUDATE
Cirrhosis	Malignancy
Constrictive pericarditis	Infection, e.g. pyogenic, tuberculous
Cardiac failure	Pancreatitis
Hypoalbuminaemia, e.g. nephrotic syndrome	Budd–Chiari syndrome
Meigs' syndrome*	Myxoedema
(ovarian tumour)	Lymphatic obstruction (chylous ascites)

*Meig's syndrome is the combination of an ovarian tumour, ascites and hydrothorax.

Management

Most patients are managed with diuretics.

DIURETICS. The management of ascites resulting from cirrhosis is based on a stepwise approach starting with bed rest, reduced salt intake (40 mmol/day) and the aldosterone antagonist, spironolactone, 50–100 mg/day. The rate of fluid loss is best assessed by changes in body weight. The aim of diuretic therapy is to produce weight loss of about 0.5 kg/day, because the maximum rate of transfer of fluid from the ascitic to the vascular compartment is only about 700 ml/day. If there is no response in a few days, spironolactone may be increased gradually to a maximum of 600 mg/day before adding 20–40 mg of frusemide. This potent loop diuretic may cause volume depletion, hypokalaemia and precipitate encephalopathy.

PARACENTESIS. All the ascites can be removed over several hours. There is therefore rapid symptom relief and reduced hospital stay compared to use of diuretics. The major danger of this approach is the production of hypovolaemia because the ascites reaccumulates at the expense of the circulating volume. This is largely overcome by the intravenous infusion of plasma expanders (albumin, Dextran-70, gelatin) administered after paracentesis.

PERITONEOVENOUS SHUNTS (Le-Veen shunts): these are catheters running subcutaneously from the peritoneal cavity to the internal jugular vein. A one-way valve allows passage of the ascites into the circulation. They are rarely used and only in resistant cases.

Complications
Spontaneous bacterial peritonitis occurs in 8% of cirrhotic patients and has a mortality rate of 50%. The most common infecting organism is *Escherichia coli*. Clinical features may be minimal, but include abdominal pain and fever. Diagnosis is made on the cell count, and Gram stain and culture of ascitic fluid (see above). Empirical therapy, e.g. intravenous ceftazidine or cefotaxime, should be started before the results of culture are available.

Portosystemic encephalopathy

The term 'portosystemic encephalopathy' (PSE) refers to a chronic neuropsychiatric syndrome which occurs with advanced hepatocellular disease, either chronic (cirrhosis) or acute (fulminant hepatic failure). It is also seen in patients following a portacaval shunt operation.

Pathophysiology
The mechanisms are unclear but are believed to involve toxic substances, normally detoxified by the liver, bypassing the liver via the collaterals and gaining access to the brain. A putative toxin is ammonia produced from dietary protein by gut bacteria. In chronic liver disease there is an acute-on-chronic course, with acute episodes precipitated by a number of possible factors (Table 3.9)

Table 3.9 Factors precipitating portosystemic encephalopathy

High dietary protein
Gastrointestinal haemorrhage (i.e. a high protein load)
Constipation
Infection
Fluid and electrolyte disturbance
Drugs, e.g. opiates, diazepam
Portosytemic shunt operations

Clinical features
The earliest features are lethargy, mild confusion, anorexia and a reversal of the sleep pattern. Later there is disorientation, a decreased conscious level and eventually coma (see Table 3.4). The signs are a flapping tremor of the

outstretched hand (asterixis), inability to draw a five-pointed star (constructional apraxia) and a prolonged trail-making test (the ability to join numbers and letters within a certain time). Serial attempts are easily compared and used to monitor patient progress.

Investigations

The diagnosis is clinical. An EEG (showing δ waves) and visual evoked potentials may aid diagnosis in difficult cases.

Management

The aims of management are to identify and treat any precipitating factors and to minimize the absorption of nitrogenous material, particularly ammonia, from the gut. This is achieved by the following:

- Laxatives and enemas: lactulose (10–30 ml three times daily) is an osmotic purgative which reduces colonic pH and increases transit. It may be given via a nasogastric tube if the patient is comatose.
- In resistant cases oral neomycin 1 g 6 hourly is given to reduce the number of bowel organisms.
- Maintenance of nutrition with a high-carbohydrate, low-protein diet.

Once the patient recovers the protein content of the diet may be increased and lactulose is continued to produce soft stools but not diarrhoea.

Prognosis

The prognosis is that of the underlying liver disease.

TYPES OF CIRRHOSIS

Alcoholic

This is discussed in the section on alcoholic liver disease (page 90).

Primary biliary cirrhosis

Primary biliary cirrhosis (PBC) is a chronic disorder in which there is progressive destruction of intrahepatic bile ducts causing cholestasis, eventually leading to cirrhosis.

Epidemiology

It affects predominantly women aged 40–50 years (female : male ratio 6 : 1).

Aetiology

The aetiology is unknown but thought to be immunologically mediated. Antimitochondrial antibodies (AMAs) are present in almost all (> 95%) patients but are not thought to play a part in the pathogenesis. Antinuclear antibodies are found less commonly.

Clinical features

Pruritus, with or without jaundice, is the single most common presenting complaint. In advanced disease there is, in addition, hepatosplenomegaly and xanthelasma (PBC is a cause of secondary hypercholesterolaemia). Asymptomatic patients may be discovered on routine examination or screening to have hepatomegaly, a raised serum alkaline phosphatase or autoantibodies.

Autoimmune disorders, e.g. Sjögren's syndrome, scleroderma and rheumatoid arthritis, are seen with increased frequency.

Investigations

LIVER BIOCHEMISTRY may show only a raised serum alkaline phosphatase.

SERUM AMAs are found in more than 95% of patients and a titre of 1 : 160 or greater makes the diagnosis very likely. The antibodies are very occasionally found in normal people or in those with autoimmune disease. The M2 subset is specific for PBC and may be useful if uncertainty exists. Other non-specific antibodies, e.g. antinuclear factor, may also be present.

SERUM IgM may be very high.

LIVER BIOPSY shows loss of bile ducts, lymphocyte infiltration of the portal tracts, granuloma formation and, at a later stage, fibrosis and eventually cirrhosis.

Management

Numerous medical treatments have been tried (e.g. steroids, immunosuppressants, ursodeoxycholic acid) and, although some may improve liver biochemistry, none has been shown to improve survival. Treatment is therefore entirely symptomatic until such time that liver transplantation is considered necessary (see later).

Pruritus may be helped by cholestyramine and malabsorption of fat-soluble vitamins (A, D, K) is treated by supplementation.

Prognosis

Asymptomatic patients may show a near-normal life expectancy. In symptomatic patients with jaundice, there is a steady downhill course with death in approximately 5 years.

Secondary biliary cirrhosis

Cirrhosis can result from prolonged (for months) large duct biliary obstruction. Causes include bile duct strictures, gallstones and sclerosing cholangitis. Ultrasonography examination followed by endoscopic retrograde cholangiopancreatography (ERCP) or percutaneous transhepatic cholangiography (PTC) is performed to outline the ducts and any remedial cause is dealt with.

Haemochromatosis

Idiopathic haemochromatosis (IHC) is an inherited disease characterized by excess iron deposition in various organs leading to eventual fibrosis and functional organ failure.

Aetiology

Failure of regulation of iron absorption from the small bowel leads to overload, with deposition in, and damage to, the cells of the liver, heart, pancreas and pituitary gland. It is inherited as an autosomal recessive with only homozygotes manifesting the clinical features of the disease. HLA-A3, -B7 and -B14 occur with increased frequency compared with the general population.

Clinical features

Most affected individuals present in their 50s. There is a reduced incidence of overt disease in women presumably because of iron lost in blood during menstruation. The classic triad of bronze skin pigmentation (caused by melanin deposition), hepatomegaly and diabetes mellitus is only present in cases of gross iron overload. Other more common features include gonadal atrophy and loss of libido secondary to pituitary dysfunction. There may be a cardiomyopathy and arthritis resulting from calcium pyrophosphate deposition in both large and small joints.

Investigations

SERUM LIVER BIOCHEMISTRY is often normal even with cirrhosis.

SERUM IRON is elevated and total iron-binding capacity reduced.*

SERUM FERRITIN reflects iron stores and is usually greatly elevated (often >500 μg/l).

LIVER BIOPSY is performed to measure the extent of tissue damage, to assess tissue iron and to measure the hepatic iron concentration.

Causes of secondary iron overload such as multiple transfusions must be excluded. In addition, in alcoholic liver disease, hepatic iron stores may increase. The precise reason is unknown but the hepatic iron concentration does not reach the very high levels seen in haemochromatosis.

Management

The aim of treatment is to remove excess tissue iron and this is best achieved by venesection; 500 ml of blood is removed twice weekly and this may need to be continued for up to 2 years. Three or four venesections per year are then required to prevent reaccumulation of iron.

*The transferrin saturation $\left(\dfrac{\text{serum iron}}{\text{total iron-binding capacity}}\right) \times 100\%$ is greater than 60% (normal about 33%).

All first-degree relatives are screened with a serum ferritin to detect and treat early disease.

Prognosis

The major complication is development of hepatocellular carcinoma in patients with cirrhosis. This can be prevented by venesection before cirrhosis develops and life expectancy is then much the same as the normal population.

Wilson's disease (hepatolenticular degeneration)

This is a rare, recessively inherited disorder in which there is failure of the normal mechanism to excrete copper in the bile, resulting in accumulation of copper and deposition in various organs to produce cirrhosis and basal ganglia degeneration.

Clinical features

Children usually present with hepatic problems ranging from fulminant hepatic failure to cirrhosis. Young adults have more neurological problems which start with a mild tremor and speech problems, and progress to involuntary movements and eventual dementia. A specific sign is the Kayser–Fleisher ring, which is caused by copper deposition in the cornea. It appears as a greenish-brown pigment at the periphery of the cornea, best seen with a slit-lamp. Additional features are haemolytic anaemia and renal tubular defects.

Investigations

The diagnosis is usually made by demonstrating the following:

- A low serum ceruloplasmin (the copper-carrying protein)
- Increased 24-hour urinary copper
- Increased hepatic copper concentration in a biopsy specimen

Management

The treatment of choice is life-long penicillamine which binds copper and is then excreted in the urine. Liver transplantation may be offered to those with end-stage liver disease. First-degree relatives are screened by slit-lamp examination and serum ceruloplasmin measurements. Asymptomatic homozygotes should be treated.

α_1-Antitrypsin deficiency

This is a rare cause of cirrhosis. Alpha-1-antitrypsin (α_1AT) is a glycoprotein and part of a family of protease inhibitors (Pi) which control various inflammatory cascades, e.g. complement and coagulation. Several forms are produced and one of them (PiZ) cannot be secreted from the liver into the blood.

Clinical features
Homozygous individuals (PiZZ) have very low circulating levels of α_1-AT associated with chronic liver disease and pulmonary emphysema (especially in smokers).

Investigations
The serum α_1AT is low. Liver biopsy demonstrates α_1AT-containing globules in the hepatocytes.

Management
There is no specific treatment. Patients should be advised to stop smoking.

Alcohol and the liver

Alcohol is the most common cause of chronic liver disease in the Western World. Alcoholic liver disease occurs more commonly in men, usually in the fourth and fifth decades, although subjects can present in their twenties with advanced disease. Although alcohol acts as a hepatotoxin, the exact mechanism leading to hepatitis and cirrhosis is unknown. As only 10–20% of people who drink excessively develop cirrhosis, genetic predisposition and immunological mechanisms have been proposed.

There are three major pathological lesions and clinical illnesses associated with excessive alcohol intake: *fatty liver, alcoholic hepatitis* and *cirrhosis.*

Fatty liver

This is the most common biopsy finding in alcoholic individuals. Fat accumulates within the hepatocyte and the cells may eventually become swollen with fat (steatosis). A similar picture can be seen in obesity, diabetes, starvation and, occasionally, chronic illnesses. Symptoms are usually absent and, on examination, there may be tender hepatomegaly. Laboratory tests are often normal, although an elevated mean corpuscular volume (MCV) often indicates heavy drinking. The γGT level is usually elevated. Patients with fatty liver alone have an excellent prognosis with complete resolution of the lesion on cessation of alcohol.

Alcoholic hepatitis

This is a more serious sequela of excessive alcohol because it may lead to hepatic failure and cirrhosis. There is necrosis of liver cells and infiltration of polymorphonuclear leukocytes, with accumulation of dense cytoplasmic material called a Mallory body in the hepatocytes. Presentation encompasses a broad spectrum of patients from those who are asymptomatic to those who are very ill with hepatic failure. Investigations show a leukocytosis with elevated bilirubin and transferases. The albumin may be low and prothrombin time prolonged. [99mTc]-labelled colloid scan is sometimes performed and shows no uptake in the liver. Treatment is supportive and adequate nutritional intake must be maintained. Corticosteroids are of benefit in some cases.

Alcoholic cirrhosis

This represents the final stage of liver disease from alcohol abuse. There is destruction and fibrosis with regenerating nodules producing a classic micronodular cirrhosis. Patients may be asymptomatic although they often present with one of the complications of cirrhosis and there are usually signs of chronic liver disease. Investigation is as for cirrhosis in general. Management is directed at the complications of cirrhosis and patients are advised to stop drinking for life. Abstinence from alcohol improves the 5-year survival rate.

LIVER TRANSPLANTATION

This is now an established treatment for end-stage chronic liver disease and in some circumstances for acute hepatic failure. Careful selection of patients is crucial. Psychological assessment and education of patients and their families are essential before transplantation. In adults, primary biliary cirrhosis is the most common indication and, in these patients where the natural history is well defined, transplantation is offered when the serum bilirubin reaches 100 μmol/l. Absolute contraindications to transplantation are active sepsis outside the liver and biliary tree, HIV positivity and metastatic malignancy. With rare exceptions, patients over 65 years are not transplanted. Early complications include haemorrhage, sepsis and acute rejection (< 6 weeks) which is reversible with intensive immunosuppression. Late complications include recurrence of disease (hepatitis B) and chronic rejection, which is not reversible and requires re-transplantation. The outcome of liver transplantation is good with an overall 5-year survival rate of 70–85%.

BUDD–CHIARI SYNDROME

Budd–Chiari syndrome is due to occlusion of the hepatic vein thus obstructing venous outflow from the liver.

Aetiology

Budd–Chiari syndrome may occur as a result of obstruction of the hepatic vein by malignancy, radiotherapy, trauma or from hypercoagulability states such as polycythaemia vera, taking the contraceptive pill or leukaemia. The cause is unknown in one-third of cases.

Clinical features

The syndrome presents acutely with abdominal pain, nausea, vomiting, hepatomegaly and ascites, or more insidiously with enlargement of the caudate lobe, splenomegaly, ascites and jaundice.

Investigations
The ascitic fluid shows a high protein content. Ultrasonography or CT scanning will show an enlarged caudate lobe, and Doppler studies will demonstrate abnormalities in the direction of blood flow.

Treatment
This is of the underlying cause though a portacaval shunt may help; alternatively, liver transplantation may be required.

LIVER ABSCESS

Pyogenic liver abscess

Aetiology
The cause of pyogenic liver abscess is often unknown, although biliary sepsis or portal pyaemia from intra-abdominal sepsis may be responsible. Other causes include trauma, bacteraemia or direct extension from, for example, a perinephric abscess. The most common causative organisms are *Escherichia coli*, but others include *Enterococcus faecalis*, *Proteus vulgaris* and *Staphylococcus aureus*.

Clinical features
Symptoms can be mild, although abdominal pain, fever, rigors, nausea and vomiting may occur. The patient may be jaundiced and the liver enlarged and tender.

Investigations
THE BLOOD COUNT usually shows a normochromic/normocytic anaemia and the ESR is elevated.

LIVER BIOCHEMISTRY shows a rise in serum alkaline phosphatase and an elevated bilirubin in 25% of cases.

ULTRASONOGRAPHY AND CT are useful for detecting fluid-filled lesions.

Management
Treatment is with broad-spectrum antibiotics and drainage of the abscess either under ultrasonic control or with surgery.

Amoebic abscess

Aetiology
An amoebic abscess results from spread of the organism *Entamoeba histolytica* from the bowel to the liver via the portal venous system (page 12). Multiple microabscesses develop which coalesce to form single or multiple large abscesses.

Clinical features
The onset is usually gradual with fever, weight loss and malaise, often with no history of dysentery. The patient looks

ill with tender hepatomegaly, and, sometimes, consolidation or an effusion in the right side of the chest.

Investigations
This is as for pyogenic abscess. Serological tests for amoeba, e.g. complement-fixation test or enzyme-linked immunosorbent assay (ELISA) are almost always positive. Aspiration of the abscess yields fluid like 'anchovy sauce'.

Management
Metronidazole 800 mg three times daily is given for 10 days. Surgical drainage is used for large abscesses or those failing to respond to medical treatment.

Hydatid disease

For details of hydatid disease see page 15.

JAUNDICE IN PREGNANCY

Viral hepatitis is the single most common cause of jaundice in pregnancy. Three types of liver disease are specific to pregnancy: acute fatty liver of pregnancy (a severe fulminating illness with jaundice, vomiting and hepatic coma), recurrent intrahepatic cholestasis (presenting with jaundice and pruritus), and haemolysis (occasionally producing jaundice) which occurs in pre-eclamptic toxaemia. The three conditions present most commonly in the third trimester and resolve with delivery of the baby.

LIVER TUMOURS

The most common malignant liver tumours are metastatic, particularly those from the gastrointestinal tract, breast or bronchus. Primary liver tumours may be benign or malignant.

Hepatocellular carcinoma (hepatoma)

Hepatocellular carcinoma (HCC) is one of the most common cancers worldwide, although it is rare in the Western hemisphere.

Aetiology
Chronic hepatitis B infection is the most important predisposing factor to HCC worldwide. Cirrhosis is present in over 90% of these patients. HCC is also related to other forms of cirrhosis, e.g. chronic hepatitis C, haemochromatosis and alcoholic cirrhosis. Other suggested aetiological factors include aflatoxin, androgenic steroids and possibly the contraceptive pill.

Clinical features
Weight loss, anorexia, fever, ascites and abdominal pain occur. The rapid development of these features in a patient with cirrhosis is suggestive of HCC.

Investigations

SERUM α-FETOPROTEIN is raised.

ULTRASONOGRAPHY OR RADIO-ISOTOPE SCANS show large filling defects in 90% of cases.

LIVER BIOPSY under ultrasonic control provides histological confirmation.

Management

Surgical resection is occasionally possible, but chemotherapy and radiotherapy are unhelpful.

Prognosis

Survival is seldom more than 6 months.

Benign liver tumours

The most common are haemangiomas, usually found incidentally on a liver ultrasonogram or CT scan. They require no treatment. Hepatic adenomas are less common and associated with use of oral contraceptives. Resection is required if there are symptoms (e.g. pain, intraperitoneal bleeding).

GALLSTONES

Gallstones are present in 10–20% of the population. They are most common in women and the prevalence increases with age.

Pathophysiology

Gallstones are of two types:

● CHOLESTEROL GALLSTONES composed mainly of cholesterol and accounting for 80% of all gallstones in the Western World. Cholesterol, insoluble in water, is held in solution by the detergent action of bile salts and phospholipids with which it forms micelles and vesicles. Cholesterol gallstones only form in bile which has an excess of cholesterol relative to bile salts and phospholipids (supersaturated or lithogenic bile) thus allowing cholesterol crystals to form and grow as stones (Table 3.10).

Table 3.10 Risk factors for cholesterol gallstones

RISK FACTOR	MECHANISM
Increased age	
Sex (F>M)	Increased cholesterol in bile
Obesity	
Contraceptive pill	
Terminal ileal disease	Decreased bile salts in bile caused by
Terminal ileal resection	interruption of enterohepatic circulation

- PIGMENT STONES consist of bilirubin polymers and calcium bilirubinate. They are seen in patients with chronic haemolysis, e.g. hereditary spherocytosis and sickle-cell disease in which bilirubin production is increased, and also in cirrhosis. Pigment stones may also form in the bile ducts after cholecystectomy and with duct strictures.

Clinical features
Most gallstones never cause symptoms and cholecystectomy is not indicated in asymptomatic cases. The complications are summarized in Figure 3.7.

Acute cholecystitis

Acute cholecystitis follows impaction of a stone in the cystic duct or neck of the gallbladder. Very occasionally acute cholecystitis may occur without stones (acalculous cholecystitis).

Clinical features
There is constant, severe pain in the epigastrium and right hypochondrium with radiation to the back and shoulder. There may be nausea, vomiting and jaundice. On examination there is fever and right hypochondrial tenderness worse on inspiration (Murphy's sign).

Investigations
WHITE CELL COUNT shows a leukocytosis.

SERUM LIVER BIOCHEMISTRY may be mildly abnormal.

RADIOLOGY. The diagnosis is made by ultrasonography examination showing gallstones and a distended gallbladder with a thickened wall. There is focal tenderness directly over the visualized gallbladder (sonographic Murphy's sign).

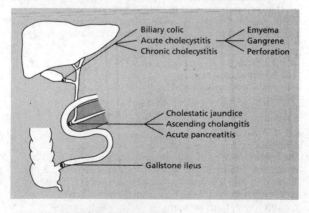

Figure 3.7 The complications of gallstones.

^{99m}Tc-HIDA (an amino-diacetic acid derivative) scan shows a blocked cystic duct. This test is gradually being superseded by ultrasonography.

Management

The initial treatment is conservative with nil by mouth, intravenous fluids, pain relief and antibiotics, e.g. amoxicillin. Cholecystectomy is usually performed within 48 hours of the acute attack and always if complications (see above) develop. Alternatively the patient may be readmitted for cholecystectomy 2–3 months later.

Chronic cholecystitis

Chronic inflammation of the gallbladder is often found in association with gallstones. There is no evidence that this produces any symptoms and cholecystectomy is not indicated. Chronic right hypochondrial pain and fatty food intolerance are likely to be functional in origin and gallstones an incidental finding.

Biliary pain

Biliary pain, at one time called biliary colic, is usually the result of stone impaction in Hartman's pouch, the cystic duct or the common bile duct (CBD).

Clinical features

Symptoms are episodes of constant (not colicky) epigastric or right hypochondrial pain lasting several hours, with often little to find on examination.

Investigations

The diagnosis is usually made on the basis of a typical history and an ultrasonogram showing gallstones. Increases of serum alkaline phosphatase and bilirubin during an attack support the diagnosis of biliary pain. The absence of inflammatory features (fever, white cell count and local peritonism) differentiates this from acute cholecystitis.

Management

The treatment is analgesia and elective cholecystectomy, unless ultrasonography shows a stone in the CBD (see below).

Common bile duct stones (cholelithiasis)

Clinical features

CBD stones may be asymptomatic. Usually one or more of the symptoms of pain, jaundice and fever are present. The jaundice is cholestatic in type and therefore the urine is dark, stools pale and the skin may itch. High fever and rigors indicate biliary tract infection (cholangitis). Charcot's triad is the three symptoms occurring together and indicates cholangitis.

Investigations

WHITE CELL COUNT shows a leukocytosis if infection is present.

BLOOD CULTURES are often positive (*E.coli, E. faecalis*) in the presence of cholangitis.

LIVER BIOCHEMISTRY shows a cholestatic picture with a raised serum bilirubin and alkaline phosphatase.

RADIOLOGY: ultrasonography may show a dilated common bile duct containing a stone.

ERCP confirms the diagnosis and allows stone removal.

Management

Treatment depends on the clinical situation but includes analgesia for pain, and antibiotics (amoxycillin, with gentamicin in severe cases) if infection is present. The stone must be removed from the duct and the preferred treatment is ERCP, sphincterotomy and extraction with a Dormia basket or balloon. Most patients with an intact gallbladder containing stones then go on to elective laparoscopic cholecystectomy.

Management of gallbladder stones

- CHOLECYSTECTOMY is the treatment of choice for symptomatic gallstones. This is almost always done via the laparoscope rather than as an open procedure.

- DISSOLUTION THERAPY: in patients who refuse or are unfit for surgery pure cholesterol gallstones are dissolved by oral bile acids (e.g. ursodeoxycholic acid). Few patients are suitable for this approach because bile acids dissolve only radiolucent stones in a functioning gallbladder. Even after 2 years of treatment, many stones have not dissolved and those that have, return when treatment is stopped.

- LITHOTRIPSY: shock-wave treatment of gallstones can be carried out using ultrasonic-guided lithotripters. The indications for treatment are the same as dissolution therapy.

PRIMARY SCLEROSING CHOLANGITIS

Primary sclerosing cholangitis results from inflammation and fibrosis of the bile ducts leading to multiple areas of narrowing throughout the biliary tree. It is of unknown cause; 50% or more cases have ulcerative colitis which may be asymptomatic. Patients with AIDS have been found to have sclerosing cholangitis that is believed to be infectious in origin. Episodes of ascending cholangitis and jaundice are common. A liver biopsy shows fibrosis around the bile ducts and ERCP shows multiple bile duct strictures. Extrahepatic strictures may be amenable to dilatation. There is no proven medical therapy of benefit and the only option is eventual liver transplantation.

PANCREATITIS

The classification of pancreatitis is difficult because of the inability to separate acute and chronic forms clearly. By definition, acute pancreatitis which can occur as isolated or recurrent attacks, is distinguished from chronic pancreatitis by the absence of continuing inflammation, irreversible structural changes and permanent loss of exocrine and endocrine pancreatic function. The causes are shown in Table 3.11.

Table 3.11 Causes of pancreatitis

ACUTE	CHRONIC
Gallstones	Alcohol (>85% of cases)
Alcohol	Idiopathic
Idiopathic	Protein–energy malnutrition
Metabolic: hypercalcaemia,	Hereditary
hyperlipidaemia	Cystic fibrosis
Iatrogenic: postsurgical, ERCP	
Drugs: azathioprine, corticosteroids	

Acute pancreatitis

This is an acute condition presenting with abdominal pain and raised pancreatic enzymes in the blood or urine, resulting from inflammatory disease of the pancreas.

Pathogenesis
The precise mechanism by which pancreatic necrosis occurs is unclear. Reflux of bile up the pancreatic duct or autodigestion of the pancreas by proteolytic enzymes may both be important in the pathogenesis.

Clinical features
Epigastric or upper abdominal pain radiating through to the back is the cardinal symptom. There is often nausea and vomiting and in severe cases, multiorgan failure may develop. On examination there is epigastric tenderness, guarding and rigidity. Rarely, ecchymoses around the umbilicus (Cullen's sign) or in the flanks (Grey Turner's sign) may occur.

Diagnosis
A raised serum amylase, in conjunction with an appropriate history and clinical signs, strongly suggests a diagnosis of acute pancreatitis. Serum amylase may also be moderately raised in other abdominal conditions such as acute cholecystitis and perforated duodenal ulcer, although very high amylase levels strongly suggest pancreatitis. In difficult

cases peritoneal lavage with estimation of amylase in the peritoneal fluid may be useful. Ultrasonography or CT scanning may reveal a swollen pancreas, sometimes with peripancreatic fluid collections.

Management
Nasogastric suction and intravenous hydration are instituted. Nothing is given by mouth, and in severe cases intravenous feeding is required. Analgesics with opiates (other than morphine) are usually required. As yet no specific drug treatment has been shown to be beneficial; surgical treatment may be required for very severe necrotizing pancreatitis, or if complications such as pancreatic abscesses or pseudocysts occur.

Complications
Local complications of acute pancreatitis are development of pseudocysts, abscesses, phlegmons (inflammatory masses) and ascites. General complications include hypoglycaemia, hypocalcaemia, renal failure and shock.

Prognosis
Mortality rate varies from 1% in mild cases to 50% in severe cases. The patients who recover may have recurrent attacks, depending on the aetiology.

Chronic pancreatitis

Chronic pancreatitis is defined as continuing inflammatory disease of the pancreas, characterized by irreversible morphological change and/or permanent impairment of function. The disease is not reversible but it is possible to arrest the disease process, particularly if the patient stops drinking alcohol.

Clinical features
There is central abdominal pain which is located in the epigastrium and characteristically radiates to the back. The pain may be intermittent or constant, and exacerbations are precipitated by an alcoholic binge. The abdominal pain is accompanied by severe weight loss as a result of anorexia.

Diabetes may develop and steatorrhoea occurs when the secretion of pancreatic lipase is reduced by 90%. Occasionally the patient presents with biliary obstruction, jaundice and cholangitis.

Investigation
The diagnosis of chronic pancreatitis is made by radiological techniques which demonstrate *structural* changes in the gland and metabolic studies which demonstrate *functional* abnormalities.

RADIOLOGY: a plain abdominal radiograph will show pancreatic calcification in some cases. ERCP demonstrates dilatation of the pancreatic duct with stenotic segments. Ultrasonography and CT scanning will show the dilated duct and demonstrate irregular consistency and outline of the gland.

FUNCTIONAL ASSESSMENT: the serum amylase is of no use in the diagnosis of chronic pancreatitis but may be raised during an acute episode of pain. A raised blood sugar indicates diabetes mellitus.

- *The Lundh test*: a tube is passed via the mouth into the duodenum and pancreatic trypsin and lipase are collected from the duodenal lumen after stimulation of secretion with a test meal.

- *PABA test:* N-benzoyl-L-tyrosyl p-aminobenzoic acid is given by mouth. Pancreatic chymotrypsin releases free p-aminobenzoic acid (PABA) which is absorbed and excreted in the urine. With pancreatic insufficiency there is reduced absorption and the amount measured in the urine is correspondingly low.

Treatment

The patients should be told to stop drinking alcohol. The pain may require opiates for control with the attendant risk of addiction. Surgical resection may be of value for severe disease with intractable pain. Pancreatic supplements (e.g. pancreatin 2–4 g with each meal) are useful for those with steatorrhoea and may reduce the frequency of attacks of pain in those with recurrent symptoms. Diabetes requires appropriate treatment with diet, oral hypoglycaemics or insulin.

Carcinoma of the pancreas

Epidemiology

Pancreatic cancer is the fourth most common cause of cancer death in the Western World and the incidence is steadily increasing. Men are affected more commonly than women and the incidence increases with age (peak in the seventh decade).

Aetiology

The aetiology is unknown but smoking, alcohol, coffee and dietary fats have all been implicated.

Clinical features

Cancer affecting the head of the pancreas presents with painless jaundice as a result of obstruction of the common duct, and weight loss. Cancer of the body or tail presents with abdominal pain, weight loss and anorexia. Diabetes may occur and there is an increased risk of thrombophlebitis. In cancer of the head of the pancreas, examination may reveal jaundice and a distended palpable gallbladder (Courvoisier's law: if, in a case of painless jaundice, the gallbladder is palpable the cause will not be gallstones). In gallstone disease chronic inflammation and fibrosis prevent distension of the gallbladder.

Investigation

The diagnosis is made with ultrasonography or CT. Duodenoscopy and ERCP may detect tumour in the head of the pancreas or at the ampulla.

Management

Curative resection is not usually possible and treatment is thus almost always palliative. Bypass of the obstructed common bile duct will relieve jaundice and this is usually performed with endoscopic placement of a stent, surgery being reserved for cases where the duodenum is obstructed. Chemotherapy and radiotherapy are of little value.

Prognosis

The prognosis is appalling; overall the 5-year survival rate is 1%, most patients being dead within a year of diagnosis.

Endocrine tumours

These tumours arise in the pancreas from APUD (*a*mine *p*recursor *u*ptake and *d*ecarboxylation) cells and are sometimes called apudomas. They usually secrete one hormone that produces the clinical effect, although other hormones are often also synthesized. Circulating hormone concentrations can be measured and high levels provide the diagnosis. Endoscopic ultrasonography is a new technique which aids in localization of the tumour before surgery.

GASTRINOMAS (ZOLLINGER–ELLISON SYNDROME)

Gastrinomas arise from the G cells of the pancreas and secrete large amounts of gastrin. This stimulates maximal gastric acid secretion resulting in the development of peptic ulcers which are often multiple, large and resistant to conventional treatment. Diarrhoea may also occur as a result of inhibition of digestive enzymes at low pH in the intestine. Treatment is with omeprazole (which inhibits the H^+/K^+ proton pump necessary for acid secretion). Surgery is reserved for removal of the primary tumour only.

VIPOMAS

These rare tumours produce vasoactive intestinal polypeptide (VIP) which stimulates intestinal water and electrolyte secretion, causing severe watery diarrhoea and dehydration. Treatment is with surgical resection or octreotide.

GLUCAGONOMAS

Glucagonomas arise from the α cells of the pancreas and produce pancreatic glucagon. Patients present with diabetes mellitus and a unique necrolytic migratory erythematous rash.

FINAL MEDICINE EXAMINATION: LIVER, BILIARY TRACT AND PANCREAS

The most common types of questions all relate to the differential diagnosis and appropriate investigations in a jaundiced patient.

1. A 50-year-old woman complains of itching, passing dark urine and pale stools, and is deeply jaundiced. What causes should be considered in the first instance and how would you investigate these?

2. A 36-year-old woman presents with a 4-day history of painless jaundice. There is no previous history of medical illness and, apart from marked jaundice, there are no abnormal physical signs. Initial investigations show:

   Hb 11.5 g/dl, WCC 36×10^9/l, MCV 106 fl, platelets 41×10^9/l.
   Serum sodium 129 mmol/l, potassium 2 mmol/l, urea 1.4 mmol/l.
   Serum bilirubin 190 µmol/l, alkaline phosphatase 350 U/l, ALT 108 U/l, γGT 250 U/l.
   Hepatitis B and A antibody titres are not elevated.
   Serum vitamin B_{12} and folate are normal.

   What is the probable diagnosis and what further tests would be useful? What is the initial management?

Other questions related to the management of complications which may develop in chronic liver disease:

3. Discuss the immediate and subsequent management of a patient with a haematemesis caused by oesophageal varices.

4. Describe the factors underlying the formation of ascites. Describe the principles of management when the ascites results from chronic liver disease.

ANSWERS

1. The jaundice is associated with pruritus, dark urine and pale stools, and is therefore *cholestatic*. The next step is to establish whether this is intrahepatic or extrahepatic. The causes are listed in Table 3.1. Information obtained from a detailed clinical history and physical examination may well point to one of these as the probable cause; ultrasonography is the initial key investigation (Figure 3.2).

2. The most probable diagnosis is alcoholic hepatitis superimposed on a background of chronic alcoholic liver disease (even in the absence of physical signs). The

raised MCV (with a normal vitamin B_{12} and folate), very high γGT and thrombocytopenia all suggest alcohol abuse. The very high WCC is typical of alcoholic hepatitis. The sodium is probably low because of inability to excrete a free water load and dilutional hyponatraemia (page 206). Further investigations and initial management are discussed on pages 90–91. In addition thiamine must be given to prevent Wernicke's encephalopathy.

3, 4. The answers to these are discussed on pages 82 and 83, respectively.

CHAPTER 4

Diseases of the Blood

[CM p. 293]

ANAEMIA

Anaemia is present when there is a decrease in the level of haemoglobin (Hb) in the blood below the reference range for the age and sex of the individual. Reduction of Hb is usually accompanied by a fall in red cell count (RCC) and packed cell volume (PCV, haematocrit), although an increase in plasma volume (as with massive splenomegaly) may cause anaemia with a normal RCC and PCV ('dilutional anaemia'). The normal values for these indices are given in Table 4.1, all of which are measured using automated cell counters as part of a routine full blood count (FBC).

Table 4.1 Normal values for adult peripheral blood

	Men	Women
Hb (g/dl)	14–17.7	12–16
PCV (l/l)	0.42–0.53	0.36–0.45
RCC ($\times 10^{12}$/l)	4.5–6.0	3.9–5.1
MCV (fl)	80–96	80–96
MCH (pg)	27–33	27–33
WCC ($\times 10^9$/l)	4.0–11.0	4.0–11.0
Platelets ($\times 10^9$/l)	150–400	150–400
ESR (mm/h)	< 20	< 20
Reticulocytes (%)	0.2–2.0	0.2–2.0

Clinical features

Symptoms depend on the severity and speed of onset of anaemia. A very slowly falling level of Hb allows for haemodynamic compensation and enhancement of the oxygen-carrying capacity of the blood. In general elderly people tolerate anaemia less well than young people. The symptoms are non-specific and include fatigue, faintness and breathlessness. Angina pectoris and intermittent claudication may occur in those with coexistent atheromatous arterial disease. On examination the skin and mucous membranes are pale; there may be a tachycardia and a systolic flow murmur. Cardiac failure may occur in elderly people or those with compromised cardiac function.

Classification of anaemias (Table 4.2)

The anaemias are classified in terms of the red cell indices, particularly the mean corpuscular volume (MCV). The mean

Table 4.2 Classification of anaemias based on the MCV

Microcytic/hypochromic	Normocytic/normochromic	Macrocytic
Low MCV and MCH	**Normal MCV and MCH**	**High MCV**
Iron deficiency	Acute blood loss	Vitamin B$_{12}$ deficiency
Thalassaemia	Anaemia of chronic disease	Folate deficiency
Anaemia of chronic disease	Aplastic anaemia	Myelodysplasia
Sideroblastic anaemia	Combined deficiency, e.g. iron and folate	Haemolysis
	Haemolytic anaemia	Other defects of DNA synthesis, e.g. chemotherapy
	Endocrine disorders	
	Hypopituitarism	
	Hypothyroidism	
	Hypoadrenalism	

MCV, mean corpuscular volume; MCH, mean corpuscular haemoglobin.

corpuscular haemoglobin (MCH) provides little additional information. This classification is useful because the type of anaemia then indicates the underlying causes and necessary investigations.

Microcytic anaemia

Iron deficiency

The most common cause of a microcytic anaemia is iron deficiency. Iron is absorbed in the duodenum and jejunum; factors that promote absorption include gastric acid, iron deficiency and active erythropoiesis. Iron is transported in the plasma bound to the protein transferrin, which is normally about one-third saturated with iron (Figure 4.1), and stored in the reticuloendothelial system as ferritin and haemosiderin. A fixed amount of iron, about 1 mg, is lost in sweat, urine and faeces each day. In women there is an additional loss during menses and premenopausal women may often border on iron deficiency.

Aetiology

The most common cause of iron deficiency is blood loss from the uterus or gastrointestinal tract. Other causes are:

● Increased demands – during growth and pregnancy

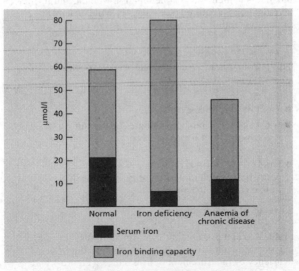

Figure 4.1 Serum iron and total iron-binding capacity in normal subjects and in iron-deficiency and anaemia of chronic disease.

- Decreased absorption with small bowel disease or after gastrectomy
- Poor intake; this is rare in developed countries

Clinical features

Symptoms and signs are the result of anaemia (see earlier) and of decreased epithelial cell iron which causes brittle hair and nails, atrophic glossitis, angular stomatitis and koilonychia (spoon-shaped nails). Rarely, pharyngeal webs cause dysphagia (Paterson–Brown–Kelly syndrome).

Investigations

BLOOD COUNT shows a low Hb with a low MCV.

BLOOD FILM: the red cells are microcytic and hypochromic with anisocytosis (variation in size) and poikilocytosis (variation in shape).

SERUM IRON is low and the total iron-binding capacity (TIBC) is high (Figure 4.1).

SERUM FERRITIN reflects iron stores and is low.

BONE MARROW EXAMINATION is only necessary in complicated cases and shows erythroid hyperplasia and absence of iron.

Iron deficiency is almost always the result of gastrointestinal blood loss in men and postmenopausal women, and further investigation is required (see page 41). Mild anaemia in premenopausal women is usually the result of menstrual blood loss.

Differential diagnosis

This is from other causes of a microcytic/hypochromic anaemia (Table 4.2).

Management

- Treat the underlying cause.
- ORAL IRON, e.g. ferrous sulphate 200 mg three times daily, is given for about 6 months to correct the anaemia and replace iron stores.
- PARENTERAL IRON is rarely necessary and used only when patients are intolerant or there is a poor response to oral iron, e.g. severe malabsorption.

Anaemia of chronic disease

This occurs in patients with a variety of chronic diseases (Table 4.3) and presents with a normochromic, normocytic or microcytic anaemia which is differentiated from iron deficiency by measurement of iron indices (Figure 4.1). It is the result of decreased release of iron from bone marrow to developing erythroblasts, inadequate erythropoietin response to the anaemia and decreased red cell survival. Treatment is of the underlying cause.

Table 4.3 Causes of anaemia of chronic disease

Chronic renal failure
Liver disease
Inflammatory disease, e.g. Crohn's disease, polymyalgia rheumatica
Chronic infections, e.g. infective endocarditis, tuberculosis
Malignancy
Myelodysplasia

Sideroblastic anaemia

Sideroblastic anaemia is a rare disorder of haem synthesis characterized by a refractory anaemia with hypochromic cells in the peripheral blood and ring sideroblasts in the bone marrow. Ring sideroblasts are erythroblasts with iron deposited in mitochondria around the nucleus. It may be congenital or acquired (secondary to myelodysplasia, alcohol, lead or isoniazid, or idiopathic). Treatment is to withdraw causative agents. Some cases respond to pyridoxine (vitamin B_6). In many cases anaemia is transfusion dependent and iron overload becomes a problem.

Megaloblastic anaemias

The megaloblastic anaemias are a group of anaemias characterized by the presence in the bone marrow of erythroblasts with delayed nuclear maturation relative to that of the cytoplasm (*megaloblasts*). The underlying defect accounting for the asynchronous maturation of the nucleus is defective DNA synthesis which may also affect the white cells (causing hypersegmented neutrophils and sometimes leukopenia) and platelets (causing thrombocytopenia). The peripheral red cells are large (macrocytic). The most common cause (see Table 4.2) of megaloblastic anaemia is deficiency of vitamin B_{12} or folate which are both necessary to synthesize DNA.

Vitamin B_{12} deficiency

Vitamin B_{12} is obtained from animal sources (meat, fish, eggs and milk). It is liberated from protein complexes in food by pancreatic and gastric enzymes and binds to *intrinsic factor* which is secreted from gastric parietal cells. This complex is delivered to the terminal ileum where vitamin B_{12} is absorbed and transported to the tissues by the carrier proteins, transcobalamin I and II. Vitamin B_{12} is stored in the liver where there is sufficient supply for 2 or more years. The causes of vitamin B_{12} deficiency are listed in Table 4.4.

Table 4.4 Causes of vitamin B$_{12}$ deficiency

Low dietary intake
Vegans

Impaired absorption
Intrinsic factor deficiency
    Pernicious anaemia
    Gastrectomy
Small bowel malabsorption
    Ileal disease or resection
    Tropical sprue
    Coeliac disease
Consumption in the small bowel
    Bacterial overgrowth
Pancreatic disease
    Chronic pancreatitis

Transcobalamin deficiency (rare)

Pernicious anaemia

Pernicious anaemia is an autoimmune condition in which there is atrophy of the gastric mucosa with consequent failure of intrinsic factor production and vitamin B$_{12}$ malabsorption. It is the most common cause of vitamin B$_{12}$ deficiency in Western countries.

Epidemiology

This is a disease of elderly people (1 in 8000 affected over the age of 60 years). It is more common in women and in people with fair hair and blue eyes. There is an association with other autoimmune diseases, e.g. hypothyroidism, vitiligo.

Pathology

There is severe atrophic gastritis causing absent acid and intrinsic factor secretion.

Clinical features

The onset of pernicious anaemia is insidious with progressively increasing symptoms of anaemia. There may be glossitis (a red sore tongue), angular stomatitis and mild jaundice. Neurological features are peripheral neuropathy, optic atrophy, dementia and subacute combined degeneration of the cord. This is characterized by demyelination of the corticospinal tracts and posterior columns, causing progressive weakness, ataxia and eventually paraplegia.

Investigations

BLOOD COUNT AND FILM: a macrocytic anaemia (MCV often > 110 fl) is often seen with hypersegmented neutrophils (nuclei with six or more lobes), and, in severe cases, leucopenia and thrombocytopenia.

SERUM VITAMIN B_{12} is low, frequently < 50 ng/l (normal > 160 ng/l).

RED CELL FOLATE may be reduced because vitamin B_{12} is necessary to convert serum folate to the active intracellular form.

SERUM BILIRUBIN is raised as a result of excess breakdown of haemoglobin because of ineffective erythropoiesis in the bone marrow.

SERUM AUTOANTIBODIES: parietal cell antibodies are present in 90% and antibodies to intrinsic factor in 50%.

THE SCHILLING TEST (Table 4.5) will differentiate pernicious anaemia from malabsorption as the cause of vitamin B_{12} deficiency. Defective vitamin B_{12} absorption is corrected by intrinsic factor in the former.

BONE MARROW EXAMINATION shows a hypercellular bone marrow with megaloblastic changes. This is not necessary in the straightforward case.

Table 4.5 Schilling test

Part I
- Give 1 µg ^{58}Co–vitamin B_{12} orally to fasting patient.
- Give 1000 µg B_{12} (non-radioactive) by intramuscular injection to saturate vitamin B_{12}-binding proteins and to flush out ^{58}Co–vitamin B_{12}.
- Collect urine for 24 h.
- Normal subjects excrete more than 10% of the radioactive dose.

If abnormal:

Part II
- Repeat part I after giving oral intrinsic factor capsules.

Result
- If excretion still abnormal, lesion is in the terminal ileum or there is bacterial overgrowth.
- If excretion now normal, diagnosis is pernicious anaemia.

Management
Treatment is with intramuscular hydroxycobalamin. Injections (1 mg) are given twice weekly for 3 weeks to replenish body stores, and then 3-monthly injections are continued for life.

Complications
There is an increased incidence of gastric carcinoma. Endoscopy or barium meal examination of the stomach is performed only if gastric symptoms are present.

Folate deficiency

Folate is found in green vegetables and offal, and absorbed in the upper small intestine. Folate deficiency, sufficient to cause anaemia, may be the result of a poor dietary intake of folate alone, but occurs more commonly in combination with malabsorption or increased folate utilization (Table 4.6).

Table 4.6 Causes of folate deficiency

Poor intake	Old age, poverty, alcohol excess (also impaired utilization), anorexia
Malabsorption	Tropical sprue, coeliac disease
Excess utilization	
Physiological	Pregnancy, lactation, prematurity
Pathological	Haemolysis, malignant disease, inflammatory disease (Crohn's disease, tuberculosis, psoriasis), haemodialysis or peritoneal dialysis
Antifolate drugs	Phenytoin, trimethoprim

Clinical features
Symptoms and signs are the result of anaemia.

Investigations
Red cell folate is low (normal range 160–640 µg/l) and is a more accurate guide of tissue folate levels than *serum folate* which is also low (normal range 3.0–15 µg/l). If the history does not suggest dietary deficiency, further investigations such as a jejunal biopsy should be performed to look for small bowel disease.

Management
The underlying cause must be treated and folate deficiency corrected by giving oral folic acid 5 mg daily. Prophylactic folate is given to patients with chronic haemolysis and to pregnant women.

In megaloblastic anaemia of undetermined cause, folic acid alone must not be given as this will aggravate the neuropathy of vitamin B_{12} deficiency.

Differential diagnosis of megaloblastic anaemias

A raised MCV with macrocytosis on the peripheral blood film can occur with a normoblastic rather than a megaloblastic bone marrow (Table 4.7). The exact mechanism for the large red cells in each of these conditions is not always clear.

Table 4.7 Causes of macrocytosis other than megaloblastic anaemia

Alcohol excess
Liver disease
Pregnancy and the newborn
Reticulocytosis
Hypothyroidism
Aplastic anaemia
Primary acquired sideroblastic anaemia
Myelodysplastic syndrome

ANAEMIA CAUSED BY MARROW FAILURE (APLASTIC ANAEMIA)

Aplastic anaemia is defined as pancytopenia with *hypocellularity* (aplasia) of the bone marrow. It is an uncommon but serious condition which may be inherited but is more commonly acquired.

Aetiology

A list of the main causes of aplasia is given in Table 4.8. Suppression of bone marrow stem cells by T-suppressor cells is responsible for many cases of idiopathic acquired aplastic anaemia. Many drugs have been associated with the development of aplastic anaemia and this occurs as a predictable dose-related effect (e.g. chemotherapeutic agents) or as an idiosyncratic reaction (e.g. chloramphenicol).

Clinical features

Symptoms are the result of the deficiency of red blood cells, white blood cells and platelets and include anaemia, increased susceptibility to infection and bleeding. Physical findings include bruising, bleeding gums and epistaxis. Mouth infections are common.

Investigations

BLOOD COUNT shows pancytopenia with low or absent reticulocytes.

BONE MARROW EXAMINATION shows hypoplasia with increased fat spaces.

Differential diagnosis

This is from other causes of pancytopenia (Table 4.8). A bone marrow trephine biopsy is essential for assessment of the bone marrow cellularity.

Table 4.8 Causes of pancytopenia

Hypocellular bone marrow	Cellular bone marrow

Aplastic anaemia
  Congenital
  Unknown (50%)
  Chemicals, e.g. benzene
  Drugs: cytotoxics,
  chloramphenicol, gold,
  Insecticides
  Ionizing radiation
  Infections, e.g. viral hepatitis,
  measles
  Pregnancy
	Bone marrow infiltration
	  Lymphoma
	  Acute leukaemia
	  Myeloma
	  Secondary carcinoma
	  Myelofibrosis

Paroxysmal nocturnal
  haemoglobinuria
  (a rare cause)
	Abnormal maturation
	  Myelodysplasia
	  Megaloblastic anaemia
	Excess destruction
	  Hypersplenism
	  Systemic lupus erythematosus
	    (antibody formation)

Management

The cause of the aplastic anaemia must be eliminated if possible. Supportive care, including transfusions of red cells and platelets and antibiotic therapy, should be given as necessary. The course of aplastic anaemia is very variable, ranging from a rapid spontaneous remission to a persistent, increasingly severe pancytopenia, which may lead to death through haemorrhage or infection. Bad prognostic features are the following:

- A peripheral blood neutrophil count $< 0.5 \times 10^9/l$
- A peripheral blood platelet count $< 20 \times 10^9/l$
- A reticulocyte count of $< 10 \times 10^9/l$ (0.1%)
- Severe hypocellularity of the bone marrow

In those patients who do not undergo spontaneous recovery the options for treatment are the following:

- BONE MARROW TRANSPLANTATION from a histocompatible sibling donor is the treatment of choice for young patients (< 20 years) and older patients (> 45 years) with very severe disease (as indicated by the presence of all the bad prognostic features).
- IMMUNOSUPPRESSIVE THERAPY is used for older patients with less severe forms of the disease and younger patients without an HLA-identical sibling. Antilymphocyte globulin, steroids and cyclosporin are used alone or in combination.

HAEMOLYTIC ANAEMIA

Haemolytic anaemia results from increased destruction of red cells with a reduction of the circulating lifespan (normally 120 days). Haemolysis may be extravascular (*within the reticuloendothelial system*) or intravascular (*within the blood vessels*). The causes of haemolytic anaemia in adults are listed in Table 4.9.

Table 4.9 Causes of haemolytic anaemia

Inherited	Acquired
Red cell membrane defect	Immune
Hereditary spherocytosis	Autoimmune haemolytic anaemia
Hereditary elliptocytosis	Haemolytic transfusion reactions
Haemoglobin abnormalities	Non-immune
Thalassaemia	Paroxysmal nocturnal haemoglobinuria
Sickle-cell disease	Microangiopathic haemolytic anaemia
	March haemoglobinuria
Metabolic defects	Miscellaneous
Glucose-6-phosphate	Infections (e.g. malaria)
dehydrogenase	Drugs/chemicals
deficiency	Hypersplenism
Pyruvate kinase deficiency	

In most haemolytic conditions, red cell destruction is extravascular and cells are removed from the circulation by macrophages in the reticuloendothelial system, particularly the spleen.

When red cells are broken down within the circulation, Hb is released and binds to plasma haptoglobins. When these become saturated, free Hb appears in the urine. Some Hb is broken down in the renal tubular cells and appears as haemosiderin in the urine. Figure 4.2 shows an approach to investigating the patient with haemolytic anaemia.

INHERITED HAEMOLYTIC ANAEMIAS

Membrane defects

Hereditary spherocytosis

Hereditary spherocytosis is the most common inherited haemolytic anaemia in northern Europeans and is inherited in an autosomal dominant manner. It is the result of a defect in the red cell membrane caused by deficiency of the structural membrane protein, *spectrin*. Red cells become spherical in shape, are more rigid and less deformable than normal red cells, and are thus destroyed prematurely in the spleen.

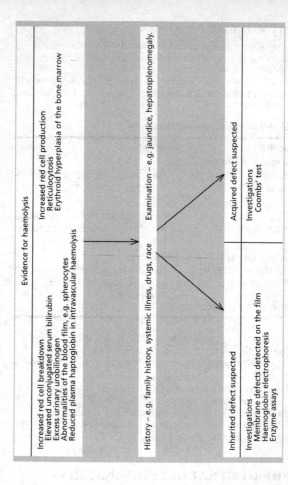

Evidence for haemolysis

Increased red cell breakdown	Increased red cell production
Elevated unconjugated serum bilirubin	Reticulocytosis
Excess urinary urobilinogen	Erythroid hyperplasia of the bone marrow
Abnormalities of the blood film, e.g. spherocytes	
Reduced plasma haptoglobin in intravascular haemolysis	

History – e.g. family history, systemic illness, drugs, race

Examination – e.g. jaundice, hepatosplenomegaly.

Inherited defect suspected

Investigations
Membrane defects detected on the film
Haemoglobin electrophoresis
Enzyme assays

Acquired defect suspected

Investigations
Coombs' test

Figure 4.2 An algorithm for investigation of suspected haemolytic anaemia.

Clinical features
Hereditary spherocytosis may present with jaundice or be asymptomatic. Patients may develop anaemia, splenomegaly and leg ulcers. As in many haemolytic anaemias, the course of the disease may be interrupted by aplastic, haemolytic and megaloblastic crises. Aplastic anaemia usually occurs after infections, particularly with parvovirus, whereas megaloblastic anaemia is the result of folate depletion caused by hyperactivity of the bone marrow. Chronic haemolysis may lead to the development of pigment gallstones.

Investigations
BLOOD COUNT demonstrates reticulocytosis and anaemia which is usually mild.

THE BLOOD FILM shows spherocytes (also seen in autoimmune haemolytic anaemia) and reticulocytes.

The diagnosis is made by demonstration of increased red cell osmotic fragility when placed in hypotonic solutions.

Management
Splenectomy should be performed in all but the mildest of cases. This is usually postponed until after childhood to minimize the risk of overwhelming pneumococcal infection. Following splenectomy, all patients should receive pneumococcal vaccine and long-term prophylactic penicillin.

Hereditary elliptocytosis

Hereditary elliptocytosis is similar to spherocytosis but the red cells are elliptical in shape. It is milder clinically and usually does not require treatment.

Haemoglobin abnormalities

Normal adult Hb is made up of haem and two polypeptide globin chains, the α and β chains. The haemoglobinopathies can be classified into two subgroups: *abnormal chain production* or *abnormal chain structure* of the polypeptide chains (Table 4.10).

Thalassaemia

In normal Hb there is a balance (1:1) in production of α and β chains. The thalassaemias are a group of disorders arising from one or multiple gene defects, resulting in reduced rate of production of one or more globin chains. The imbalanced globin chain production leads to precipitation of globin chains within red cells or precursors. This results in ineffective erythropoiesis and haemolysis.

There are two main types:

Table 4.10 Types of haemoglobin

	Haemoglobin	Structure	Comment
Normal	A	$\alpha_2\beta_2$	92% of adult haemoglobin
	A_{1c}	$\alpha_2\beta_2$	5% of adult haemoglobin (glycosylated Hb)
	A_2	$\alpha_2\delta_2$	2% of adult haemoglobin; elevated in β-thalassaemia
	F	$\alpha_2\gamma_2$	Normal haemoglobin in fetus from 3rd to 9th month; increased in β-thalassaemia
Abnormal chain production	H	β_4	Found in α-thalassaemia
	Barts	γ_4	Found in homozygous α-thalassaemia
Abnormal chain structure	S	$\alpha_2\beta_2$	Substitution of valine for glutamic acid in position 6 of the β chain
	C	$\alpha_2\beta_2$	Substitution of lysine for glutamic acid in position 6 of the β chain

1. α-Thalassaemia – reduced α-chain synthesis.
2. β-Thalassaemia – reduced β-chain synthesis.

β-THALASSAEMIA
In homozygous β-thalassaemia there is little or no β-chain production, resulting in excess α chains. These combine with whatever δ and γ chains are produced leading to increased Hb A$_2$ and Hb F. There are three main clinical forms of β-thalassaemia:

1. *β-Thalassaemia trait*: this is the asymptomatic heterozygous carrier state. Anaemia is mild or absent with a low MCV and MCH. Iron stores are normal.

2. *β-Thalassaemia intermedia*: this includes patients with moderate anaemia (Hb 7–10 g/dl) that does not require regular blood transfusions. Splenomegaly, bone deformities, recurrent leg ulcers and gallstones are other features. This may be caused by a combination of homozygous β- and α-thalassaemia.

3. *β-Thalassaemia major*: this presents in the first year of life with severe anaemia *(Cooley's anaemia),* failure to thrive, recurrent infections and extramedullary haemopoiesis, leading to hepatosplenomegaly and thalassaemic facies (enlarged maxilla with prominent frontal and parietal bones).

Investigations
BLOOD COUNT AND FILM show a hypochromic/microcytic anaemia, raised reticulocyte count and nucleated red cells in the peripheral circulation.

THE DIAGNOSIS is made by haemoglobin electrophoresis which shows an increase in Hb F and absent or markedly reduced Hb A.

Management
The mainstay of treatment is blood transfusion, aiming to keep the haemoglobin above 10 g/dl thus suppressing ineffective erythropoiesis, preventing bony abnormalities and allowing normal development. Iron overload caused by repeated transfusions may lead to damage to endocrine glands, liver, pancreas and heart, with death in the second decade from cardiac failure. Treatment with the iron-chelating agent, desferrioxamine, may prevent iron loading. Bone marrow transplantation has been used in some cases of thalassaemia.

α-THALASSAEMIA
The clinical manifestations of this disorder vary from a mild anaemia with microcytosis to a severe condition incompatible with life. There are four α-globin genes per cell. The manifestations depend on whether one, two, three or all four of the genes are deleted and thus whether α-chain synthesis is

partial or completely absent. In the most severe form where there is complete absence of α-globin (Hb Barts) infants are stillborn (hydrops fetalis).

Antenatal diagnosis of haemoglobin abnormalities

It is possible to identify a fetus with β-thalassaemia major by DNA analysis of chorionic villous samples taken in the first trimester, or by testing umbilical cord blood in the second trimester. Abortion is offered if the fetus is found to be affected. This examination is appropriate if the mother is found to have a thalassaemia trait during antenatal testing and on subsequent screening her partner is also affected.

Sickle-cell disease

Sickle-cell disease results from the production of an abnormal haemoglobin, haemoglobin S, as a result of the substitution of the amino acid valine for glutamic acid in position 6 of the β chain. It is found most commonly in people of African origin (25% carry the gene). In the deoxygenated state, Hb S molecules link to form chains and this results in increased rigidity of the red cells causing the classic sickle appearance. Sickling produces a shortened red cell survival and obstruction of the microcirculation, and is often precipitated by infection, dehydration, cold or hypoxia. As the production of Hb F is normal, the disease is usually not manifest until Hb F decreases to adult levels at about 6 months of age.

Clinical features

In the heterozygous state, Hb AS (*sickle-cell trait*), there are usually no symptoms unless the patient is exposed to extreme hypoxia, e.g. poor anaesthesia.

Symptoms of the homozygous state, Hb SS (*sickle-cell anaemia*), vary from mild anaemia to severe haemolysis with recurrent sickle-cell crises. A *painful crisis* may be precipitated by infection, cold and dehydration. It is caused by sickling with occlusion of small vessels and characterized by severe pain, often in the bones. Other features are indicated in Table 4.11. Children may develop the hand and foot syndrome caused by recurrent infarcts of the small bones which result in digits of varying length. An *aplastic crisis* is usually associated with parvovirus infection – patients have a sudden fall in haemoglobin with a low reticulocyte count. *Sequestration crises* are uncommon and produce a rapid fall in Hb as a result of red cell trapping in the liver and spleen.

In the long term, patients are more prone to infections (*Streptococcus pneumoniae*, salmonella osteomyelitis), chronic leg ulcers, pigment gallstones and aseptic necrosis of the femoral head.

Table 4.11 Features of a sickle-cell crisis

Bone pain
Pleuritic chest pain
Cerebral infarction causing fits and hemiparesis
Renal papillary necrosis
Liver and splenic infarction
Priapism (prolonged erections)

Investigations

BLOOD COUNT: in sickle-cell disease there is a low haemoglobin (8–9 g/dl) with a high reticulocyte count. Patients with sickle-cell trait are not anaemic.

DIAGNOSIS is made with Hb electrophoresis showing 80–90% Hb SS and absent Hb A. In addition sickling can be induced *in vitro* with sodium metabisulphite.

Treatment

Asymptomatic anaemia requires no treatment. Acute attacks require intravenous fluids, analgesia, oxygen and antibiotics if infection is present. The pain during a sickling crisis is very severe and opiate analgesia is often required in those admitted to hospital. Exchange transfusions may be used to reduce the frequency of crises or as prophylaxis in pregnancy or before surgery.

Bone marrow transplantation is currently being assessed as a potential treatment for severe disease.

Metabolic red cell disorders

A number of red cell enzyme deficiencies may produce haemolytic anaemia, the most common of which is glucose-6-phosphate dehydrogenase (G6PD) deficiency.

Glucose-6-phosphate dehydrogenase deficiency

G6PD is a vital enzyme in the hexose monophosphate shunt which maintains glutathione in the reduced state. Glutathione is important in combating oxidative stress in the red cell. G6PD deficiency is a common heterogeneous X-linked trait found predominantly in African, Mediterranean and Middle Eastern populations.

The cardinal clinical manifestation is haemolysis, which occurs as a consequence of oxidative stress on the erythrocyte. Important precipitants are oxidizing drugs (e.g. quinine, sulphonamides, nitrofurantoin), oxidants in food (e.g. fava bean constituents) and infection. Other clinical features are neonatal jaundice and chronic haemolysis.

Table 4.12 Features of autoimmune haemolytic anaemia

	Warm antibody	Cold antibody
Temperature at which antibody attaches best to red cell	37°C	Lower than 37°C
Type of antibodies	IgG	IgM
Direct Coombs' test	Strongly positive	Positive
Cause of primary condition	Idiopathic	Idiopathic
Causes of secondary condition	Autoimmune disorders, e.g. SLE Lymphomas Hodgkin's disease Drugs, e.g. methyldopa	Infections *Mycoplasma* sp. Infectious mononucleosis Viruses Lymphomas Paroxysmal cold haemoglobinuria (very rare)

ACQUIRED HAEMOLYTIC ANAEMIA

Autoimmune haemolytic anaemia

Autoimmune haemolytic anaemia is classified according to whether the antibody reacts best at body temperature *(warm antibodies)* or at lower temperatures *(cold antibodies)* (Table 4.12). IgG or IgM antibodies attach to the red cell resulting in extravascular haemolysis through sequestration in the spleen or in intravascular haemolysis through activation of complement.

Warm antibody haemolysis

Clinical features

This anaemia occurs at all ages in both sexes with a variable clinical picture ranging from mild haemolysis to life-threatening anaemia. About 50% are associated with other autoimmune disorders or lymphoma.

Investigation

There is evidence of haemolysis (page 116) and the direct antiglobulin test *(Coombs' test)* is positive (Figure 4.3).

Management

High-dose steroids induce remission in 80% of cases. Splenectomy is useful in those failing to respond to steroids. Occasionally immunosuppressive drugs such as azathioprine and cyclophosphamide are beneficial.

Cold antibody haemolysis

Clinical features

IgM antibodies *(cold agglutinins)* attach to red cells in the cold peripheral parts of the body and cause agglutination and complement-mediated intravascular haemolysis. Infection with mycoplasmas or Epstein–Barr virus may lead to increased synthesis of cold agglutinins (normally produced in insignificant amounts) and produce transient haemolysis. A chronic idiopathic form occurs in elderly people with recurrent haemolysis and peripheral cyanosis.

Investigation

There is evidence of haemolysis and the direct antiglobulin test is positive. Red cells agglutinate in the cold or at room temperature.

Management

This usually does not require treatment other than treating the underlying condition and avoiding exposure to cold.

Drug-induced haemolysis

Drug-induced haemolysis may occur through one of the following mechanisms.

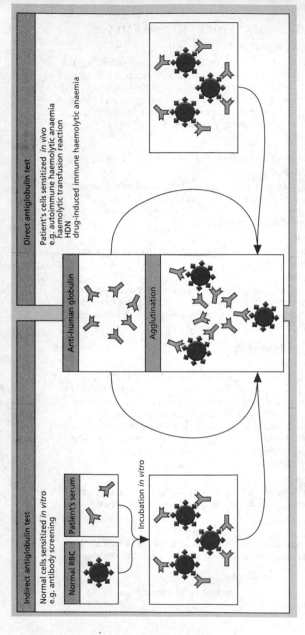

Figure 4.3 Antiglobulin (Coombs') test: the human antiglobulin forms bridges between the sensitized cells causing visible agglutination. The direct test detects patient's cells sensitized *in vivo* and the indirect test detects normal cells sensitized *in vitro*.

IMMUNE COMPLEX

A drug–antibody immune complex forms which attaches to the red cell inducing complement and red cell destruction (e.g. *quinine*).

MEMBRANE ADSORPTION

An antigenic drug–red cell complex is formed stimulating the adsorption and production of antibodies which results in red cell destruction (e.g. *penicillin*).

AUTOANTIBODY

The drug induces production of a red cell autoantibody (e.g. *methyldopa*).

Non-immune haemolytic anaemia

Paroxysmal nocturnal haemoglobinuria

Paroxysmal nocturnal haemoglobinuria (PNH) is a rare disease in which a clone of red cells is unduly sensitive to complement-mediated lysis in the absence of antibody. There is intravascular haemolysis and episodes of thrombosis. Aplastic anaemia and acute myeloid leukaemia develop in some patients. Diagnosis is by *Ham's test* (*in vitro* lysis of the red cells in acidified serum). There is no specific treatment for PNH and management is supportive.

Mechanical haemolytic anaemia

Red cells may be injured by physical trauma in the circulation. Examples of this form of haemolysis include the following:

- PROSTHETIC HEART VALVES: damage to red cells in passage through heart.
- MARCH HAEMOGLOBINURIA: damage to red cells in the feet from prolonged marching.
- MICROANGIOPATHIC HAEMOLYSIS: fragmentation of red cells in abnormal microcirculation.

MYELOPROLIFERATIVE AND MYELODYSPLASTIC DISORDERS

Myeloproliferative and myelodysplastic syndromes are both clonal haemopoietic stem cell disorders which arise from a single abnormal multipotential cell in the bone marrow. Both disorders have the potential to transform into acute leukaemia. *Myelodysplastic syndromes* are characterized by ineffective erythropoiesis and peripheral blood cytopenias. *Myeloproliferative disorders* are characterized by over-production of one or more cell lines (myeloid, erythroid or megakaryocyte) and comprise chronic granulocytic leukaemia (CGL), polycythaemia vera, essential thrombocythaemia and myelofibrosis. These disorders differ from the acute

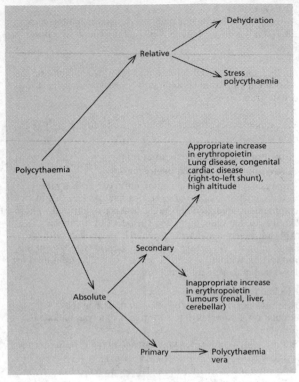

Figure 4.4 The causes of polycythaemia.

leukaemias (also clonal proliferation of a single cell line) where the cells also do not differentiate normally but there is progressive accumulation of *immature* cells.

Polycythaemia

Polycythaemia is defined as an increase in Hb, PCV and red cell count (RCC). The production of red cells by the bone marrow is normally regulated by the hormone erythropoietin produced in the kidney. The stimulus for erythropoietin production is tissue hypoxia. *Absolute polycythaemia* (Figure 4.4) is therefore the result of an appropriate increase in erythropoietin secondary to hypoxia, an inappropriate increase in erythropoietin resulting from abnormal production by certain tumours or escape by marrow stem cells from erythropoietin control (polycythaemia vera). Absolute polycythaemia must be differentiated from *relative polycythaemia* where PCV is normal but plasma volume is decreased. Relative polycythaemia usually affects middle-aged obese men who are smokers (stress polycythaemia). When associated with hypertension it is termed Gaisböck's syndrome. The causes of polycythaemia are shown in Figure 4.4.

Primary polycythaemia

Clinical features

Polycythaemia vera, like the other myeloproliferative disorders, occurs principally in middle-aged and elderly people. Symptoms and signs are the result of hypervolaemia and hyperviscosity. Typical symptoms include headache, dizziness, tinnitus, visual disturbance, angina pectoris, intermittent claudication, pruritus and venous thrombosis. Physical signs include a plethoric complexion and hepatosplenomegaly as a result of extramedullary haemopoiesis. There is an increased risk of haemorrhage as a result of friable haemostatic plugs and gout caused by increased cell turnover and uric acid production.

Investigations

BLOOD COUNT shows a high Hb and PCV. The WCC is raised in 70% and the platelet count in 50% of patients; such abnormalities are rarely present in polycythaemia from other causes.

RED CELL VOLUME measured with ^{51}Cr-labelled red cells is increased.

PLASMA VOLUME measured using ^{131}iodine-labelled-albumin dilution is normal or increased (compare with reactive).

BONE MARROW shows erythroid hyperplasia with increased numbers of megakaryocytes.

Differential diagnosis

This is from secondary and relative polycythaemia. An abdominal ultrasound, arterial P_aO_2 and measurement of serum erythropoietin may be necessary to differentiate. Erythropoietin is low or normal in polycythaemia vera and usually high in secondary polycythaemia.

Management

There is no cure; treatment is symptomatic.

- VENESECTION to maintain PCV < 0.45 l/l. Regular venesection (e.g. three monthly) may be all that is needed in many patients.

- CHEMOTHERAPY: hydroxyurea and busulphan are particularly useful to reduce the platelet count.

- RADIOACTIVE PHOSPHOROUS (^{32}P) is used for severe disease.

Prognosis

Median survival in untreated patients is 1–2 years and may be increased to approximately 14 years with treatment. Thirty per cent will develop myelofibrosis and 5% acute leukaemia. The risk of acute myeloid leukaemia is marginally increased by treatment with busulphan or phosphorus-32.

Secondary polycythaemia

Secondary polycythaemia presents with similar clinical features to primary polycythaemia, although the white cell and platelet count are normal and the spleen is not enlarged. In patients with tumours the primary disease must be treated to lower the level of erythropoietin. In hypoxic patients, oxygen therapy (page 334) may reduce the Hb and a small volume phlebotomy (400 ml) may help those with severe symptoms.

Essential thrombocythaemia

Essential thrombocythaemia is characterized by very high platelet counts (usually > 1000 × 10^9/l). Platelet size and function is abnormal and presentation may be with bleeding or thrombosis. Busulphan and hydroxyurea are used to reduce platelet production. Differential diagnosis is from secondary causes of a raised platelet count: connective tissue disorders, chronic infections, malignancy, other myeloproliferative disorders, haemorrhage, surgery and splenectomy.

Primary myelofibrosis (myelosclerosis)

Myelofibrosis is characterized by haemopoietic stem-cell proliferation associated with marrow fibrosis (abnormal megakaryocyte precursors release growth factors which stimulate fibroblasts).

Clinical features

There are constitutional symptoms of fever, weight loss and lethargy.

Bleeding occurs in the thrombocytopenic patient. There is hepatomegaly and massive splenomegaly caused by extramedullary haemopoiesis.

Investigations

BLOOD COUNT shows anaemia. The white cell and platelet count are high initially, but fall with disease progression as a result of marrow fibrosis.

BLOOD FILM examination shows a leukoerythroblastic picture (immature red cells caused by marrow infiltration) and 'tear drop'-shaped red cells.

BONE MARROW is usually unobtainable by aspiration (dry tap); trephine biopsy shows increased fibrosis.

Management

● TRANSFUSIONS for anaemia.

● BUSULPHAN OR HYDROXYUREA are used to reduce the raised white cell and platelet count.

- SPLENIC IRRADIATION may be useful to reduce a large painful spleen.
- SPLENECTOMY is performed if the spleen is very large and painful and the transfusion requirements are high.

Prognosis

The median survival is 3 years. Transformation to acute myeloid leukaemia occurs in 10–20%.

THE SPLEEN

The spleen, situated in the left hypochondrium, is the largest lymphoid organ in the body. Its main functions are phagocytosis of old red blood cells, immunological defence and as a 'pool' of blood from which cells may be rapidly mobilized. Pluripotential stem cells are present in the spleen and proliferate in severe haematological stress (*extramedullary haemopoiesis*), e.g. haemolytic anaemia.

Hypersplenism

Hypersplenism can result from splenomegaly of any cause (Table 4.13). It results in pancytopenia, increased plasma volume and haemolysis caused by increased destruction of red cells.

Table 4.13 Causes of splenomegaly

Sometimes massive (extending into right iliac fossa)	Moderate

Haematological
  Chronic myeloid leukaemia
  Myelofibrosis
	Haematological
	  Lymphomas
	  Leukaemias
	  Myeloproliferative disorders
	  Haemolytic anaemia

Infections
  Chronic malaria
  Schistosomiasis
  Kala-azar
	Infection
	  Septicaemia
	  Infectious mononucleosis
	  Infective endocarditis
	  Tuberculosis
	  Brucellosis

Other
  Tropical splenomegaly
	Inflammation
	  Rheumatoid arthritis
	  Sarcoidosis
	  Systemic lupus erythematosus

	Others
	  Portal hypertension, e.g. cirrhosis
	  Amyloidosis
	  Gaucher's disease

Splenectomy

This is performed mainly for:

- Trauma
- Idiopathic thrombocytopenic purpura
- Haemolytic anaemias
- Hypersplenism

The main complications are thrombophilia in the short term and overwhelming infection in the longer term. The main infecting organisms are *Strep. pneumoniae*, *H. influenzae* and the meningococci. Vaccines against these three bacteria should be given routinely to patients about to undergo splenectomy. In addition, antibiotic prophylaxis (phenoxymethylpenicillin, twice daily) should be given for the first two years after splenectomy and continued in children up to the age of 16 years. Some authorities recommend lifelong penicillin for all patients after splenectomy.

BLOOD PRODUCTS AND TRANSFUSION

Blood collected from donors is either used 'whole' or processed into blood components and blood products (Figure 4.5).

Blood groups

The blood groups are determined by antigens on the surface of red cells; more than 400 blood groups have been found. The ABO (Table 4. 14) and rhesus (Rh) systems are the two most important blood groups, but incompatibilities involving many other blood groups (such as Kell and Duffy) may cause haemolytic transfusion reactions and/or haemolytic disease of the newborn.

Table 4.14 Antigens and antibodies in the ABO system

Blood group	Serum antibody	UK frequency (%)	Comment
O	Anti-A and anti-B	44	'Universal donors' are O Rh negative
A	Anti-B	45	
B	Anti-A	8	
AB	None	3	Universal recipients

Complications of transfusing red blood cells

- ABO incompatibility is the most serious complication and often results from simple clerical errors, leading to the incorrect labelling and identification of blood and patient's blood sample for cross-matching. There is an immediate

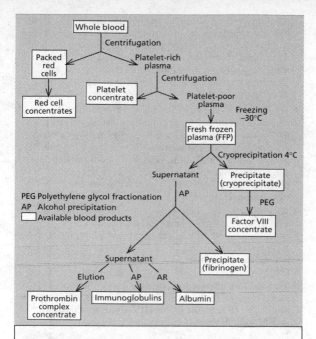

Whole blood is used for the correction of acute massive blood loss.

Packed red cells and red cell concentrates are used for acute bleeds and correction of anaemia.

Platelet concentrates are used to treat or prevent bleeding in patients with severe thrombocytopenia.

Fresh frozen plasma contains all the coagulation factors and is used in acquired coagulation factor deficiencies.

Albumin is sometimes given to patients with acute severe hypoalbuminaemia.

Immunoglobulins are used in patients with hypogammaglobulinaemia to prevent infection and in patients with idiopathic thrombocytopenic purpura. Specific immunoglobulin, e.g. anti-hepatitis B is used after exposure of a non-immune patient to infections.

Figure 4.5 Blood fractionation. (Adapted and reproduced with permission from Hayes, P. and Mackay, T., 1992, *Churchill's Pocketbook of Medicine*, Edinburgh, Churchill Livingstone.)

reaction, starting within minutes of the transfusion, leading to intravascular haemolysis, rigors, lumbar pain, dyspnoea and hypotension. The transfusion must be stopped and the donor units returned to the blood transfusion laboratory for testing with a new blood sample from the patient. Emergency treatment may be needed to maintain the blood pressure (page 367).

- Febrile reactions are usually the result of antileukocyte antibodies in the recipient acting against transfused leukocytes, leading to release of pyrogens. Typical signs are flushing, fever and tachycardia which may respond to slowing of the transfusion. Leukocyte-poor red-cell concentrates may be used in patients who have had febrile reactions or who are likely to receive repeated transfusions.

- Anaphylactic reactions are seen in patients lacking IgA but who produce anti-IgA that reacts with IgA in the transfused blood. This is a medical emergency (page 369). Urticarial reactions are treated by slowing of the infusion and giving intravenous antihistamines, e.g. chlorpheniramine.

- Transmission of infection is reduced now that donated blood is tested for hepatitis B surface antigen and antibodies to hepatitis C and HIV. Cytomegalovirus and Epstein–Barr virus may cause post-transfusion hepatitis.

- Heart failure may occur particularly in elderly people and with those having large transfusions.

- Complications of massive transfusion include hypocalcaemia, hyperkalaemia and hypothermia. Bleeding may occur as a result of depletion of platelets and clotting factors in stored blood.

BLEEDING DISORDERS

A bleeding disorder is suggested when the patient has unexplained (i.e. no history of trauma) bruising or bleeding, or prolonged bleeding in response to injury or surgery, e.g. after tooth extraction.

Reactions involved in haemostasis

When a blood vessel is damaged the exposed collagen sets in motion a series of events leading to haemostasis. Haemostasis depends on the interactions of the vessel wall, platelets and coagulation factors.

- Blood vessel damage leads to immediate vasoconstriction reducing blood flow to the injured area and allowing contact activation of platelets and coagulation factors.

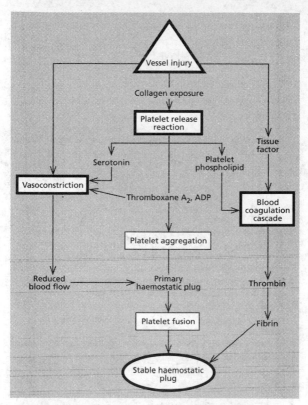

Figure 4.6 Reactions involved in haemostasis. (Adapted from Hoffbrand and Pettit, *Essential Haematology*, 2nd ed., Oxford, Blackwell Science Ltd.)

- Platelets *adhere* to the exposed subendothelial connective tissue; adherence is potentiated by a portion of the factor VIII protein, von Willebrand's factor (VIII:vWF). Collagen activates platelet prostaglandin synthesis leading to the formation of thromboxane A_2 which causes vasoconstriction, and lowers cyclic AMP, thereby initiating release of platelet granules (Figure 4.6). *Aggregation* of platelets is facilitated by thromboxane A_2 and ADP released from platelet granules. During aggregation platelet membrane receptors are exposed allowing a surface for the interaction of coagulation factors and ultimately the formation of a stable haemostatic plug.

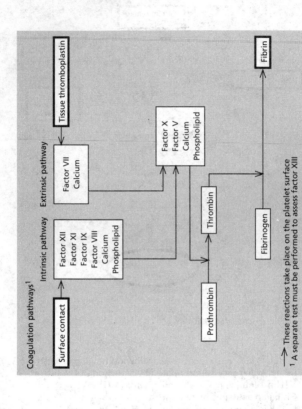

Figure 4.7 The coagulation cascade. (Adapted from Castaldi, 1992, The patient with easy bruising and bleeding. *Medicine International*, p. 4062.)

- Coagulation involves a series of enzymatic reactions leading to the conversion of soluble plasma fibrinogen to fibrin clot (Figure 4.7).

Limitation of coagulation

Coagulation would lead to dangerous occlusion of blood vessels if it were not limited to the site of injury by protective mechanisms.

RAPID BLOOD FLOW

Rapid blood flow at the periphery of the damaged area dilutes and removes coagulation factors.

CIRCULATING INHIBITORS OF THE COAGULATION FACTORS

- Antithrombin III binds to and forms stable complexes with coagulation factors. Activity is increased by heparin
- Active protein C destroys factors V and VIII
- Protein S is a cofactor for protein C

THE FIBRINOLYTIC SYSTEM

The plasma protein, plasminogen, is converted to plasmin by activators present in the tissue and endothelial cells. Plasmin breaks down fibrin and fibrinogen into smaller fragments known as fibrinogen degradation products (FDPs).

Bleeding disorders are therefore the result of a defect in *vessels*, *platelets* or the *coagulation pathway* (Table 4.15).

Table 4.15 Classification of bleeding disorders

Blood vessel defect
Hereditary
    Hereditary haemorrhagic telangiectasia (rare)
    Connective tissue disorders: Marfan's and Ehlers–Danlos syndromes
Acquired
    Severe infections: meningococcal, typhoid
    Drugs: steroids
    Allergic: Henoch–Schönlein purpura (mainly children)
    Others: scurvy, senile purpura
    Easy bruising syndrome

Platelet defect
Decreased platelet number or decreased function

Coagulation defect
Hereditary
    Haemophilia A or B, von Willebrand's disease
Acquired
    Anticoagulant treatment, liver disease, disseminated intravascular coagulation

Investigation of bleeding disorders

The nature of the defect and therefore the most appropriate initial investigations may be suggested by the history and examination, e.g family history, intercurrent disease, alcohol consumption, drugs. *Vascular/platelet bleeding* is characterized by bruising of the skin and bleeding from mucosal membranes. The *inherited coagulation disorders* are typically associated with haemarthroses (bleeding into joints) and muscle haematomas. The most common cause of abnormal bleeding is thrombocytopenia.

- PLATELET COUNT AND BLOOD FILM. This is the initial investigation.
- COAGULATION TESTS. Coagulation tests are abnormal with *deficiencies* or *inhibitors* of the clotting factors. If the abnormal result is corrected by the addition of normal plasma to patient's plasma in the assay then the result is abnormal as a result of deficiency and not of inhibitors.

Prothrombin time (PT) or *internationalized normalized ratio* (INR) is prolonged with abnormalities of the extrinsic and common pathways of the coagulation cascade.

Partial thromboplastin time with kaolin (PTTK) is prolonged with abnormalities of the intrinsic or common pathways.

Thrombin time (TT) is prolonged with fibrinogen deficiency, dysfibrinogenaemia (normal levels, abnormal function), heparin treatment or disseminated intravascular coagulation (DIC).

- THE BLEEDING TIME is abnormal with von Willebrand's disease, with blood vessel defects and when there is a decrease in the number or function of platelets.

These tests will localize the site of the problem. Further specialized investigations, e.g. platelet aggregation studies and measurement of individual clotting factors, will be necessary to identify the exact haemostatic defect correctly.

Platelet defects

Platelet defects are the result of thrombocytopenia (Table 4.16) or disorders of platelet function, e.g. those occurring with aspirin treatment and uraemia. Spontaneous bleeding from skin and mucous membranes is unlikely to occur with platelet counts above 20×10^9/l. Increased destruction or decreased production can be differentiated by bone marrow examination which will show increased or decreased number of megakaryocytes respectively.

Table 4.16 Causes of thrombocytopenia

Decreased marrow production
Leukaemia, myelofibrosis, aplastic anaemia, megaloblastic anaemia, alcohol, drugs (e.g. co-trimoxazole), viral infections

Increased destruction
Immune
    Autoimmune, postincompatible transfusion
Consumption
    Disseminated intravascular coagulation, hypersplenism, infections

Sequestration
Hypersplenism

Autoimmune thrombocytopenic purpura

Thrombocytopenia results from immune destruction of platelets. *Acute* autoimmune thrombocytopenic purpura (AITP) is seen in children, often following a viral infection. There is rapid onset of purpura which is usually self-limiting and becomes chronic in only about 5% of cases. *Chronic* AITP is more commonly seen in adults and is associated with platelet autoantibodies in 60–70%.

Aetiology
Chronic AITP is usually idiopathic but may occur with autoimmune disorders, e.g. SLE, thyroid disease, chronic lymphatic leukaemia and some viral infections, e.g. HIV. The same drugs that cause autoimmune haemolytic anaemia may also cause thrombocytopenia (and neutropenia).

Clinical features
The condition is characteristically seen in young women. There is a fluctuating course with skin and mucosal bleeding.

Investigation
There is thrombocytopenia with increased megakaryocytes on bone marrow examination. The detection of antiplatelet autoantibodies is unnecessary in a straightforward case.

Management
Platelet transfusion and/or high-dose intravenous immunoglobulin produce a rapid but transient rise in the platelet count and may be useful in severe haemorrhage. Prednisolone (60 mg/day) is the initial treatment of choice and 20% will have a complete and sustained response. Splenectomy, which has a 60% cure rate, is indicated in those with moderate-to-severe thrombocytopenia who fail medical treatment. Immunosuppressive drugs (e.g. azathioprine) are indicated in refractory cases.

Inherited coagulation disorders

Inherited disorders usually involve deficiency of only one coagulation factor whereas acquired disorders involve deficiency of several factors.

Haemophilia A

This is the result of a deficiency of factor VIII:C which is one part of the factor VIII molecule. It is inherited as an X-linked recessive, affecting 1 in 10 000 males.

Clinical features

Clinical features depend on the factor VIII plasma levels. If more than 5% of the normal level is present the disease is mild with post-traumatic bleeding only. Levels of less than 1% are associated with frequent spontaneous bleeding from early life. Bleeding is often into joints and muscles. The joints most frequently involved are the knees, elbows, ankles, shoulders and hips.

Investigations

The PTTK is prolonged and plasma factor VIII:C levels are reduced.

Management

- Intravenous injection of factor VIII concentrates are the mainstay of treatment. They are given as *prophylaxis*, e.g. before and after surgery, or to *treat* an acute bleeding episode. Many patients have a supply of factor VIII concentrates at home and inject themselves at the first sign of bleeding.

- Desmopressin (DDAVP), which is injected or inhaled, raises the level of factor VIII and may be used to treat mild haemophiliacs.

- Treatment with recombinant factor VIII:C is currently under trial.

- The cloning of the factor VIII gene and progress in the development in the retroviral-vector delivery systems have led to considerable interest in the possibility that haemophilia A could be 'cured' by gene therapy.

Complications

Recurrent bleeds into joints may lead to deformity and arthritis. There is a risk of acquiring transfusion-associated infection and many severe haemophiliacs who have had multiple transfusions are infected with hepatitis C and HIV, with some dying from AIDS. This risk has been eliminated because of the exclusion of high-risk blood donors, screening of donors and heat treatment of factor VIII concentrates. Ten per cent of severe haemophiliacs develop antibodies to factor VIII and may need massive doses to overcome this.

Haemophilia B (Christmas disease)

This is the result of deficiency of factor IX and affects 1 in 30 000 males. Inheritance and clinical features are the same as for haemophilia B. Treatment is with factor IX concentrates.

Von Willebrand's disease

Von Willebrand's disease is an inherited deficiency of von Willebrand's factor, which is an essential cofactor for normal platelet adhesion to damaged subendothelium. This factor also serves as a carrier for factor VIII:C to form the whole VIII complex.

Clinical features

Types I and II are mild forms, inherited as autosomal dominant and characterized by mucosal bleeding and prolonged bleeding after dental treatment or surgery.

Type III is the severe form, recessively inherited, with clinical features resembling haemophilia A.

Investigations

Prolonged bleeding time reflects a defect in platelet adhesion. There is a prolonged PTTK and decreased plasma levels of VIII:C and VIII:vWF.

Management

This is with factor VIII concentrates and desmopressin (DDAVP).

Acquired coagulation disorders

Disseminated intravascular coagulation

There is widespread generation of fibrin within blood vessels caused by initiation of the coagulation pathway. There is consumption of platelets and coagulation factors, and secondary activation of fibrinolysis leading to production of fibrin degradation products (FDPs) which contribute to coagulation by inhibiting fibrin polymerization.

Aetiology

Intravascular coagulation is initiated by release of procoagulant substances into the blood (amniotic fluid embolism, abruptio placentae, snake bite and malignancy), by contact of blood with an abnormal surface (burns, infection and grafts) or by generation of procoagulant substances in the blood (promyelocytic leukaemia, haemolytic transfusion reaction).

Clinical features

The presentation varies from no bleeding at all to complete haemostatic failure with bleeding from venepuncture sites and the nose and mouth. Thrombotic events may occur as a result of vessel occlusion by platelets and fibrin.

Investigations
There is thrombocytopenia, prolonged PT, PTTK and TT, decreased fibrinogen and elevated FDPs. The blood film shows fragmented red cells. In mild cases with compensatory increase of coagulation factors the only abnormality may be an increase in the FDPs.

Management
- Treat the underlying condition.
- Platelets, red cell concentrates and fresh frozen plasma may be necessary in patients who are bleeding.
- The use of heparin remains controversial.

Vitamin K deficiency
Vitamin K is needed for the formation of active factors II, VII, IX and X. Deficiency which occurs in malabsorption of vitamin K and with warfarin treatment (an inhibitor of vitamin K synthesis) leads to an increase in PT. Treatment, if required, is with parenteral phytomenadione (vitamin K).

Liver disease
Liver disease results in a number of defects of haemostasis: vitamin K deficiency in cholestasis, reduced synthesis of clotting factors, thrombocytopenia and functional abnormalities of platelets. DIC may occur in acute liver failure.

THROMBOSIS

A thrombus is defined as a solid mass formed in the circulation from the constituents of the blood, usually resulting from a complex series of events involving coagulation factors, platelets, red blood cells and the vessel wall.

Arterial thrombosis
Arterial thrombosis is usually the result of atheroma which forms particularly at areas of turbulent blood flow such as the bifurcation of arteries. Platelets adhere to the damaged vascular endothelium and aggregate in response to ADP and TxA_2. This may stimulate blood coagulation leading to complete occlusion of the vessel, or embolization resulting in distal obstruction.

Prevention and treatment of arterial thrombosis
Prevention of thrombosis is with antiplatelet drugs:
- Aspirin which inhibits production of thromboxane A_2
- Dipyridamole which potentiates prostacyclin

Treatment (thrombolytic therapy):
- Streptokinase is a purified fraction of the filtrate which is obtained from cultures of haemolytic streptococci. It forms

a 1:1 complex with plasminogen which activates other plasminogen molecules to form plasmin. The dose in myocardial infarction is 1 500 000 units given by infusion over one hour. The main disadvantage of streptokinase is the indiscriminate activation of plasminogen both in clots and in the circulation, leading to an increased risk of haemorrhage. Nevertheless this is currently the thrombolytic agent of choice.

- Anisoylated plasminogen streptokinase activator complex (APSAC) is a complex of plasminogen and an anisoylated form of streptokinase which has a more sustained duration of action than streptokinase and is more specific for fibrin-bound plasminogen.

- Tissue-type plasminogen activator (tPA) is produced using recombinant gene technology, and was claimed to be more specific for clot-bound plasminogen. However, tPA has not been shown to produce fewer bleeding episodes than streptokinase.

The use of thrombolytic therapy with myocardial infarction is discussed on page 291. The main risk of thrombolysis is bleeding. Contraindications are recent major bleed, stroke (within 2 months), uncontrolled hypertension, surgery or other invasive procedure (within 10 days), and bleeding disorders.

Venous thrombosis

Unlike arterial thrombosis, venous thrombosis usually occurs in normal vessels, often in the deep veins of the leg. They originate around the valves as red thrombi consisting of red cells and fibrin. Propagation occurs inducing a risk of embolization to the pulmonary vessels. Chronic venous obstruction in the leg results in a permanently swollen leg which is prone to ulceration (*postphlebitic syndrome*). Factors predisposing to venous thromboembolism are displayed in Table 4.17.

Table 4.17 Risk factors for venous thromboembolism

Patient factors	Disease or surgical procedure
Age	Trauma or surgery, especially pelvis or hip
Obesity	Malignancy
Varicose veins	Cardiac failure
Immobility (bed rest > 4 days)	Recent myocardial infarction
Pregnancy and puerperium	Infection
High doses of oestrogens	Inflammatory bowel disease
Previous deep vein thrombosis	Nephrotic syndrome
Thrombophilia	Polycythaemia, thrombocythaemia
	Paraproteinaemia

Prevention and treatment of venous thromboembolism

Heparin and warfarin are the two drugs used most frequently in the prevention and treatment of thromboembolism (Table 4.18). In general, prophylaxis of venous thromboembolism relies on measures that prevent stasis, such as early mobilization, elevation of the legs and compression stockings, with heparin reserved for higher-risk patients. These higher-risk patients should receive specific prophylaxis such as low-dose heparin subcutaneously (5000 units twice daily) until the patient is ambulatory; no laboratory monitoring is required. Recently low-molecular-weight heparins (M_r 2000–8000 daltons), produced by the enzymatic or chemical breakdown of the conventional heparin molecule (M_r 12 000–15 000 daltons), have been developed. These can be administered on a once-daily basis, have greater efficacy than conventional heparin in high-risk patients, but are considerably more expensive. Fixed-dose low-molecular-weight heparin regimens are being studied for the treatment of established thrombosis.

In established thromboembolism, full anticoagulation should be undertaken as follows:

- Heparin 5000 units unfractionated is given intravenously as a loading dose
- Heparin is continued as an intravenous infusion of 1000–2000 units/hour or as subcutaneous injections of 15 000 units every 12 hours
- The dose of heparin is adjusted to maintain the PTTK at between 1.5 and 2.5 times the control value
- Warfarin 5–10 mg orally is started at the same time as the heparin
- The dose of warfarin is adjusted to maintain the INR usually at two to three times the control value
- Heparin can be discontinued when the INR is in the therapeutic range

THE HAEMATOLOGICAL MALIGNANCIES

The leukaemias

The leukaemias are malignant neoplasms of the haemopoietic stem cells, characterized by diffuse replacement of the bone marrow by neoplastic cells. In most cases, the leukaemic cells spill over into the blood where they may be seen in large numbers. The cells may also infiltrate the liver, spleen, lymph nodes and other tissues throughout the body.

Leukaemias are classified on the basis of the cell type involved and the state of maturity of the leukaemic cells.

Table 4.18 Anticoagulant treatment

	Heparin	Warfarin
Route of administration	i.v./s.c.	Orally
Half-life	2 hours	2 days
Mode of action	Binds to antithrombin III	Interferes with vitamin K metabolism
Monitoring	PTTK	PT / INR
Treatment of overdose if serious bleeding	Intravenous protamine (rarely needed)	Fresh frozen plasma Intravenous vitamin K

Thus *acute leukaemias* are characterized by the presence of very immature cells (blast cells) and by a rapidly fatal course in untreated patients. *Chronic leukaemias* are associated, at least initially, with more mature leukocytes and a relatively indolent course. Acute and chronic leukaemias are further subdivided into the cell type involved:

- Acute myelogenous leukaemia (AML)
- Acute lymphoblastic leukaemia (ALL)
- Chronic myeloid leukaemia (CML)
- Chronic lymphocytic leukaemia (CLL)

Aetiology

In most cases the aetiology is unknown.

GENETIC FACTORS

Genetic factors are suggested by the increased incidence in patients with chromosomal disorders (e.g. Down's syndrome) and in the identical twin of an affected patient. Chromosomal abnormalities have been described in patients with leukaemia. The earliest described was the Philadelphia (Ph) chromosome found in 95% of cases with CML and some patients with ALL. In the Ph chromosome the long arm of chromosome 22 is shortened by reciprocal translocation to the long arm of chromosome 9. It is unclear how these molecular events contribute to the disease process.

ENVIRONMENTAL FACTORS

- Chemicals, e.g. benzene compounds used in industry
- Drugs, e.g. chemotherapy using chlorambucil and procarbazine
- Radiation exposure, e.g. nuclear generators and treatment for Hodgkin's disease

Treatment of haematological malignancies

The treatment of the haematological malignances is based on the use of chemotherapy drugs and radiotherapy. Surgery and other treatments (e.g. steroids and interferon) are used less often.

CHEMOTHERAPEUTIC AGENTS

There are many chemotherapy drugs in common use. They act in a number of different ways; however, the end result is to inhibit the process of cell division. They therefore not only affect tumour cells but also rapidly dividing *normal* cells of the bone marrow, gastrointestinal tract and germinal epithelium. The principal side effects are the following:

- Bone marrow suppression leading to anaemia, thrombocytopenia and infection
- Mucositis causing mouth ulceration

- Loss of hair (alopecia)
- Sterility which can be irreversible

To minimize these side effects, chemotherapy is given at intervals to allow some recovery of normal cell function between cycles. Nausea and vomiting may be severe with some drugs, such as cisplatin, and is related to the direct actions of cytotoxic agents on the brain-stem chemoreceptor trigger zone. Antiemetics such as metoclopramide and domperidone are used initially, but the serotonin $5HT_3$ antagonists (ondansetron and granisetron) have revolutionized management of severe vomiting. Finally, chemotherapy drugs may themselves cause cancer, particularly acute leukaemia presenting years after treatment.

RADIOTHERAPY

Radiation damages nuclear DNA and thus impairs the ability of cells to divide. The complications of radiotherapy depend on the radiosensitivity of normal tissue in the path of the radiation field. General side effects are lethargy and loss of energy. There may be damage to the skin (erythema and desquamation), gut (nausea, mucosal ulceration and diarrhoea), testes (sterility) and bone marrow (anaemia, leukopenia).

Acute leukaemia

Epidemiology

Both types of acute leukaemia can occur in all age groups, but ALL is predominantly a disease of childhood, whereas AML is seen most frequently in older adults (middle-aged and elderly).

Clinical features

These are the result of marrow failure: anaemia, bleeding and infection, e.g. sore throat and pneumonia. Sometimes there is peripheral lymphadenopathy and hepatosplenomegaly.

Investigations

Definitive diagnosis is made on the peripheral blood film and a bone marrow aspirate. The various subtypes (Table 4.19) are classified on the basis of morphology and immunophenotyping, and cytogenetic studies of blast cells. If the patient has a fever, blood cultures and chest radiograph are essential.

BLOOD COUNT shows anaemia and thrombocytopenia. The white cell count is usually raised but may be normal or low.

THE PERIPHERAL BLOOD FILM shows characteristic leukaemic blast cells.

BONE MARROW ASPIRATE usually shows increased cellularity with a high percentage of abnormal lymphoid or myeloid blast cells.

Table 4.19 The FAB (French, American, British) classification of acute leukaemia

Lymphoblastic

L1	Homogeneous population of small cells (childhood ALL)
L2	Heterogeneous population of cells (more often seen in adults)
L3	Rare – cells such as those seen in Burkitt's lymphoma

Myeloid

M1	Myeloblastic (no maturation)
M2	Myeloblastic (with maturation)
M3	Promyelocytic*
M4	Myelomonocytic
M5	Monoblastic †
M6	Erythroblastic
M7	Megakaryoblastic

* Associated with disseminated intravascular coagulation.
† Characterized by leukaemic skin nodules, gum hypertrophy and CNS infiltration.

Management

The aim of treatment is to achieve complete remission (defined as a normal full blood count and less than 5% of blasts in the bone marrow) and restore the patient to a normal state of health.

GENERAL

Before starting treatment the following need to be considered:

- Correction of anaemia and thrombocytopenia by administration of blood and platelets.
- Treatment of infection with intravenous antibiotics.
- Prevention of the acute tumour lysis syndrome (ATLS) with adequate hydration and allopurinol. ATLS results from a massive release of cellular breakdown products consequent upon tumour cell death following effective therapy. The biochemical disturbances include hyperkalaemia, hyperuricaemia, hyperphosphataemia and hypocalcaemia.

TREATMENT OF AML

This is in two parts: induction of remission and post-remission/consolidation.

Induction of remission is achieved with an aggressive combination of intravenous chemotherapy (e.g. cytosine, arabinoside and daunorubicin) given at intervals to allow marrow recovery in between.

Postremission therapy. The options are further courses of chemotherapy *or* myeloablative therapy with allogeneic/autologous bone marrow transplantation (see page 151).

Chemotherapy achieves an initial remission rate of 70% although long-term cure is only around 35% with chemotherapy alone. BMT improves long-term remission to 50%.

TREATMENT OF ACUTE PROMYELOCYTIC LEUKAEMIA (APML)
It has recently been demonstrated that the use of a differentiating agent, all-*trans*-retinoic acid, given orally can lead to remission in some patients with APML. It does not appear to be effective in other subtypes of AML. Unfortunately such remissions do not last and need to be consolidated with conventional chemotherapy.

TREATMENT OF ACUTE LYMPHOBLASTIC LEUKAEMIA
The principles of treatment are similar to those for AML; cyclical combination chemotherapy (vincristine, prednisolone and daunorubicin) is given to induce a remission and for postremission therapy. However, ALL has a propensity for involvement of the CNS, so treatment also includes prophylactic intrathecal drugs (methotrexate or cytosine arabinoside) with or without prophylactic cranial radiotherapy. Most patients also receive oral maintenance chemotherapy for 2–3 years. Relapse may occur in the blood, testes and CNS.

Overall 90% of children with ALL respond to treatment and 50–60% are cured. The results in adults are not so good, with only about 30% being cured.

Chronic myeloid leukaemia

Clinical features
Chronic myeloid leukaemia (CML) occurs most commonly in middle age. There is an insidious onset with fever, weight loss, sweating and symptoms of anaemia. Massive splenomegaly is characteristic.

Investigations
BLOOD COUNT usually shows anaemia and a raised white cell count (often $> 100 \times 10^9/l$). The platelet count may be low, normal or raised.

BONE MARROW ASPIRATE shows a hypercellular marrow with an increase in myeloid progenitors. On cytogenetic analysis, the Ph chromosome is present in most patients.

Management
Hydroxyurea (or busulphan) is given orally to control the white cell count. Interferon is currently under investigation. Curative treatment with bone marrow transplantation should be considered in younger patients.

Prognosis
The chronic phase described above lasts 3–4 years. This is followed by blast transformation with the development of

acute leukaemia (usually acute myeloid) and commonly rapid death. Less frequently, CML transforms into myelofibrosis, death ensuing from bone marrow failure.

Chronic lymphocytic leukaemia

CLL is an incurable disease of older people characterized by an uncontrolled proliferation and accumulation of mature B lymphocytes (although T-cell CLL does occur).

Clinical features

Symptoms are a consequence of bone marrow failure: anaemia, infections and bleeding. An autoimmune haemolysis contributes to the anaemia. Some patients may be asymptomatic, the diagnosis being a chance finding on the basis of a blood count done for a different reason. There may be lymphadenopathy and, in advanced disease, hepato-splenomegaly.

Investigations

BLOOD COUNT shows a raised white cell count $> 15 \times 10^9/l$ of which at least 40% are lymphocytes. There may be anaemia and thrombocytopenia.

BONE MARROW ASPIRATE shows infiltration by lymphocytes with variable reduction in normal haemopoietic tissue.

Management

Treatment, usually with oral chlorambucil, is indicated only for those with symptomatic disease.

Prognosis

The median survival is 8 years for those with only lymphocytosis. The prognosis is much worse (median survival 2 years) for those patients with marrow failure at presentation.

THE LYMPHOMAS

The lymphomas represent abnormal proliferation of different parts of the lymphoid system and are currently classified on the basis of histological appearance into:

- Hodgkin's disease
- Non-Hodgkin's lymphoma (NHL)

Hodgkin's disease

Clinical features

Hodgkin's disease is primarily a disease of young adults. The most common presentation is painless lymph node enlargement (most often cervical nodes). Systemic symptoms, known as 'B' symptoms, are fever, night sweats and weight loss. Other constitutional symptoms may occur, such as pruritus, fatigue, anorexia and alcohol-induced pain at the site of the enlarged lymph nodes.

On examination enlarged nodes are typically non-tender, discrete and with a rubbery consistency. There may be hepatosplenomegaly.

Investigations

BLOOD COUNT often shows a normochromic/normocytic anaemia with a raised ESR.

LIVER BIOCHEMISTRY may be abnormal with liver involvement.

RADIOLOGY: chest radiography and CT are important for staging and may show mediastinal, intrathoracic or abdominal lymphadenopathy.

LYMPH NODE BIOPSY and histological examination is required for definitive diagnosis. Classically, Sternberg–Reed (binucleate or multinucleate cells) are present with a characteristic admixture of lymphocytes and histiocytes.

BONE MARROW ASPIRATE AND TREPHINE BIOPSY may show involvement in patients with advanced disease.

Differential diagnosis

This includes any other cause of lymphadenopathy (Table 4.20).

Table 4.20 Differential diagnosis of lymphadenopathy

Localized	Generalized

Local infection
  Pyogenic infection, e.g. tonsillitis
  Tuberculosis
	Infection
	  Epstein–Barr virus
	  Cytomegalovirus
	  Toxoplasma sp.
	  Tuberculosis
	  HIV infection

Secondary carcinoma	Lymphoma
Lymphoma	Leukaemia

	Systemic disease
	  Systemic lupus erythematosus
	  Sarcoidosis
	  Rheumatoid arthritis

	Drug reaction, e.g. phenytoin

Management

Treatment is always given with a curative intent and consists of radiotherapy, cyclical combination chemotherapy or both.

The choice of treatment depends on:

- Stage (Table 4.21)
- Involved sites

- Bulk of lymph nodes involved
- Presence or absence of 'B' symptoms

Stage IA and stage IIA disease are treated with radiotherapy. All other stages are usually treated with combination chemotherapy. The prognosis is related to the stage of the disease with a 5-year survival rate of approximately 90% in stage I disease. The presence of B symptoms indicates more severe disease with a worse prognosis.

Table 4.21 Staging classification of Hodgkin's disease*

Stage	Definition
I	Involvement of a single lymph node region or a single extralymphatic organ or site
II	Involvement of two or more lymph node regions on the same side of the diaphragm, or localized involvement of an extralymphatic organ or site and of one or more lymph node regions on the same side of the diaphragm
III	Involvement of lymph node regions on both sides of the diaphragm, which may also be accompanied by involvement of the spleen or by localized involvement of an extralymphatic organ or site or both
IV	Diffuse or disseminated involvement of one or more extralymphatic organs or tissues, with or without associated lymph node involvement

* Each stage is subdivided into A (no systemic symptoms) or B (unexplained fever, night sweats and weight loss > 10% of body weight).

Non-Hodgkin's lymphoma

This is a heterogeneous group of disorders which encompasses many different histological subtypes. Several rather confusing classifications have been suggested, based on parameters such as histological type, rate of cell division or B- or T-cell origin. The simplest classification is the working classification which is based primarily on how the lymphomas behave clinically (Table 4.22).

Table 4.22 Working formulation for non-Hodgkin's lymphoma

Low grade		High grade	
A	Small lymphocytic	G	Diffuse large-cell
B	Follicular small-cleaved	H	Immunoblastic
C	Follicular mixed histiocytic	I	Lymphoblastic
D	Follicular large-cell	J	Small non-cleaved
E	Diffuse small-cleaved		
F	Diffuse mixed histiocytic		

Clinical features

Non-Hodgkin's lymphoma (NHL) is rare before the age of 40 years. The presentation can be very varied and almost any organ in the body can be involved. Peripheral lymph node enlargement is the most common clinical presentation. Systemic symptoms as in Hodgkin's disease may occur. Bone marrow infiltration leading to anaemia, recurrent infections and bleeding is often seen in low-grade lymphoma.

Investigations

BLOOD COUNT may show anaemia. An elevated WCC or thrombocytopenia suggests bone marrow involvement.

LIVER BIOCHEMISTRY may be abnormal if the liver is involved.

RADIOLOGY such as a chest radiograph and CT will show involvement of mediastinal, intrathoracic or intra-abdominal lymph nodes.

LYMPH NODE BIOPSY is required for definitive diagnosis.

BONE MARROW ASPIRATION AND TREPHINE BIOPSY will confirm marrow involvement.

Management

Treatment depends on the grade and histological subtypes.

LOW-GRADE DISEASE in general is not curable. However, patients may survive for many years and usually experience several remissions with relatively simple treatment such as chlorambucil or radiotherapy in localized disease.

HIGH-GRADE DISEASE requires combination chemotherapy. Modern regimens, e.g. cyclophosphamide, vincristine and prednisolone (CHOP) achieve a 60–70% response rate, and cure in about one-third. Some patients with localized disease can be cured with local radiotherapy.

Mycosis fungoides and Sézary's syndrome
[CM pp. 1032–1033]

These are rare cutaneous T-cell lymphomas that may spread in the later stages to involve lymph nodes and other organs.

Burkitt's lymphoma

This is a form of NHL occurring mainly in African children and is associated with Epstein–Barr virus infection. Jaw tumours are common, usually with gastrointestinal involvement. Treatment is with radiotherapy and chemotherapy.

MYELOABLATIVE THERAPY WITH BONE MARROW TRANSPLANTATION

Myeloablative therapy is a term used for treatment that employs high-dose chemotherapy or chemotherapy plus radiation, with the aim of clearing the bone marrow completely of both benign and malignant cells. Without bone marrow replacement or 'transplantation', the patient would die of bone marrow failure. Approaches to restore bone marrow function include the following:

- ALLOGENEIC BONE MARROW TRANSPLANTATION (BMT): bone marrow, usually from an HLA-identical sibling, is infused intravenously following myeloablative therapy. Immunosuppression is required to prevent host rejection and graft-versus-host disease (GVHD). The latter is a syndrome in which donor T lymphocytes infiltrate the skin, gut and liver causing a maculopapular rash, diarrhoea and liver necrosis. Following allogeneic BMT, the blood count usually recovers within 3–4 weeks. The mortality rate is 25–40% depending on the person's age and is often a result of infection or GVHD.

- AUTOLOGOUS BMT: part of the patient's own marrow is removed, following induction of remission, and usually cryopreserved. Following myeloablative therapy, the marrow is reinfused. The time for blood count recovery is somewhat longer than with an allograft although mortality is considerably lower, GVHD not being a problem.

- USE OF PERIPHERAL BLOOD PROGENITOR CELLS (PBPCs): it is possible by using chemotherapy followed by the growth factor, colony-stimulating factor (G-CSF), to stimulate haemopoietic progenitor cells in the marrow to proliferate so that they can be collected from the peripheral blood. They are stored and reinfused after myeloablative therapy. The main advantage is the short time for blood count recovery because PBPCs are more differentiated. This technique has predominantly been used in patients with Hodgkin's disease and NHL in an experimental setting.

The paraproteinaemias
Multiple myeloma

Multiple myeloma is a neoplastic clonal proliferation of bone marrow plasma cells usually capable of producing abnormal immunoglobulins (*paraproteins*) which are IgG or IgA in most cases. The paraprotein may be associated with excretion of light chains in the urine, which are either κ (kappa) or λ (lambda); the excess light chains are known as *Bence-Jones protein*.

Clinical features

The peak age of presentation is 60 years. The neoplastic clone of cells induces excess osteoclastic activity which results in osteoporosis, osteolytic lesions, pathological fractures and hypercalcaemia. Bone pain is the most common presenting symptom. Progressive marrow infiltration results in anaemia, infections and bleeding. Renal failure has multiple causes:

deposition of light chains in the tubules, hypercalcaemia, hyperuricaemia and amyloid deposition in the kidneys. Paraproteins may form aggregates in the blood which greatly increase the viscosity, leading to blurred vision, gangrene and bleeding.

Investigations
The diagnosis is made by demonstrating the following:

- Plasma cell infiltration on bone marrow aspirate or trephine biopsy
- Osteolytic bone lesions (often in the skull) on skeletal survey
- Monoclonal ('M') bands on serum protein electrophoresis or Bence-Jones protein in the urine

Other essential investigations are the following.

BLOOD COUNT which may show anaemia, thrombocytopenia and leukopenia. The ESR is almost always high.

SERUM BIOCHEMISTRY may show evidence of renal failure and hypercalcaemia. The alkaline phosphatase is usually normal.

Management
Combination chemotherapy with doxorubicin–carmustine–cyclophosphamide–melphalan produces better results than melphalan and prednisolone, which has been the standard treatment for years. Newer treatments including bone marrow transplantations, PBPCs and adjuvant interferon therapy are currently being evaluated. Localized bone pain can be helped by radiotherapy and pathological fractures prevented by pinning of lytic bone lesions. Renal failure and hypercalcaemia will often be corrected by adequate hydration. Hyperviscosity is treated by plasmapheresis together with systemic therapy.

Prognosis
The median survival with treatment is about 2 years.

Waldenström's macroglobulinaemia

As in myeloma the neoplastic B cells secrete a monoclonal immunoglobulin. However, unlike myeloma, but similar to lymphoma, the tumour infiltrates the lymphoid tissues including bone marrow, spleen and lymph nodes.

Clinical features
The most common features are malaise, weight loss, lymph node enlargement and symptoms of hyperviscosity.

Investigations
BLOOD COUNT may show a normal or low Hb and WCC although the ESR is almost always high.

PROTEIN ELECTROPHORESIS shows an IgM paraprotein.

BONE MARROW ASPIRATE shows infiltration with lymphoplasmacytoid cells.

Management

Treatment is with alkylating agents or doxorubicin-containing regimens. Hyperviscosity is treated with plasmapheresis.

Monoclonal gammopathy of undetermined significance

This is usually seen in older patients, where a raised level of paraprotein (usually IgA) is found in the blood, but without other features of myeloma. Patients are often asymptomatic and no treatment is required. Regular follow-up is usually indicated in case they later develop lymphoma or myeloma.

A DICTIONARY OF TERMS: DISEASES OF THE BLOOD

ERYTHROCYTE SEDIMENTATION RATE (ESR) measures the speed of sedimentation of red cells in plasma over 1 hour. The speed is mainly determined by the concentration of large proteins, e.g fibrinogen. The ESR is higher in women and rises with age. It is raised in a wide variety of systemic inflammatory and neoplastic diseases. The highest values (> 100 mm/hour) are found in chronic infections (e.g. TB), myeloma, connective tissue disorders and cancer. The *C-reactive protein* (CRP) is synthesized in the liver and produced during the acute phase response. It is quick and easy to measure and is replacing measurement of the ESR in some centres.

BONE MARROW is obtained for examination by *aspiration* from the anterior iliac crest or sternum. In many cases a *trephine biopsy* (removal of a core of bone marrow tissue) is also necessary.

PANCYTOPENIA is deficiency of all cell elements of the blood.

LEUKOERYTHROBLASTIC REACTION: immature red and white cells appearing in the peripheral blood. It occurs in marrow infiltration (e.g. malignancy), myeloid leukaemia and severe anaemia.

PROMYELOCYTES, MYELOCYTES AND METAMYELOCYTES: these are immature white cells seen in the peripheral blood in leukoerythroblastic anaemia.

NORMOBLASTS are immature nucleated red blood cells (RBCs) seen in the peripheral blood with a leukoerthyro-blastic reaction and severe anaemia.

RETICULOCYTES (normal range 0.2–2% of RBCs) are young red cells, recently released from the bone marrow, which still contain RNA. The reticulocyte count gives a guide to the erythroid activity in the bone marrow and is increased with haemorrhage, haemolysis and after the response to treatment with a specific haematinic.

POLYCHROMASIA: blue tinge to RBCs in the blood film caused by the presence of young red cells.

HOWELL JOLLY BODIES: DNA remnants in peripheral RBCs seen postsplenectomy, in leukaemia and megaloblastic anaemia.

TARGET CELLS ('MEXICAN HAT CELLS'): RBCs with central staining surrounded by a ring of pallor and an outer ring of staining. They occur in thalassaemia, sickle-cell disease and liver disease.

LEUKOCYTOSIS: an increase in the total circulating white cells ($> 11 \times 10^9$/l).

LEUKOPENIA: a decrease in the total circulating white cells ($< 4.0 \times 10^9$/l).

NEUTROPHIL LEUKOCYTOSIS (normal range $2–7.5 \times 10^9$/l, 40–75% of total white cells) occurs in bacterial infection, tissue necrosis, inflammation, corticosteroid therapy, myeloproliferative disease, leukaemoid reaction, leukoerythroblastic anaemia, acute haemorrhage and haemolysis.

NEUTROPENIA: causes include racial (in black African individuals), viral infection, severe bacterial infection, megaloblastic anaemia, pancytopenia and drugs (marrow aplasia or immune destruction).

LEFT SHIFT: immature white cells appear in the peripheral blood, e.g. with infection.

LEUKAEMOID REACTION: a reactive but excessive leukocytosis characterized by the presence of immature cells in the peripheral blood.

EOSINOPHILIA (normal range $0.04–0.44 \times 10^9$/l, 1–6% of total white cells) occurs in asthma and allergic disorders, parasitic infections (e.g. ascaris), skin disorders (urticaria, pemphigus and eczema), malignancy and the hypereosinophilic syndrome (restrictive cardiomyopathy, hepatosplenomegaly and very high eosinophil count).

MONOCYTOSIS (normal range $0.04–0.44 \times 10^9$/l, 1–6% of total white cells) occurs in chronic bacterial infections (e.g. TB), myelodysplasia and malignancy, particularly chronic myelomonocytic leukaemia.

FINAL MEDICINE EXAM: HAEMATOLOGY

The most common questions relate to the investigation and differential diagnosis of patients presenting with anaemia, usually microcytic or macrocytic. The anaemia of chronic disease frequently appears but the emphasis in these questions is usually on the investigation of the underlying pathology (Q4).

1. Discuss the causes of hypochromic/microcytic anaemia.

2. You are asked to assess a 25-year-old woman who is found to have a low haemoglobin at her first antenatal booking clinic. There are no physical abnormalities. The values are as follows: Hb 10.7 g/dl, MCV 64 fl, WBC 7.2 × 10^9/l, platelets 202 × 10^9/l.

   What diagnoses do you consider and what simple investigations would you request in the first instance? Why are they important ?

3. A 36-year-old woman complains of being easily tired over 6 months and her stools have become more frequent. An FBC shows a Hb of 8 g/dl, MCV 110 fl. Describe your investigations and treatment.

4. A 65-year-old woman comes to see you complaining of severe headaches for several weeks, and of now having lost vision in one eye. Initial investigations show: Hb 10.5 g/dl, WBC 8.0 × 10^9/l, ESR 90 mm.

   (a) What features would you pay attention to in the physical examination?

   (b) What is the probable diagnosis?

   (c) What further diagnostic investigation would you arrange?

   (d) What treatment would you give?

   (e) What possible complications of this treatment would concern you in a patient of this age?

Other common questions are listed below.

5. Discuss the diagnostic considerations in investigating an adult presenting with non-accidental bruising.

6. Discuss the investigation and management of a 50-year-old man found to have a raised haematocrit (packed cell volume or PCV) on routine blood count.

7. Discuss the causes and investigation of persistent enlargement of the cervical lymph nodes in a man aged 25 years.

8. A 60-year-old woman with repeated sore throats has a blood count carried out by her general practitioner who

seeks your advice. Investigations reveal: Hb 9.1 g/dl, WBC 2.0×10^9/l, platelets 80×10^9/l.

What does it show and what causes should you consider?

ANSWERS

1. The causes of hypochromic/microcytic anaemia are discussed on page 107–109. Iron deficiency is the most common cause.

2. This woman has a mild microcytic anaemia. The most probable causes are thalassaemia trait (particularly with the very low MCV) and iron-deficiency anaemia. Iron requirements increase during pregnancy (2 mg/day) as a result of transfer of iron to the fetus and an increased red cell mass. These processes occur largely in the second trimester and therefore it is likely that she was iron deficient before pregnancy (if this is the cause of the anaemia). In a young woman the most probable cause of iron deficiency is heavy menstrual blood loss (suggested by frequent periods, passage of clots and frequent change of pads/tampons). Investigations are Hb electrophoresis and iron studies (page 108). It is important to know the cause for (a) treatment (page 108) and (b) antenatal diagnosis of thalassaemia (page 120).

3. Anaemia with an MCV of > 100 fl is most probably the result of vitamin B_{12} or folate deficiency. The frequent stools suggest gastrointestinal disease. Taking these two together the most likely diagnosis is small bowel disease – either Crohn's or coeliac disease (pages 42 and 48). Initial investigations are measurement of serum vitamin B_{12}, red cell folate, small bowel follow-through, jejunal biopsy. There may also be malabsorption of iron and iron deficiency must be excluded (page 108). Treatment is that of the underlying disease and replacement of haematinics (pages 43, 50, 111 and 112).

4. The most probable diagnosis is giant cell arteritis (page 494) causing central retinal artery occlusion and anaemia of chronic disease.

   Examine the temporal arteries, the eyes (milky-white fundus as a result of oedema) and general examination (fever, weight loss). The diagnosis and treatment are discussed on pages 494–495. Complications of steroid treatment are: osteoporosis and fractures, diabetes mellitus, hypertension, depression, psychosis and risk of peptic ulceration particularly when together with NSAIDs.

5. The causes and investigation of a bleeding disorder are discussed on pages 135–136. Bruising suggests a platelet or vascular problem. Inherited clotting factor deficiency usually presents with mucosal bleeding, bleeding after surgery and haemarthroses. The probable cause may be suggested after thorough history and examination (e.g. female or male patient, age, family history, concomitant disease, drugs, alcohol).

6. This is polycythaemia and is discussed on page 126.

7. *Persistent* enlargement of a group of nodes makes most infections unlikely. In a young man this is most probably the result of Hodgkin's disease, leukaemia or possibly TB. Non-Hodgkin's lymphoma is uncommon in a young person. If there are risk factors HIV infection (usually generalized lymphadenopathy) must be considered. Initial investigations: FBC and blood film, ESR, lymph node biopsy for histological examination. Further investigation which includes chest radiograph, CT, bone marrow, HIV test, would depend partly on initial results.

8. This elderly woman has pancytopenia the causes of which are listed in Table 4.8. The probable cause may be suggested by a detailed history (particularly drugs) and physical examination. A bone marrow trephine biopsy is the key investigation.

CHAPTER 5

Rheumatology

Musculoskeletal problems are common and account for about one in six GP consultations. Most of these are non-articular problems (see below). Osteoarthritis and rheumatoid arthritis are more commonly seen in hospital clinics. Pain is the most common presenting symptom and may be localized to a single joint or affect many joints.

Arthralgia is the term used to describe joint pains when the joint appears normal on examination. *Arthritis* is the term used when there is objective joint abnormality (swelling, deformity or an effusion). In a patient presenting with joint pains, the history and examination must assess the distribution of joints affected (symmetrical?, axial or peripheral?), the presence of morning stiffness (common in inflammatory arthropathies), aggravating and relieving factors, past medical history and family history. Table 5.1 is a guide to the approach to a patient with joint pains based on the age and sex of the patient and the presence of associated features.

Pain in or around a single joint may arise from the joint itself (articular problem) or from structures surrounding the joint (periarticular problem). Enthesitis (inflammation at the site of attachment of ligaments, tendons and joint capsules), bursitis and tendinitis are all causes of periarticular pain. Pain arising from the joint may be the result of a mechanical problem (e.g. torn meniscus) or an inflammatory problem. The causes of a large joint monoarthritis include gout, pseudogout, osteoarthritis, trauma and septic arthritis. The key investigation is synovial fluid aspiration with Gram stain and culture, and analysis for crystals (in gout and pseudogout). Less common causes are rheumatoid arthritis, the spondyloarthropathies, tuberculous infection and haemarthrosis (e.g. in haemophilia).

ARTHRITIS

Osteoarthritis

Radiological changes of osteoarthritis may be seen in about 10% of the population as a whole and in 50% of those aged over 60 years, although only a proportion of these have symptoms.

Epidemiology

Osteoarthritis occurs throughout the world although it is uncommon in the black population. It is twice as common in women as in men and there is a marked familial tendency.

Table 5.1 Differential diagnosis of polyarticular disease in adults in the UK

Age	Predominantly males	Predominantly females
Young	Reiter's syndrome (urethritis, conjunctivitis) Reactive arthritis Ankylosing spondylitis (back pain, iritis) Psoriatic arthropathy (psoriatic rash, nail pitting) Enteropathic arthropathy (ulcerative colitis, Crohn's disease)	Systemic lupus erythematosus (facial rash, Raynaud's, depression) Rheumatoid arthritis (nodules, anaemia) Sjögren's disease
Middle age	Gout (obesity, alcohol, thiazides)	Rheumatoid arthritis Sjögren's syndrome Generalized osteoarthritis
Elderly	Polymyalgia rheumatica (malaise, weight loss, temporal arteritis) Pseudogout Malignancy presenting with joint pains	
Uncommon arthropathies	e.g. sarcoidosis (page 346), malignant disease (e.g. hypertrophic pulmonary osteoarthropathy), Lyme disease, rheumatic fever (page 294), Henoch–Schönlein purpura (page 180), Behçet's syndrome	

Pathology and pathogenesis

Osteoarthritis is characterized by a progressive destruction and loss of articular cartilage. The exposed subchondral bone becomes sclerotic with increased vascularity and cyst formation. Attempts at repair produce cartilaginous growths at the margins of the joint which later become calcified (osteophytes). [CM p. 385]

It is probable that different stimuli can initiate this degenerative process, but the two most obvious are mechanical insults and biochemical abnormalities of cartilage.

Most osteoarthritis is primary. Secondary osteoarthritis occurs in joints that have been damaged in some way (e.g. intra-articular fractures, avascular necrosis) or are congenitally abnormal (e.g. slipped femoral epiphysis).

Clinical features

The main symptom of osteoarthritis is pain, made worse by movement and relieved by rest. Stiffness occurs after sitting down and for a short period ($< \frac{1}{2}$ h) on waking in the morning. The joints most commonly involved are the distal interphalangeal joints (DIPJ) and first carpometacarpal joint of the hands, first metatarsophalangeal joint of the foot and the weight-bearing joints – vertebrae, hips and knees. On examination there is deformity and bony enlargement of joints, limited joint movement and muscle wasting of surrounding muscle groups. There may occasionally be a joint effusion. Heberden's nodes are bony swellings at the distal interphalangeal joints. Bouchard's nodes are similar but occur at the proximal interphalangeal joint.

Differential diagnosis

Osteoarthritis is differentiated from rheumatoid arthritis by the pattern of joint involvement (Figure 5.1) and the absence of the systemic features that occur in rheumatoid arthritis. Pyrophosphate arthropathy (page 182) affects a similar age group as osteoarthritis but the wrists are usually involved. Chronic tophaceous gout (page 180) and psoriatic arthritis affecting the DIPJ (page 170) may mimic osteoarthritis.

Investigations

RADIOLOGY. Radiographs of affected joints show narrowing of the joint space (resulting from loss of cartilage), osteophytes, subchondral sclerosis and cyst formation.

OTHER TESTS. The FBC and ESR are both normal. Rheumatoid factor is negative but low titre tests may occur incidentally in elderly people.

Management

There are three main types of treatment: drugs, physical measures and surgery. Obese patients should be encouraged to lose weight, particularly if weight-bearing joints are affected.

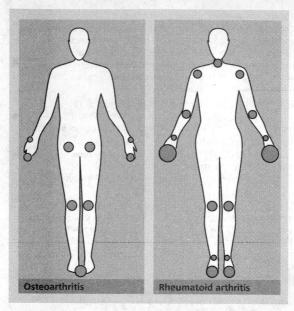

Figure 5.1 The pattern of joint involvement in osteoarthritis compared with rheumatoid arthritis. Both conditions are usually bilateral and symmetrical in distribution.

- DRUGS. Paracetamol and NSAIDs are used to control symptoms. Intra-articular steroids can be used for inflammatory exacerbations but systemic corticosteroid therapy is not used.
- PHYSICAL THERAPY. The application of heat to an affected joint may provide pain relief. Exercises maintain muscle power and improve mobility of weight-bearing joints.
- SURGERY. Replacement of the joint is indicated if pain and loss of function have failed to respond to drugs and physical therapy.

Rheumatoid arthritis

Rheumatoid arthritis is a chronic, inflammatory arthritis associated with systemic disturbance and extra-articular involvement, e.g. the lungs and many other organs.

Epidemiology

Rheumatoid arthritis affects about 2% of the population worldwide with a peak prevalence between the ages of 30 and 40 years. Women are affected three times more often than men. There is an increased incidence in those with a family history of rheumatoid arthritis and an association with HLA-DR4 in most ethnic groups.

Aetiology

The cause of rheumatoid arthritis is unknown. The most widely held view is that interplay of genetic factors, sex hormones and an infectious agent initiates an autoimmune mechanism with inflammatory and destructive features. [CM pp. 387–388]

Pathology

Rheumatoid arthritis is a disease of the synovium. There is infiltration by chronic inflammatory cells: lymphocytes, plasma cells and macrophages. The synovium then proliferates and grows out over the surface of cartilage producing a tumour-like mass called 'pannus'. Pannus destroys the articular cartilage and subchondral bone producing bony erosions.

Subcutaneous nodules (rheumatoid nodules) have a characteristic appearance with a central area of necrosis surrounded by macrophages and fibrous tissue. Similar lesions occur in the pleura, pericardium and lung.

Clinical features

The typical presentation is with an insidious onset of pain, stiffness and swelling in the small joints of the hands and feet, which is most marked on waking in the mornings. Early in the disease there is spindling of the fingers caused by swelling of the proximal but not the distal interphalangeal joints; the metacarpophalangeal joints and wrist joints are also swollen. As the disease progresses there is weakening of joint capsules causing joint instability, subluxation (partial dislocation) and deformity. The characteristic deformities of the rheumatoid hand are shown in Figure 5.2. Most patients eventually have many joints involved, including the wrists, elbows, shoulders, cervical spine, knees, ankles and feet. The dorsal and lumbar spine are not involved. Joint effusions and wasting of muscles around the affected joints are early features. Later there is joint deformity, subluxation and instability.

Less common presentations are 'explosive' (sudden onset of widespread arthritis), palindromic (relapsing and remitting monoarthritis of different large joints) or with a systemic illness with few joint symptoms initially. [CM pp. 388–391]

EXTRA-ARTICULAR MANIFESTATIONS

Periarticular features of rheumatoid arthritis include bursitis, tenosynovitis, muscle wasting and nodule formation. Rheumatoid nodules are found in about 20% of cases, usually on the ulnar surface of the forearm just below the elbow. Patients with nodules are usually seropositive (see later).

Other extra-articular disease manifestations are summarized in Table 5.2. The most common manifestations are

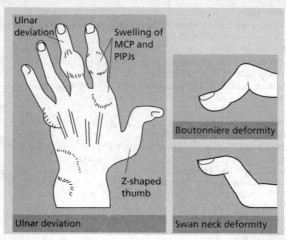

Figure 5.2 Characteristic hand deformities in rheumatoid arthritis. MCP, metacarpophalanges; PIPJs, proximal interphalangeal joints. (Adapted from Read *et al.*, 1992, *Essential Medicine*, Edinburgh, Churchill-Livingstone.)

highlighted; these may be present but cause few symptoms, e.g. a pericardial rub is often heard (up to 30%) but pericarditis is seldom a clinical problem. Atlantoaxial subluxation is commonly seen on a cervical radiograph but much less commonly causes problems.

Table 5.2 Extra-articular manifestations of rheumatoid arthritis

Systemic	Fever
	Fatigue
	Weight loss
Eyes	Secondary Sjögren's syndrome
	Scleritis
	Scleromalacia perforans
Neurological	Carpal tunnel syndrome
	Atlantoaxial subluxation and cord compression
	Polyneuropathy, predominantly sensory
	Mononeuritis multiplex
Reticuloendothelial	Lymphadenopathy
	Felty's syndrome (rheumatoid arthritis, splenomegaly, neutropenia)
Blood	Anaemia caused by:
	Chronic disease
	NSAID-induced gastrointestinal blood loss
	Haemolysis
	Hypersplenism
	Thrombocytosis ➤

➤ Pulmonary	Pleural effusion
	Diffuse fibrosing alveolitis
	Rheumatoid nodules
	Rheumatoid pneumoconiosis (Caplan's syndrome)
	Small airway disease
Heart	Pericarditis
	Pericardial effusion
Kidneys	Amyloidosis
	Analgesic nephropathy
Vasculitis	Leg ulcers
	Nail fold infarcts
	Gangrene of fingers and toes

The most common manifestations are highlighted.

Investigations

BLOOD COUNT. There is a normochromic/normocytic anaemia and thrombocytosis which correlates with disease activity. Other forms of anaemia may also occur (Table 5.2). The ESR and CRP are raised in proportion to the activity of the inflammatory process.

SERUM AUTOANTIBODIES. Rheumatoid factor is positive in 80% of cases and antinuclear factor in 30% (page 196).

RADIOLOGY. Radiographs of affected joints may show joint narrowing, erosions at the joint margins, porosis of periarticular bone and cysts.

SYNOVIAL FLUID is sterile with a high neutrophil count in uncomplicated disease.

Differential diagnosis

In the patient with symmetrical peripheral arthritis, nodules and positive rheumatoid factor, the diagnosis is straight-forward. Rheumatoid must be distinguished from the symmetrical seronegative arthropathy occurring in psoriasis and severe rheumatoid from 'arthritis mutilans' (page 170). In a young woman presenting with joint pains, SLE must be considered; characteristically the joints are normal on examination.

Management

Effective management of rheumatoid arthritis requires a multidisciplinary approach, with input from rheumatologists, orthopaedic surgeons (joint replacement, arthroplasty), occupational therapists (aids to reduce disability) and physiotherapists (teaching of exercises to improve muscle power and to maintain mobility to prevent flexion deformities).

NSAIDs are effective in relieving the joint pain and stiffness of rheumatoid arthritis, but they do not slow disease progression or alter inflammatory markers. Slow-release indomethacin taken at night may produce dramatic relief of symptoms on the following day. The main side effects are peptic ulceration, with the risk of bleeding and perforation, fluid retention and chronic tubulointerstitial nephritis.

Second-line drug treatment should be considered in patients with progressive disease, troublesome non-articular symptoms or when there is a poor symptomatic response to NSAIDs. This group of drugs slows down the disease process but may take up to 6 months for maximum effect. The most effective drugs are penicillamine, azathioprine and methotrexate. Hydroxychloroquine, sulphasalazine and auranofin are a little less effective but safer. Penicillamine is often the first choice of drug for younger patients and methotrexate is in other circumstances. The exact mode of action of these drugs is unknown; they can have serious side effects (Table 5.3) so careful monitoring with blood tests is necessary. The antimalarial drug, hydroxychloroquine, may produce corneal deposits (which disappear when treatment is stopped) and more rarely retinopathy which may be permanent. Visual acuity must be checked and ophthalmoscopy performed 6 monthly.

Table 5.3 Drugs used in long-term suppressive therapy for rheumatoid arthritis

Drug	Side effects
Penicillamine	Rash
	Thrombocytopenia
	Proteinuria
Intramuscular gold (sodium aurothiomalate)	Rash
	Thrombocytopenia
Oral gold (auranofin)	Diarrhoea
	Rash
Azathioprine	Neutropenia
	Nausea and vomiting
Methotrexate	Neutropenia
	Liver fibrosis
Hydroxychloroquine	Retinopathy
Sulphasalazine	Nausea
	Male infertility (reversible)

Corticosteroids suppress disease activity but the dose required is often large, with the considerable risk of long-term toxicity (osteoporosis, diabetes mellitus, hypertension and myopathy). They are seldom used except in the elderly patient with explosive rheumatoid arthritis. Local injection of a troublesome joint (see below) with a long-acting corticosteroid improves pain, synovitis and effusion. Repeated injections into an individual joint are possible but this is usually limited to four a year because too frequent injections may accelerate joint damage.

In patients presenting with disproportionate involvement of a single joint, septic arthritis (page 171) must be considered and excluded before the symptoms are attributed to a disease flare-up.

Prognosis

The prognosis is variable. After 10 years, 10% of patients will be severely crippled and 25% will have minimal, if any, symptoms. Other patients lie between these two extremes.

THE SPONDYLOARTHROPATHIES

This term describes a family of diseases with common features which are summarized in Figure 5.3. The same patient may have several different syndromes from the group either simultaneously or at different times; thus a patient with enteropathic arthritis may also have anterior uveitis. There is a

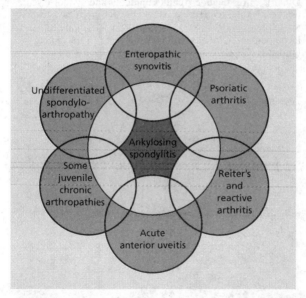

- Inflammatory back pain
- Synovitis – lower limbs and asymmetrical
- Sacroiliitis on radiograph
- Overlap of features
- Familial aggregation
- HLA-B27
- Absence of rheumatoid factor and nodules ('seronegativity')
- Anterior uveitis

Figure 5.3 The spondyloarthropathies: clinical and laboratory features.

common genetic basis to these conditions: HLA-B27 (page 195) is found in all of them but more frequently in ankylosing spondylitis (95% of cases). The explanation for the link of HLA-B27 with the spondyloarthropathies is not known.

Ankylosing spondylitis
Clinical features
The typical patient with ankylosing spondylitis is a young man (late teens, early twenties) who presents with increasing pain and morning stiffness in the lower back. There is a progressive loss of spinal movement. Inspection of the spine reveals two characteristic abnormalities:

● Loss of lumbar lordosis and increased kyphosis (Figure 5.4)
● Variable limitation of spinal flexion and a reduction in chest expansion

Other features include Achilles tendinitis and plantar fasciitis (enthesitis) and tenderness around the pelvis and chest wall.

Non-articular features are iritis (in 25%) and, rarely, aortic incompetence, cardiac conduction defects and apical lung fibrosis.

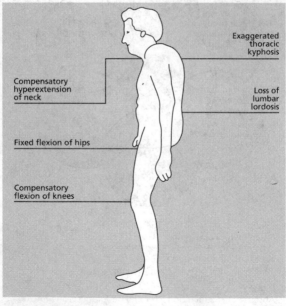

Figure 5.4 Ankylosing spondylitis – the typical posture in advanced cases. (Adapted from Calin, 1994, Seronegative spondylarthritides. *Medicine International*, vol. 22.4, p. 148.)

Investigations
BLOOD COUNT. The ESR and CRP are often raised.

RADIOLOGY. Radiographs may be normal or show erosion and sclerosis of the margins of the sacroiliac joints, proceeding to ankylosis (immobility and consolidation of the joint). In the spinal column, squaring of the vertebrae (caused by erosion of the corners) and progressive calcification of the interspinous ligaments produce the 'bamboo spine'.

Management
REGULAR EXERCISES (twice daily) are essential to maintain posture and mobility.

DRUGS. Slow-release indomethacin taken at night is particularly effective in relieving night pain and morning stiffness. Sulphasalazine is useful as a long-term suppressive drug in difficult cases.

Prognosis
Most patients are able to lead a normal active life and remain at work. In severe cases the spine becomes completely fused and brittle with a risk of fracture (on minimal trauma) and cord compression. The fixed kyphosis of the cervical and thoracic spine may impair ventilation.

Reiter's syndrome

Reiter's syndrome consists of the triad of a seronegative reactive arthritis, non-specific urethritis and conjunctivitis. Two types are recognized:

1. Following a gastrointestinal infection with *Shigella, Salmonella, Yersinia* or *Campylobacter* (enteric).

2. Following non-specific urethritis.

Clinical features
ARTHRITIS. The typical case is a young man who presents with an acute arthritis shortly (within 4 weeks) after an enteric or venereal infection which may have been mild or asymptomatic. The joints of the lower limbs are particularly affected in an asymmetrical pattern; the knees, ankles and feet are the most common sites.

URETHRITIS is associated with a sterile urethral discharge and dysuria.

CONJUNCTIVITIS occurs in one-third of patients and is usually mild and bilateral.

Occasional, additional features are iritis, enthesiopathy (plantar fasciitis, Achilles tendinitis), circinate balanitis (superficial ulceration around the penile meatus) and keratoderma blenorrhagica, an intense scaling of the soles of the feet resembling pustular psoriasis.

Investigations
The diagnosis is clinical. The ESR is raised in the acute stage. Aspirated synovial fluid is sterile with a high neutrophil count.

Management
Treatment is with NSAIDs together with local joint
aspiration and injection of corticosteroid. In chronic cases
sulphasalazine or azathioprine may be necessary.

Prognosis
The acute arthritis resolves within a few months. However,
50% of patients develop recurrent arthritis, iritis or
ankylosing spondylitis.

Reactive arthritis

The full triad of Reiter's syndrome is rare but a large joint
arthritis following enteric or venereal infection is common
and is the most common cause of arthritis in young men.

Psoriatic arthritis

This is a seronegative arthritis occurring in up to 10% of
patients with psoriasis, particularly in those with nail disease
(page 54).

Clinical features
There are several types:

- Asymmetrical involvement of the small joints of the hand,
  including the distal interphalangeal joints
- Symmetrical polyarthritis resembling rheumatoid arthritis
- Arthritis mutilans, a severe form with destruction of the
  small bones in the hands and feet
- Ankylosing spondylitis occurs with increased frequency in
  patients with psoriasis

Investigations
BLOOD COUNT. Routine blood tests are unhelpful in the
diagnosis. The ESR is often normal.

RADIOLOGY. Radiographs may show erosions and periarticular
osteoporosis in the terminal interphalangeal joint.

Treatment
This is with analgesia and NSAIDs. Gold and azathioprine
are useful in severe cases.

Enteropathic arthritis

Enteropathic arthritis is a large joint mono- or asymmetrical
oligoarthritis, occurring in patients with ulcerative colitis and
Crohn's disease. It parallels the activity of the inflammatory
bowel disease and consequently improves as bowel symptoms
improve. Ankylosing spondylitis occurs in 5% of patients
with inflammatory bowel disease but is not related to disease
activity.

INFECTIVE ARTHRITIS

Joint infection is uncommon but is important because it can
lead to considerable joint destruction. Infection of the joints
may be caused by the following:

- Bacteria (see below)
- Viruses: rubella, mumps and hepatitis B virus infection are associated with a mild self-limiting arthritis. HIV infection is associated with an intermittent arthritis
- Spirochaetes and fungi (rare)

Septic arthritis

Septic arthritis results from infection of the joint with pyogenic organisms, most commonly *Staphylococcus aureus*. The organism reaches the joint through the blood stream from a distant site of infection, from local spread of adjacent osteomyelitis or through direct injury or trauma.

Clinical features
Classically there is a hot painful red joint, often the knee, which has developed acutely. There may be fever and evidence of infection elsewhere. Fever and systemic reactions may be absent in those with rheumatoid arthritis or in patients taking corticosteroids.

Investigations
JOINT ASPIRATION is the single most important diagnostic procedure. The synovial fluid is usually purulent with > 50 000 × 10^6/l white blood cells, predominantly neutrophils. Gram staining may show the presence of organisms which may be confirmed by culture.

BLOOD CULTURES may be positive.

RADIOLOGY: Radiographs play little role in the diagnosis because these only become abnormal when joint destruction has occurred.

Management
Treatment should be started immediately because joint damage can occur rapidly. The joint should be rested and immobilized. Appropriate antibiotics should be given parenterally for the first 2 weeks followed by oral antibiotics for the following 4 weeks. Treatment depends on the organism concerned, but a suitable 'blind' regimen would be flucloxacillin together with clindamycin or fusidic acid. Adequate joint drainage usually with needle aspiration is also required as long as the effusion is detectable.

Tuberculous arthritis

Approximately 1% of patients with TB have skeletal involvement which is usually caused by haematogenous spread from pulmonary or renal disease.

Clinical features
Spinal involvement is particularly common (50%) but the knee, hip, sacroiliac and other joints may be involved. There is an insidious onset of pain, swelling and dysfunction, often associated with general symptoms of malaise, anorexia and night sweats.

Diagnosis
Culture of the synovial fluid may give the diagnosis.
Occasionally, synovial biopsy is required.

Treatment
Treatment is as for tuberculosis elsewhere (see page 344), in addition to joint rest and immobilization.

Meningococcal arthritis

Meningococcal arthritis usually occurs as part of a meningococcal septicaemia and results from deposition of circulating immune complexes containing meningococcal antigens. It is a migratory polyarthritis, not associated with joint destruction. Treatment is with penicillin.

Gonococcal arthritis

Gonococcal arthritis occurs secondary to genital or oral infection (often asymptomatic) and presents with a mild inflammatory polyarthritis. Concomitant skin involvement is common (maculopapular pustules). It affects particularly young women and homosexual men. The organism can usually be cultured from the blood stream, and from the joints in 25% of cases. Treatment is with penicillin.

Salmonella arthritis

Salmonella arthritis presents as a mild polyarthritis and occurs with types of salmonellae that invade the blood stream rather than staying within the gastrointestinal tract. Gastrointestinal symptoms may therefore be minor or absent. Treatment is with amoxycillin.

CONNECTIVE TISSUE DISEASE

The term 'connective tissue disease' is used for three diseases: (1) systemic lupus erythematosus (SLE), (2) systemic sclerosis, and (3) polymyositis and dermato-myositis. Their relationship is illustrated in Figure 5.5.

These diseases have a number of features in common, including arthritis, immune complex deposition and vasculitis. Features of all three occur in mixed connective tissue disease.

Systemic lupus erythematosus

SLE is the most common of the connective tissue disorders and is characterized by the presence of serum antibodies against nuclear components. It is a multisystem disease and has a varied clinical presentation.

Epidemiology
SLE is mainly a disease of young women with a peak age of onset between 20 and 40 years. It affects about 0.1% of the population but is much more common in Afro-Caribbean individuals.

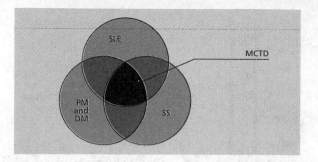

Figure 5.5 The family of connective tissue diseases. MCTD, mixed connective tissue disorders; PM, DM, poly- and dermatomyositis; SLE, systemic lupus erythematosus; SS, systemic sclerosis.

Aetiology

The cause of the disease is unknown but is probably multifactorial. Factors that are thought to play a role include the following:

- GENETIC FACTORS: there is a 70% concordance for SLE between identical twins and an increased incidence of HLA-B8 and -DR3
- IMMUNOLOGICAL FACTORS: antinuclear antibodies are present which are thought to result from polyclonal activation of B cells by an antigenic stimulus, possible viral antigens. This may be associated with impaired T-cell regulation and deficiencies in complement. Most of the visceral lesions are mediated by vascular immune complex (DNA–anti-DNA) deposition
- DRUGS: hydralazine and procainamide may cause a mild lupus-like syndrome which often resolves after the drug is withdrawn
- INFECTION: viral infections may be responsible
- HORMONAL FACTORS: the high incidence in women suggests that female hormones may modify the immune response

Clinical features

These are illustrated in Figure 5.6. A migratory asymmetrical arthralgia is one of the most common presenting features. Synovitis and joint effusions are uncommon and joint destruction is very rare. Non-specific features such as fever, malaise and depression may dominate the clinical picture.

Discoid lupus is often a benign variant of the disease in which skin involvement may be the only feature. There is a characteristic facial rash with erythematous plaques which progress to scarring and pigmentation. Sunlight is an exacerbating factor in most patients.

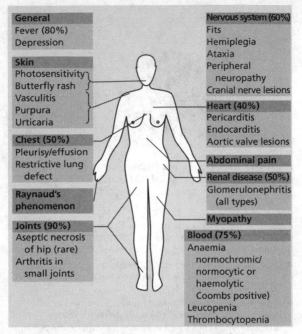

Figure 5.6 Clinical features of systemic lupus erythematosus.

Investigations
BLOOD COUNT usually shows a normochromic/normocytic anaemia often with neutropenia and thrombocytopenia. The ESR is raised but the CRP is usually normal.

SERUM AUTOANTIBODIES: antinuclear antibodies are positive in almost all cases. Double-stranded DNA (dsDNA) binding is specific for SLE but is positive in only 50% of cases. Rheumatoid factor is positive in 50% of cases.

SERUM COMPLEMENT LEVELS are reduced in active disease.

HISTOLOGICAL INVESTIGATION, for example, of a renal biopsy, shows a vasculitis.

Management
Treatment depends on the symptoms and severity of disease.

- NSAIDs are useful for patients with mild disease and with arthralgia
- Hydroxychloroquine is used for mild disease when symptoms cannot be controlled with NSAIDs or for cutaneous disease
- Corticosteroids form the mainstay of treatment,

particularly in moderate-to-severe disease. The aim is to control disease activity (e.g. prednisolone 30 mg/day for 4 weeks) before gradually reducing the dose

- Immunosuppressives (e.g. azathioprine, chlorambucil), usually in combination with corticosteroids, are used for patients with severe manifestations, e.g. renal disease. Cyclophosphamide is reserved for patients with life-threatening disease
- Topical steroids are used for discoid lupus. These patients should also avoid excessive sunlight

Prognosis

The disease is characterized by relapses and remissions even in severe disease. The overall 5-year survival is about 95%. Infection has replaced renal failure as the most common cause of death in SLE.

Antiphospholipid syndrome

This syndrome is characterized by the presence of antiphospholipid antibodies which are thought to play a role in thrombosis by an effect on platelet membranes, endothelial cells and clotting compounds such as prothrombin, protein C and protein S (page 135). It was first described in patients with SLE, but it has become clear that it is much more common than SLE and most patients (often young women) with the syndrome do not have SLE.

Clinical features

The major clinical features are the result of thrombosis:

- In arteries, e.g stroke, transient ischaemic attacks, myocardial infection
- In veins, e.g. deep vein thrombosis, Budd–Chiari syndrome
- In the placenta: recurrent abortions

Other features include valvular heart disease, migraine, epilepsy and thrombocytopenia.

Investigations

Anticardiolipin antibodies are diagnostic.

Management

Small doses of aspirin are used in mild cases; warfarin is used in more severe cases.

Systemic sclerosis

Systemic sclerosis (scleroderma) is a chronic multisystem disease which predominantly affects the skin and is usually accompanied by Raynaud's phenomenon (page 316). It is three to five times more common in women than men and presents before the age of 50 years.

Aetiology

The cause of systemic sclerosis is unknown although many abnormalities in both cellular and humoral immunity have been documented. There is an increase in dermal collagen and a decrease in elastic tissue which leads to the typical thickening and immobility.

Clinical features

Cutaneous manifestations dominate this disease although multiple organs may be involved. Typically the skin is thickened, bound down to underlying structures and the fingers taper (sclerodactyly). There is often a characteristic facial appearance with beaking of the nose, a fixed expression, radial furrowing of the lips and limitation of mouth movements. There may be telangiectasia and palpable subcutaneous nodules of calcium deposition in the fingers (calcinosis). Table 5.4 shows the other main clinical features and their relative frequency.

The CREST syndrome (**C**alcinosis, **R**aynaud's phenomenon, o**E**sophageal involvement, **S**clerodactyly, **T**elangiectasia) and *morphoea* (dermal fibrosis producing plaques of thickened skin) are variants of systemic sclerosis which carry a better prognosis.

Table 5.4 Major clinical features of scleroderma

Organ	Clinical manifestation	Involved in (%)
Skin	Thickened skin, sclerodactyly, telangiectasia, calcinosis	90
Vascular	Raynaud's phenomenon	80
Oesophagus	Impaired peristalsis, stricture formation	80
Lungs	Fibrosis, pulmonary hypertension	45
Heart	Myocardial fibrosis with arrhythmias and conduction defects	40
Kidney	Obliterative endarteritis of renal vessels with renal failure and malignant hypertension	35
Eyes	Sjögren's syndrome	
Joints/Muscle	Joint deformity, myopathy, myositis	20–25

Investigations

BLOOD COUNT shows a normochromic/normocytic anaemia and the ESR may be raised.

SERUM AUTOANTIBODIES: antinuclear antibodies are often positive. Specific types are antinucleolar and anti-Scl 70. Anticentomere antibodies occur in the CREST syndrome.

RADIOLOGY: a radiograph of the hands may show deposits of calcium around the fingers, and there may be erosion and resorption of the tufts of the distal phalanges.

Management

Management is symptomatic. There is no specific treatment.

Prognosis

Mean 5-year survival rate is 50%. Lung disease is now the major cause of death (previously accelerated hypertension and renal failure).

Polymyositis and dermatomyositis

Polymyositis is a muscle disorder of unknown aetiology in which there is inflammation and necrosis of muscle fibres. When accompanied by a rash it is called *dermatomyositis*.

Clinical features

Peak ages of onset are in childhood and in the fifth and sixth decades. Muscle weakness affecting the proximal muscles of the shoulder and pelvic girdle is the chief symptom. This may be accompanied by pain, tenderness and muscle wasting. The skin changes of dermatomyositis are characteristic: a purple (heliotrope) periorbital skin rash, a photosensitive scaling rash on the face and erythematous plaques over the dorsal aspects of the fingers and knuckles. Other features include arthralgia or arthritis, dysphagia resulting from oesophageal muscle involvement and Raynaud's phenomenon. Dermatomyositis is associated with an increased incidence of underlying malignancy particularly in the older age groups.

Investigations

The diagnosis is confirmed if at least two of the following three tests are positive:

- Elevated muscle enzymes (aldolase or creatinine kinase) in the serum
- An abnormal EMG which shows characteristic changes
- Muscle biopsy showing inflammation and necrosis of muscle cells

Management

Oral prednisolone (40–60 mg/day) reducing to a lower maintenance dose is the treatment of choice. Sometimes immunosuppressive therapy with azathioprine or methotrexate is required.

Prognosis

Fifty per cent of affected children die within 2 years. In adults the prognosis is better except in association with malignancy.

Mixed connective tissue disease

This rare disorder combines features of more than one of the connective tissue diseases. Cerebral and renal disease are unusual and the prognosis is good. High titres of antibodies to extractable nuclear antigens such as ribonucleoprotein (RNP) are commonly found.

Sjögren's syndrome

Sjögren's syndrome is a chronic autoimmune disorder predominantly affecting middle-aged women. It is characterized by immunologically mediated destruction of epithelial exocrine glands.

Clinical features
The main features are dry eyes (keratoconjunctivitis sicca) and dry mouth (xerostomia). It occurs as an isolated disorder (*primary Sjögren's syndrome*), also known as the sicca syndrome, or more often in association with another autoimmune disease (*secondary Sjögren's syndrome*) which is rheumatoid arthritis in 50% of cases. Other features of primary Sjögren's syndrome are arthritis, Raynaud's phenomenon and interstitial nephritis. Six per cent develop lymphomas.

Investigations
Anti-Ro and anti-La antibodies are present in 70% of patients with primary Sjögren's syndrome. Labial gland biopsy shows characteristic changes of lymphocyte infiltration and destruction of acinar tissue. A positive Schirmer test confirms defective tear production. (Schirmer test: a standard strip of filter paper is placed on the inside of the lower eyelid; wetting of less than 10 mm in 5 min is positive.)

Management
Treatment is aimed at symptomatic relief with artificial tears.

VASCULITIS

Vasculitis is inflammation of blood vessel walls and may be associated with SLE, rheumatoid arthritis and some allergic drug reactions. The term 'systemic vasculitides' describes a group of multisystem disorders in which vasculitis is the principal feature. These disorders are all rare except giant cell (temporal) arteritis. Classification of the systemic vasculitides is based on the size of the vessels affected (Table 5.5).

Table 5.5 Classification of vasculitis

Large vessel vasculitis*	Giant cell arteritis
	Takayasu's arteritis (affects young women, causing coronary and CNS ischaemia)
Medium-sized vessel vasculitis†	Polyarteritis nodosa (classic polyarteritis nodosa)
	Kawasaki's disease (affects young children)
Small vessel vasculitis‡	Wegener's granulomatosis
	Churg–Strauss syndrome
	Microscopic polyangiitis (microscopic polyarteritis)
	Henoch–Schönlein purpura

* Large artery refers to the aorta and its major branches.
† Medium-sized artery refers to the main visceral vessels, e.g. renal, coronary.
‡ Small artery refers to the smallest arteries that connect with arterioles.

Polymyalgia and giant cell arteritis

Polymyalgia and giant cell arteritis (temporal arteritis) are conditions of unknown aetiology, probably representing different clinical manifestations of the same disease. They occur most commonly in elderly women.

Clinical features
Polymyalgia is characterized by an abrupt onset of stiffness and pain in the proximal muscles of the shoulder and pelvic girdle. Significant objective weakness is uncommon. There may be constitutional symptoms with malaise, fever, weight loss and anorexia. Localized headache, particularly with temporal artery tenderness and loss of pulsation, suggests temporal arteritis (page 494).

Investigations
The diagnosis is usually based on clinical findings.

BLOOD COUNT shows a very high ESR (around 100 mm/h) and a normochromic/normocytic anaemia.

TEMPORAL ARTERY BIOPSY may be performed if arteritis is suspected.

Management
Treatment is with corticosteroids 15 mg/day for 4 weeks and then a gradual reduction over 2 years. If temporal arteritis is suspected, treatment should be started rapidly with a higher dose of steroids (30 mg/day) to prevent irreversible blindness.

Polyarteritis nodosa (classic polyarteritis nodosa)

Polyarteritis nodosa (PAN) predominantly affects middle-aged men. Hepatitis B surface antigen detected in some patients and may be involved in the pathogenesis. There is a necrotizing arteritis associated with microaneurysm formation, thrombosis and infarction. Clinical features include fever, malaise, weight loss, mononeuritis multiplex, abdominal pain (resulting from visceral infarcts), renal impairment and hypertension. Diagnosis is made on histological investigations and angiography (often of renal vessels showing aneurysms).

Microscopic polyangiitis

A necrotizing focal segmental glomerulonephritis causes haematuria, proteinuria and sometimes progressive renal failure. Other features include arthralgia and purpuric rashes. Diagnosis is by renal biopsy and measurement of serum perinuclear antineutrophil cytoplasmic antibodies (pANCA) (present in 70%, see page 196).

Churg–Strauss syndrome

This is characterized by a triad of asthma, eosinophilia and a systemic vasculitis. Treatment of Churg–Strauss syndrome, PAN and microscopic polyangiitis is similar, using prednisolone, azathioprine and cyclophosphamide.

Henoch–Schönlein purpura

This condition is most commonly seen in children and presents as a purpuric rash, mainly on the legs and buttocks. The rash is caused by a vasculitis with intradermal bleeding. Abdominal pain, arthritis, haematuria and nephritis also occur. It is the result of a type III hypersensitivity reaction which is often preceded by an acute upper respiratory tract infection. Recovery is usually spontaneous.

Arthritis in children

There are three main types: juvenile chronic arthritis, juvenile rheumatoid arthritis, juvenile ankylosing spondylitis. [CM pp. 407–408]

CRYSTAL DEPOSITION DISEASES

Gout

Gout is an abnormality of uric acid metabolism resulting in deposition of sodium urate crystals in:

- Joints causing arthritis
- Soft tissue causing tophi and tenosynovitis
- Urinary tract causing urate stones and renal failure

Epidemiology

The prevalence varies from 0.2% in Europeans to about 10% in New Zealand Maoris. The disease is ten times more common in men and is more prevalent in the upper social classes. One-third have a positive family history.

Pathogenesis

The biochemical abnormality is hyperuricaemia resulting from overproduction or renal underexcretion of uric acid. Urate is derived from the breakdown of purines (adenine and guanine in DNA and RNA) which are synthesized in the body or ingested (a minor component). In idiopathic (*primary*) gout, the most common form, impaired renal excretion, is the most common cause of hyperuricaemia. The causes of hyperuricaemia are shown in Table 5.6.

Clinical features

The typical patient is an obese middle-aged man who presents with acute gout, characterized by the sudden onset of severe pain and swelling, most frequently in the metatarsophalangeal joint of the big toe. The joint becomes red, hot, swollen and exquisitely tender. The attack may be precipitated by a surgical operation, dietary or alcoholic excess, starvation or drugs, particularly thiazide diuretics. With persisting hyperuricaemia, there is recurrent acute arthritis affecting more joints, associated with the permanent deposition of urate in and around joints (chronic tophaceous gout). Tophaceous urate deposits may also occur in cartilage, particularly the pinna of the ear.

Table 5.6 Causes of hyperuricaemia

Impaired excretion of uric acid	Increased production of uric acid
Idiopathic (primary) gout	Idiopathic (primary) gout
Chronic renal disease	Increased *de novo* purine synthesis (very rare)
Drug therapy, e.g. thiazides	HGPRT deficiency (Lesch–Nyan syndrome)
Hypertension	PPS overactivity
Lead toxicity	Increased turnover of purines:
Primary hyperparathyroidism	Myeloproliferative disorders, e.g. polycythaemia vera
Alcohol	Lymphoproliferative disorders, e.g. leukaemia
	Others, e.g. carcinoma, severe psoriasis

HGPRT, hypoxanthine–guanine phosphoribosyltransferase.
PPS, phosphoribosyl-pyrophosphate synthetase.

Investigations
SYNOVIAL FLUID EXAMINATION reveals long needle-shaped crystals which are negatively birefringent under polarized light.

SERUM URIC ACID should be measured but this may be normal in acute gout. Conversely asymptomatic hyperuricaemia is common.

Management
ACUTE ATTACKS are treated with anti-inflammatory drugs:

- NSAIDs, e.g. indomethacin, are the treatment of choice.
- Local corticosteroid injection after aspiration of effusion.
- Other treatments: intramuscular ACTH is very effective for difficult cases. Oral colchicine may be useful if NSAIDs are contraindicated, e.g. active peptic ulceration.

LONG-TERM THERAPY is considered when the acute attack subsides. Obese patients should lose weight, alcohol consumption should be reduced, and drugs such as thiazides and salicylates should be withdrawn. Drugs used to reduce serum uric acid include:

- Allopurinol inhibits xanthine oxidase (an enzyme in the purine breakdown pathway) and is the drug of choice but may precipitate an acute attack – thus it should be used initially in conjunction with a non-steroidal anti-inflammatory drug.
- Probenecid, a uricosuric agent, may be used in those allergic to allopurinol.

Pyrophosphate arthropathy

This condition is associated with the deposition of calcium pyrophosphate dihydrate in articular cartilage and periarticular tissue. The acute attacks of synovitis that occur in 25% of patients are known as *pseudogout*. The aetiology is unknown but it occurs in older people and is equally common in men and women. It may occur secondary to other diseases including primary hyperparathyroidism, haemochromatosis, hypothyroidism and gout.

Clinical features
The clinical picture is similar to primary osteoarthritis with acute attacks most commonly involving the knee. There is often polyarticular involvement or involvement of unusual joints such as the wrist.

Investigations
SYNOVIAL FLUID EXAMINATION reveals small brick-shaped pyrophosphate crystals which are positively birefringent under polarized light (compare uric acid).

RADIOGRAPH OF THE KNEE may show linear calcification parallel to the articular surfaces (chondrocalcinosis).

SERUM CALCIUM is normal.

Table 5.7 Causes of lumbar back pain

		Relevant points in the history and examination
Mechanical	Prolapsed intervertebral disc Osteoarthritis Fractures Spondylolisthesis Spinal stenosis	Often sudden onset Pain worse in the evening Morning stiffness is absent Exercise aggravates pain
Inflammatory	Ankylosing spondylitis Infection (see below)	Gradual onset Pain worse in the morning Morning stiffness is present Exercise relieves pain
Serious cause	Metastatic carcinoma Myeloma Tuberculosis osteomyelitis Bacterial osteomyelitis Cord or cauda equina compression	Constant pain without relief Systemically unwell: fever, weight loss Localized bone tenderness Bilateral signs in the legs Neurological deficit involving more than one root level
Others	Osteomalacia, Paget's disease, referred pain from pelvic/abdominal disease	

Management

Rest with joint aspiration and injection of local corticosteroids forms the mainstay of treatment. NSAIDs may also be useful.

Acute calcific periarthritis

This is the least common crystal deposition disease and is associated with deposition of hydroxyapatite in the soft tissues around joints. It results in an acute, self-limiting but recurrent arthritis most commonly affecting the shoulder joint but also the small joints of the hands and feet as well as other joints. Radiographs typically show a rounded radio-opaque deposit in the soft tissue adjacent to the joint. Treatment is with NSAIDs and local corticosteroid injection.

Unusual arthropathies [CM pp. 412–414]

BACK PAIN

Lumbar back pain

Lumbar back pain is an extremely common symptom experienced by most people at some time in their lives. In many patients (33%) no cause will be found and the term 'non-specific back pain' is used. Mechanical back pain is common and may be differentiated from inflammatory back pain by the clinical history. The history, physical examination and simple investigations will also often identify the minority of patients with a more sinister cause of back pain (Table 5.7).

The age of the patient is important in deciding the aetiology of back pain because certain causes are more common in particular age groups. These are illustrated in Table 5.8.

Table 5.8 Disorders most commonly found in specific age groups

15–30 years	30–50 years	50 years and over
Ankylosing spondylitis	Degenerative joint disease	Degenerative joint disease
Prolapsed intervertebral disc	Prolapsed intervertebral disc	Osteoporosis
Fractures	Malignancy	Paget's disease
Spondylolisthesis		Malignancy
Postural pain		Myeloma

Investigations

A detailed history and physical examination (Table 5.7) will lead to the diagnosis in many cases. The key points are age, speed of onset, presence of motor or sensory symptoms, involvement of the bladder or bowel, and the presence of stiffness and effect of exercise. In young patients with no physical signs further investigation is often not necessary.

BLOOD COUNT is usually normal. The ESR may be raised with inflammatory back pain and tumours.

SERUM BIOCHEMISTRY. A raised calcium and alkaline phophatase suggest metastases. Typically with myeloma the calcium is raised with a normal alkaline phosphatase. A raised alkaline phosphatase with a normal calcium occurs with metabolic bone disease. Prostatic specific antigen should be measured if secondary prostatic disease is suspected.

RADIOLOGY: Radiographs may be useful for excluding serious disease although they may be misleading, e.g. degenerative disease is virtually always present in older people.

TECHNECTIUM BONE SCAN will show increased uptake with infection or malignancy.

MRI is often only performed if surgery is being considered. It is useful for the detection of disc and cord lesions and has largely taken over from CT and myelography.

Management
The treatment depends on the cause. Non-specific back pain should be treated with exercise, NSAIDs and avoidance of precipitants such as lifting heavy objects.

Intervertebral disc disease

Acute disc disease

Acute disc disease is a syndrome in which there is prolapse of the intervertebral disc resulting in acute back pain (*lumbago*) with or without radiation of the pain to areas supplied by the sciatic nerve (*sciatica*). It is a disease of younger people (20–40 years) because the disc degenerates with age and is no longer capable of prolapse in elderly people. In older patients sciatica is more likely to be the result of compression of the nerve root by osteophytes in the lateral recess of the spinal canal.

Clinical features
There is a sudden onset of severe back pain often following a strenuous activity. The pain is often clearly related to position and is aggravated by movement. The radiation of the pain and the clinical findings depend on the disc affected (Table 5.9), the lowest three discs being those most commonly affected.

Investigations
Investigations are of very limited value in acute disc disease and radiographs are often normal. Myelography or MRI is usually reserved for patients in whom surgery is being considered (see later).

Management
Treatment is aimed at relief of symptoms and has little effect on the duration of the disease. In the acute stage, treatment consists of bed rest on a firm mattress, analgesia and occasionally epidural corticosteroid injection in severe

Table 5.9 Symptoms and signs of common root compression syndromes produced by lumbar disc prolapse

Root lesion	Pain	Sensory loss	Motor weakness	Reflex lost	Other signs
S1	From buttock down back of thigh and leg to ankle and foot	Sole of foot and posterior calf	Plantar flexion of ankle and toes	Ankle jerk	Diminished straight leg raising
L5	From buttock to lateral aspect of leg and dorsum of foot	Dorsum of foot and anterolateral aspect of lower leg	Dorsiflexion of foot and toes	None	As above
L4	Lateral aspect of thigh to medial side of calf	Medial aspect of calf and shin	Dorsiflexion and inversion of ankle; extension of knee	Knee jerk	Positive femoral stretch test

disease. Surgery is only considered for severe or increasing neurological impairment, e.g. foot drop or bladder symptoms. Physiotherapy plays an important role in the recovery phase, helping to correct posture and restore movement.

Chronic disc disease

This common syndrome is characterized by the presence of chronic lower back pain associated with 'degenerative' changes in the lower lumbar discs and apophyseal joints. Pain is usually of the mechanical type (see above). Sciatic radiation may occur and there may be a history of acute disc prolapse. Usually the pain is long-standing and the prospects for cure are limited. However, measures that have been found useful include NSAIDs, physiotherapy and weight reduction. Surgery can be considered when pain arises from a single identifiable level which has failed to respond to conservative measures. Fusion at this level with decompression of affected nerve roots can be successful.

Mechanical problems

Spondylolisthesis

Spondylolisthesis is characterized by a slipping forward of one vertebra on another, most commonly at L4/L5. It arises because of a defect in the pars interarticularis of the vertebra and may be either congenital or acquired (e.g. trauma). The condition is associated with mechanical pain which worsens throughout the day. The pain may radiate to one or other leg and there may be signs of nerve root irritation. Small spondylolistheses, often associated with degenerative disease of the lumbar spine, may be treated conservatively with simple analgesics. A large spondylolisthesis causing severe symptoms should be treated with a spinal fusion.

Spinal stenosis

Narrowing of the lower spinal canal compresses the cauda equina resulting in back pain typically coming on after a period of walking and easing with rest. Accordingly it is sometimes called spinal claudication. Causes include disc prolapse, degenerative osteophyte formation, tumour and congenital narrowing of the spinal canal. CT and MRI will demonstrate cord compression and treatment is by surgical decompression.

Neck pain

Pain in the neck may be caused by rheumatoid arthritis, ankylosing spondylitis or fibrositis (chronic muscle pain in young women with no underlying cause, large psychological overlay in some patients). In addition, disc disease, both acute and chronic, the latter in association with osteoarthritis, may occur in the neck as well as in the lumbar spine. The three lowest cervical discs are most often affected and there is pain and stiffness of the neck with or without root pain radiating to the arm. Chronic cervical disc disease is known as cervical spondylosis.

BONE DISEASE

Bone normally consists of 70% mineral and 30% organic matrix. The mineral component consists mostly of a complex crystalline salt of calcium and phosphate called hydroxyapatite.

Control of calcium and bone metabolism [CM pp. 422–424]

Vitamin D and parathyroid hormone (PTH) are the major factors that control plasma calcium concentration and turnover of bone. Bone metabolism is also controlled by calcitonin, glucocorticoids, sex hormones, growth hormone and thyroid hormone.

Vitamin D

The metabolism and actions of vitamin D are shown in Figure 5.7.

Parathyroid hormone

PTH levels rise as plasma calcium falls. The effects are several, all serving to increase plasma calcium and decrease plasma phosphate.

- Increased tubular reabsorption of calcium
- Increased renal excretion of phosphate
- Increased osteoclastic resorption of bone
- Increased intestinal absorption of calcium
- Increased synthesis of $1,25(OH)_2D_3$

Osteomalacia

Inadequate mineralization of the osteoid framework, leading to soft bones, produces rickets during bone growth and osteomalacia following epiphyseal closure.

Aetiology
- Deficiency of vitamin D as a result of a combination of poor diet and inadequate sunlight. This is seen in immobile elderly people and female Asian immigrants
- Malabsorption, e.g. coeliac disease and bile salt deficiency
- Renal disease leading to inadequate conversion of $25(OH)D_3$ to $1,25(OH)_2D_3$ (see Figure 5.7)
- Other causes include liver failure, renal phosphate loss and anticonvulsant therapy (caused by increased vitamin D inactivation)

Clinical features
In the adult, osteomalacia produces muscle and bone pain and fractures. In addition a proximal myopathy leads to a 'waddling gait' and difficulty in rising from a chair.

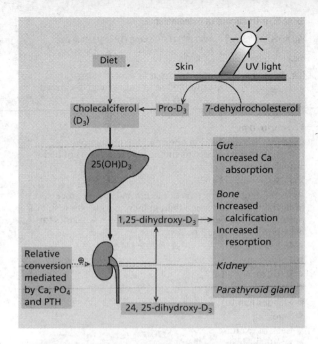

Figure 5.7 The metabolism and actions of vitamin D. Cholecalciferol is predominantly formed from photoactivation of 7-dehydrocholesterol in the skin. In the liver, cholecalciferol is converted to 25-hydroxy-cholecalciferol which is then converted to the much more active form, 1,25-dihydroxycholecalciferol in the kidney. PTH, parathyroid hormone.

Investigations
SERUM BIOCHEMISTRY shows a low phosphate, low or low–normal calcium and increased alkaline phosphatase.

RADIOLOGY: radiographs are characteristic, showing defective mineralization and Looser's zones (low density bands extending from the cortex inwards in the shafts of the long bones).

Definitive diagnosis can only be made by bone biopsy with demonstration of increased non-mineralized bone. This procedure is uncomfortable and rarely necessary.

Management
The treatment is with oral vitamin D; the dose and formulation depends on the cause (Table 5.10). Treatment is monitored by measurement of serum alkaline phosphatase and calcium.

Table 5.10 Treatment of osteomalacia

Vitamin D deficiency	Vitamin D_2 0.25 mg (10 000 units) daily
Malabsorption	Vitamin D_2 1 mg daily
Renal disease	1α-Hydroxycholecalciferol (alfacalcidol or $1\alpha(OH)D_3$) or 1,25-dihydroxycholecalciferol (calcitriol or $1,25(OH)_2D_3$)

Osteoporosis

Osteoporosis means thin bone and the term implies a reduction in bone mass, including all components of bone, not just calcium.

Aetiology

Resorption of bone is part of the normal ageing process, occurring more in women than in men, largely as a result of postmenopausal oestrogen deficiency. The risk factors for osteoporosis are listed below:

- Increasing age
- Female sex
- Early menopause
- Oophorectomy
- Slender habitus
- Smoking
- Lack of exercise
- Family history
- Excess alcohol

Classification

There are two types of osteoporosis:

- Type 1 (postmenopausal) is the result of oestrogen deficiency. Trabecular bone loss leads to vertebral fractures between the ages of 50 and 75 years.
- Type 2 (senile) affects the over 70s. Reduced intake of calcium and vitamin D lead to increased parathyroid hormone activity. This results in cortical bone resorption and hip fractures.

Osteoporosis may also occur secondary to endocrine disease (Cushing's disease, thyrotoxicosis and hypogonadism), drugs (corticosteroids) and systemic disease (e.g. rheumatoid arthritis and chronic renal failure).

Clinical features

Symptoms of osteoporosis are the result of fractures which typically occur at three sites: vertebrae, neck of femur and wrist (Colles' fracture). Vertebral fractures may lead to kyphosis and loss of height.

Investigations

SERUM BIOCHEMISTRY: calcium, phosphate and alkaline phosphatase are normal.

RADIOLOGY: radiographs will demonstrate fractures and may show reduced bone density (osteopenia).

BONE DENSITOMETRY (dual-energy X-ray absorptiometry (DEXA) scanning) is of increasing importance in screening people at risk and in monitoring the effects of treatment.

BONE BIOPSY is occasionally needed.

Management

Prevention is better than treatment of established disease, which is largely irreversible.

- Oestrogen therapy should be considered for women at high risk (see list on page 190) to reduce bone loss during the postmenopausal years. Oestrogens are combined with progestogens in women with an intact uterus because oestrogens alone increase the risk of developing endometrial cancer

- Calcium intake should be maintained and regular exercises may retard bone loss

- Bisphosphonates, which inhibit bone resorption, are often given to older patients with late-stage disease. Cyclic intermittent etidronate is given with calcium supplements

- This is an area of change and indications and treatment protocols may alter as more studies are completed

Paget's disease

Paget's disease is characterized by excessive osteoclastic bone resorption followed by disordered osteoblastic activity, leading to abundant new bone formation which is structurally abnormal and weak.

Aetiology

Osteoclasts contain viral inclusion bodies suggesting a possible 'slow viral' aetiology.

Epidemiology

The incidence increases with age; it is rare in the under 40s and affects up to 10% of adults by the age of 90 years.

Clinical features

The most common sites are the femur, pelvis, tibia, skull and lumbosacral spine, although any bone can be involved. Most cases are asymptomatic but features include the following:

- Bone pain
- Apparent joint pain when involved bone is close to a joint
- Deformities: enlargement of the skull, bowing of the legs

- Complications:
  - nerve compression (deafness, paraparesis)
  - fractures
  - rarely cardiac failure, osteogenic sarcoma

Investigations

SERUM BIOCHEMISTRY shows a markedly raised alkaline phosphatase (often > 1000 U/l) with a normal calcium and phosphate.

URINARY HYDROXYPROLINE is increased and reflects bone turnover.

RADIOLOGY shows typical osteolytic lesions and sclerosis with bony distortion.

Treatment

When asymptomatic, Paget's disease requires no treatment. Pain is the usual indication for treatment.

- Bisphosphonates (e.g. oral disodium etidronate) reduce osteoclastic activity and are used if pain does not respond to simple analgesia. The main side effect is the development of osteomalacia when used at high doses
- Calcitonin (salmon or porcine) administered intramuscularly or subcutaneously inhibits bone resorption and turnover. It is extremely expensive with troublesome side effects (nausea, flushing and antibody formation)
- Mithramycin is used in severe cases

CALCIUM AND THE PARATHYROIDS

Total plasma calcium is normally 2.2–2.6 mmol/l. Usually only 40% of total plasma calcium is ionized and physiologically relevant; the remainder is bound to albumin and is thus unavailable to the tissues. Routine analytical methods measure total plasma calcium and this must be corrected for the serum albumin concentration: add or subtract 0.02 mmol/l for every g/l by which the simultaneous albumin lies below or above 40 g/l. For critical measurements samples should be taken in the fasting state without the use of a cuff, because this affects the protein concentration.

Hypocalcaemia and hypoparathyroidism

Aetiology

The causes of hypocalcaemia are listed in Table 5.11. Renal failure is the most common cause of hypocalcaemia which results from inadequate production of active vitamin D and renal phosphate retention, leading to microprecipitation of calcium phosphate in the tissues. Mild transient hypocalcaemia often occurs after parathyroidectomy and a few patients develop long-standing hypoparathyroidism.

Table 5.11 Causes of hypocalcaemia

Hyperphosphataemia	Chronic renal failure
	Phosphate therapy
Drugs	Bisphosphonates
	Calcitonin
Hypoparathyroidism	Congenital deficiency (DiGeorge's syndrome)
	Idiopathic hypoparathyroidism (autoimmune)
	Post-thyroidectomy and parathyroidectomy
	Severe hypomagnesaemia (inhibits PTH release)
Resistance to PTH	Pseudohypoparathyroidism
Vitamin D	Deficiency
	Resistance
Miscellaneous	Acute pancreatitis
	Citrated blood in massive transfusion

Clinical features

Hypocalcaemia causes numbness around the mouth and in the extremities followed by cramps, tetany, convulsions and death if untreated. Two important signs are *Chvostek's sign* (tapping over the facial nerve causes twitching of the facial muscles) and *Trousseau's sign* (carpopedal spasm when the brachial artery is occluded with a blood pressure cuff). With prolonged hypocalcaemia there may be cataract formation and rarely papilloedema.

Investigations

The clinical picture is usually diagnostic and is confirmed by a low serum calcium. Additional tests identify the cause.

SERUM BIOCHEMISTRY: phosphate, urea and creatinine.

SERUM VITAMIN D METABOLITE LEVELS.

SERUM PARATHYROID HORMONE LEVELS.

Management

ACUTE (e.g. with tetany) 10 ml of 10% calcium gluconate intravenously and repeated as necessary as an infusion over 4 hours.

MAINTENANCE therapy is with 1α (OH)D$_3$ or $1,25(OH)_2D_3$.

Hyperparathyroidism and hypercalcaemia

Mild asymptomatic hypercalcaemia occurs in about one in 1000 of the population, especially elderly women, and is usually the result of primary hyperparathyroidism.

Aetiology

Most cases are the result of primary hyperparathyroidism or malignancy (Table 5.12). Tumour-related hypercalcaemia is caused by secretion of a peptide with PTH-like activity or direct invasion of bone and production of local factors that mobilize calcium. Ectopic PTH secretion by tumours is very rare.

Hyperparathyroidism may be primary, secondary or tertiary.

PRIMARY HYPERPARATHYROIDISM is usually caused by a single adenoma, occasionally hyperplasia and rarely carcinoma.

SECONDARY HYPERPARATHYROIDISM is a physiological response to hypocalcaemia (e.g. in renal failure or vitamin D deficiency). Calcium is low or low–normal.

TERTIARY HYPERPARATHYROIDISM is the development of apparently autonomous parathyroid hyperplasia after long-standing secondary hyperparathyroidism, most often in renal disease. Plasma calcium and PTH are both raised. Treatment is parathyroidectomy.

Table 5.12 Causes of hypercalcaemia*

Excess PTH	Primary hyperparathyroidism	
	Tertiary hyperparathyroidism	
	Ectopic PTH (very rare)	
Excess action of vitamin D	Self-administered vitamin D	
	Sarcoidosis	
Excess calcium intake	'Milk-alkali' syndrome	
Drugs	Thiazides	
Malignant disease	Bronchus	Thyroid
	Breast	Prostate
	Renal cell carcinoma	Lymphoma
	Myeloma	
Other endocrine disease	Thyrotoxicosis	
	Addison's disease	
Miscellaneous	Long-term immobility	

* The conditions causing severe hypercalcaemia (> 3.5 mmol/l) are highlighted.

Clinical features
Mild hypercalcaemia is often asymptomatic and discovered on biochemical screening. Symptoms are general malaise and depression, bone pain, abdominal pain, nausea and constipation. Calcium deposition in the renal tubules cause polyuria and nocturia. Renal calculi and renal failure may develop. With very high levels there is confusion, clouding of consciousness and a risk of cardiac arrest.

Investigations
SERUM BIOCHEMISTRY: calcium is raised; low phosphate, low bicarbonate and raised chloride support primary hyperparathyroidism.

SERUM PTH LEVELS: detectable levels during hypercalcaemia are inappropriate and imply hyperparathyroidism.

RADIOLOGY: subperiosteal erosions in the phalanges are seen in hyperparathyroidism.

HYDROCORTISONE SUPPRESSION TEST is often helpful; plasma calcium in hyperparathyroidism and some malignancies are resistant to suppression by steroids (10 days of hydrocortisone; 40 mg three times daily). Suppression is seen in most other causes of hypercalcaemia.

OTHER INVESTIGATIONS: protein electrophoresis for myeloma, thyroid function tests and investigations (e.g. MRI, selective venous sampling) to localize parathyroid adenomas before surgery.

Management
This involves lowering of the calcium levels to near normal and treatment of the underlying cause. Severe hypercalcaemia (>3.5 mmol/l) is a medical emergency which must be aggressively treated (Table 5.13).

Table 5.13 The treatment of acute hypercalcaemia

- Rehydration in all patients
  4 litres of intravenous saline over 24 hours
- Bisphosphonates intravenously (e.g. pamidronate disodium)
  treatment of choice for hypercalcaemia of malignancy
- Prednisolone (30–60 mg daily orally)
  useful in myeloma, sarcoid and vitamin D excess
- Intravenous phosphates
  rapidly lower calcium levels but may be dangerous

TREATMENT OF PRIMARY HYPERPARATHYROIDISM
The treatment of a symptomatic parathyroid adenoma is surgical removal. Conservative therapy may be indicated in asymptomatic patients with mildly raised calcium levels (2.65–3 mmol/l). In those with parathyroid hyperplasia all four glands are removed.

DICTIONARY OF TERMS: RHEUMATOLOGY

HISTOCOMPATIBILITY ANTIGENS are genetically determined isoantigens present on the membranes of nucleated cells. They incite an immune response when grafted on to genetically disparate individuals and thus determine compatibility of cells in transplantation.

HUMAN LEUKOCYTE ANTIGENS (HLA) are human histocompatibility antigens determined by a region on chromosome 6. There are several genetic loci, each having multiple alleles, designated HLA-A, HLA-B, HLA-C,

HLA-DP, -DQ and -DR. The susceptibility to some diseases is associated with certain HLA alleles (e.g. HLA-B27 in 95% of patients with ankylosing spondylitis), although their exact role in aetiology is unclear.

RHEUMATOID FACTORS (RhF) are autoantibodies found in the serum, usually of the IgM class, which are directed against human IgG. They are found in high titre in most patients with rheumatoid arthritis, in other related and unrelated diseases and in elderly people at low titres.

ANTINUCLEAR ANTIGENS (ANAs) represent a wide spectrum of autoantibodies. They are non-specific and may occur at low titre (e.g. 1:10) in healthy individuals.

EXTRACTABLE NUCLEAR ANTIGENS (ENAs) are nuclear components that are soluble in saline. Examples are Sm, Ro, La and ribonucleoprotein (RNP) antigen. The presence of serum anti-Sm antibodies is highly specific for SLE. Anti-Ro and anti-La occur in patients with Sjögren's syndrome and in some patients with SLE.

ANTINEUTROPHIL CYTOPLASMIC ANTIBODIES (ANCAs) are directed against neutrophil granule enzymes. There are two types:

- Serum that produces a cytoplasmic ANCA (cANCA) pattern is most commonly associated with Wegener's granulomatosis (90%).
- Serum that produces a perinuclear ANCA (pANCA) pattern is found in a wide variety of inflammatory conditions.

FINAL MEDICINE EXAMINATION: RHEUMATOLOGY

1. Describe a typical attack of gout. How would you confirm the diagnosis and treat the patient?

2. Write short notes on the investigation and treatment of an acute arthritis of one ankle in a man aged 50 years.

3. A 45-year-old woman with a long-standing history of rheumatoid arthritis presents with a 6-month history of increasing dyspnoea. She does not experience orthopnoea. The venous pressure is not elevated and her heart sounds are normal. Her electrocardiogram is normal. Blood gases on air show an arterial P_{O_2} 7.7 kPa, venous P_{CO_2} 4.9 kPa, pH 7.45.

   (a) What is the probable diagnosis?

   (b) What other physical signs would you look for?

   (c) What other investigations would be helpful and what would you expect the results to show?

4. Write short notes on the management of severe hypercalcaemia.

5. Write short notes on the causes of tetany in a 23-year-old woman.

6. A woman of 55 presents with backache which proves to be osteoporotic in origin. What features would lead to this diagnosis, what are the predisposing factors and how would you treat her?

7. A 60-year-old woman with a long history of alcohol abuse presents because she can no longer climb stairs or rise from chairs. She has recently begun treatment with NSAIDs given by her general practitioner for presumed osteoarthritis of both hips.

   Biochemical investigations reveal the following data: serum sodium 142 mmol/l, potassium 4.2 mmol/l, chloride 102 mmol/l, urea 8 mmol/l, creatinine 60 μmol/l, corrected calcium 2.2 mmol/l, phosphate 0.5 mmol/l, alkaline phosphatase 1000 U/l.

   Discuss these biochemical results. What do you consider to be the most probable diagnosis? Describe appropriate investigations to support your diagnosis and discuss what might be the best treatment.

ANSWERS: RHEUMATOLOGY

1. A typical attack of gout is described on page 180. The diagnosis is confirmed by joint aspiration (page 182). The serum uric acid is measured but may be normal in an acute attack. Radiographs are rarely helpful; they are normal in the early stages, in chronic disease there may be periarticular erosions. Treatment is (a) of the acute attack, (b) general advice, and (c) consideration for long-term therapy if there have been many previous attacks or evidence of chronic gouty tophi on physical examination (page 182).

2. The causes and immediate investigation of a large joint monoarthritis are discussed on page 159. Subsequent tests would depend on the findings on joint aspiration and may include radiograph of the joint and measurement of serum uric acid concentration.

3. The probable diagnosis is fibrosing alveolitis, a rare complication of rheumatoid arthritis. Less probably, it is drug induced (rare side effects of gold and methotrexate). She has type I respiratory failure (page 370). Physical signs to look for are central cyanosis, clubbing, reduced chest expansion and end-expiratory

crackles at the lung bases. Investigations to confirm the diagnosis are listed on page 349.

4. This is described on page 193. The most important initial treatment is rehydration. A diuresis obtained with physiological saline will augment the urinary excretion of calcium and this can be further increased with frusemide when the patient is adequately rehydrated. For hypercalcaemia of malignancy the treatment of choice is the bisphosphonate, pamidronate (single dose 30 mg over 8 hours) which will bring the serum calcium down over the next 5 days.

5. In a 23-year-old, presumably otherwise healthy, girl, the most probable cause is respiratory alkalosis secondary to hyperventilation. Alkalosis causes tetany by reducing ionization of calcium salts (ionized calcium is physiologically active). Other causes of tetany – hypocalcaemia (page 192), hypokalaemia (page 208) and hypomagnesaemia (page 210) – are much less likely but must be considered.

6. Backache occurs in osteoporosis as a result of vertebral collapse or a crush fracture (not osteoporosis *per se*) which is seen on plain radiograph. Bone densitometry is used to confirm the diagnosis and measure the response to treatment. The predisposing factors are listed on page 190; of these the most important is early menopause. The treatment is analgesia in the short term and, in the long term, hormone replacement therapy (HRT, page 398) and maintenance of calcium intake.

7. There is a borderline low serum calcium, a very low serum phosphate and markedly raised alkaline phosphatase. The diagnosis is probably osteomalacia (resulting from vitamin D deficiency), causing a proximal myopathy. Against this is the very high alkaline phosphatase which is usually only moderately raised in osteomalacia. The myopathy may be the result of alcohol but this does not explain the very high alkaline phosphatase. The serum urea is raised and the creatinine is at the lower end of the normal range. This picture is seen with dehydration or a gastrointestinal bleed (possibly related to ingestion of NSAIDs).

CHAPTER 6

Water and Electrolytes

Body fluid compartments

A 75-kg man contains approximately 45 litres of water (i.e. about 50–60% of total body weight is water) and 3000 mmol of osmotically active sodium. Maintenance of the total amount depends on the balance between intake and loss. Water and electrolytes are taken in as food and water, and lost in urine, sweat and faeces (Table 6.1). In addition, about 500 ml water is lost daily in expired air.

Table 6.1 The normal daily water and sodium balance in a 75-kg man

Input		Output	
Water (ml)			
Drink	1500	Urine	1500
Food	800	Insensible loss	800
Metabolism	200	(skin, lungs)	
		Faeces	200
Total	**2500**	**Total**	**2500**
Sodium (mmol)			
Food and drink	140	Urine	140
		Sweat	Negligible
		Faeces	Negligible

Body water is distributed between several compartments as shown in Figure 6.1. Two-thirds are intracellular (ICF) and the remaining one-third is extracellular, which comprises the interstitial and vascular compartment.

Water moves freely between compartments and the distribution is determined by the osmotic equilibrium between them. Osmolality is determined by the concentration of osmotically active particles. Thus 1 mole of sodium chloride dissolved in 1 kg of water has an osmolality of 2 osmol/kg, as sodium chloride freely dissociates into two particles – the sodium ion and the chloride ion. One mole of urea (which does not dissociate) in 1 kg of water has an osmolality of 1 osmol/kg. Sodium is the major extracellular ion and therefore the main determinant of plasma osmolality.

Calculated plasma osmolality (mmol) = $(2 \times [Na^+]) + [Urea] + [Glucose]$.

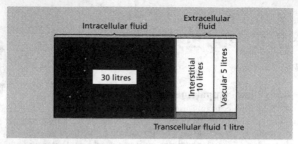

Figure 6.1 Distribution of body water in a 75-kg man.

The factor of 2 applied to sodium concentration allows for associated anions. The other extracellular solutes, e.g. calcium, potassium and magnesium, and their associated anions exist in very low concentrations and contribute so little to osmolality that they can be ignored when calculating the osmolality. The normal plasma osmolality is 285–300 mosmol/kg.

The *calculated* osmolality is the same as the osmolality *measured* by the laboratory, unless there is an unmeasured, osmotically active substance present. For instance, plasma alcohol or ethylene glycol concentration (substances sometimes taken in cases of poisoning) can be estimated by subtracting the calculated from the measured osmolality.

The distribution of extracellular water between the vascular and extravascular (interstitial space) is determined by the equilibrium between hydrostatic and plasma oncotic pressures (Starling's law, Figure 6.2).

Regulation of extracellular volume

Extracellular volume is controlled by the total body content of sodium. Control of body sodium is exerted by tight control over renal excretion. This is achieved by activation of 'volume' receptors (which respond to extracellular volume rather than changes in sodium concentration). There are two types of volume receptors:

● Extrarenal: in the large vessels near the heart
● Intrarenal: in the afferent renal arteriole which controls the renin–angiotensin system via the juxtaglomerular apparatus

A decreased effective circulating volume leads to activation of these volume receptors which leads to an increase in sodium (and hence water) reabsorption by the kidney and expansion of the extracellular volume via stimulation of the sympathetic nervous system. In contrast, atrial natriuretic

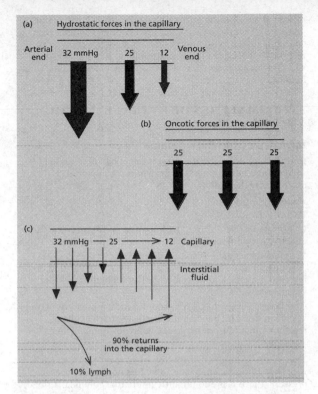

Figure 6.2 Starling's hypothesis. (a) Capillary hydrostatic forces (i.e. the pressure driving blood flow onwards) are balanced by (b) equal and opposing oncotic forces (i.e. the oncotic pressure of plasma proteins). (c) Water leaves the capillary at the arterial end (high hydrostatic pressure) but returns at the venous end (low hydrostatic pressure). Interstitial water accumulates (oedema) if hydrostatic pressures are high, e.g. with salt and water retention in heart failure or if oncotic pressure is low as a result of hypoalbuminaemia.

peptide (ANP), produced by the atria of the heart in response to an increase in blood volume, increases sodium excretion.

Regulation of body water content

Body water is controlled mainly by changes in the plasma osmolality. An increased plasma osmolality, sensed by osmoreceptors in the hypothalamus, causes thirst and the release of antidiuretic hormone (ADH) from the posterior pituitary, which increases water reabsorption from the renal collecting ducts. In addition non-osmotic stimuli may cause release of ADH even if serum osmolality is normal or low. These include hypovolaemia, stress (surgery and trauma) and nausea.

ABNORMALITIES OF EXTRACELLULAR VOLUME

Increased extracellular volume

Extracellular volume expansion is the result of increased sodium (and hence water) reabsorption or impaired excretion by the kidney.

Aetiology

RENAL IMPAIRMENT.

CARDIAC FAILURE - caused by impaired perfusion (therefore effective hypovolaemia) of the volume receptors.

HYPOALBUMINAEMIA. Loss of plasma oncotic pressure (Figure 6.2) leads to loss of water from the vascular to the interstitial space, and therefore activation of intravascular volume receptors.

CIRRHOSIS. This is through a complex mechanism, but there is vasodilatation and hence underperfusion of the volume receptors. In addition there may be hypoalbuminaemia.

Clinical features

These depend on the distribution of extracellular water, e.g. with hypoalbuminaemia caused by loss of plasma oncotic pressure, there is predominantly interstitial volume overload. Cardiac failure leads to expansion of both compartments.

INTERSTITIAL VOLUME OVERLOAD – ankle oedema, pulmonary oedema, pleural effusion and ascites.

INTRAVASCULAR VOLUME OVERLOAD – raised jugular venous pressure, cardiomegaly and a raised arterial pressure in some cases.

This must be differentiated from local causes of oedema (e.g. ankle oedema as a result of venous damage following thrombosis) which do not reflect a disturbance in the control of extracellular volume.

Management

The underlying cause must be treated. The cornerstone of treatment is diuretics which increase sodium and water excretion in the kidney. There are a number of different classes of diuretic of which the most potent are the loop diuretics, e.g. frusemide (Table 6.2).

Table 6.2 The main classes of diuretics in clinical use

Class	Example	Mechanism of action	Relative potency
Loop diuretics	Frusemide	Reduce Na$^+$ and Cl$^-$ reabsorption in ascending limb of loop of Henle	++++
Thiazides	Bendrofluazide	Reduce sodium reabsorption in distal convoluted tubule	++
Potassium-sparing diuretics	Spironolactone	Aldosterone antagonist	+
	Amiloride	Prevents potassium exchange for sodium in distal tubule	

Decreased extracellular volume

This may be the result of loss of sodium and water, plasma or blood.

Aetiology

Volume depletion occurs in haemorrhage, plasma loss in extensive burns or loss of salt and water from the kidneys, gastrointestinal tract or skin (Table 6.3).

Table 6.3 Causes of extracellular volume depletion

Haemorrhage	External
	Concealed e.g. leaking aortic aneurysm
Burns	
Gastrointestinal losses	Vomiting, diarrhoea, ileostomy losses
Renal losses	Diuretic use,
	Impaired tubular sodium conservation e.g. reflux nephropathy, papillary necrosis

Clinical features

Symptoms include thirst, nausea and postural dizziness. Interstitial fluid loss leads to loss of skin elasticity ('turgor'). Loss of circulating volume causes peripheral vasoconstriction and tachycardia, a low jugular venous pressure and postural hypotension. Severe depletion of circulating volume causes hypotension which may impair cerebral perfusion, resulting in confusion and eventual coma.

Investigations

The diagnosis is usually made clinically. A central venous line allows measurement of central venous pressure which helps in assessing the response to treatment. Blood urea may be raised because of increased urea reabsorption and, later, to prerenal failure (when the creatinine rises as well). This is, however, very non-specific. Urinary sodium is low (< 20 mmol/l) if the kidneys are working normally, which can be misleading if the cause of the volume depletion involves the kidneys (e.g. diuretics or intrinsic renal disease).

Management

The overriding aims of treatment are to replace what is missing:

- Haemorrhage involves the loss of whole blood. The rational treatment of acute haemorrhage is therefore whole blood, or a combination of red cells and a plasma substitute.
- Loss of plasma, as in burns or severe peritonitis should be treated with human plasma or a plasma substitute (see page 367).

- Loss of sodium and water as in vomiting, diarrhoea or excessive renal losses should be treated with replacement of water and electrolytes. This is best done orally if possible with an increased intake of water and salt. Glucose–electrolyte solutions are often used to restore fluid balance in patients with diarrhoeal diseases. This is based on the fact that the presence of glucose stimulates intestinal absorption of salt and water (page 14).

  In the acute situation if there have been large losses of sodium and water patients are usually treated with intravenous physiological saline (Tables 6.4 and 6.5) and replacement assessed clinically and by measurement of serum electrolytes.

- Loss of water alone, e.g. diabetes insipidus, only causes extracellular volume depletion in severe cases because the loss is spread evenly over all the compartments of body water. The correct treatment is to give water. If intravenous treatment is required, water is given as 5% dextrose (pure water is not given because it would cause osmotic lysis of blood cells).

Table 6.4 Intravenous fluids in general use*

	Na^+	K^+	HCO_3^-	Cl^-
Plasma constituents	142	4.5	26	103
Sodium chloride 0.9% (isotonic physiological saline)	150	–	–	150
Glucose 5%	–	–	–	–
Sodium chloride (0.18%) + glucose 4% (1/5 physlo-logical saline)	30	–	–	30

*Accounting for 95% of the fluids used in clinical practice.

Table 6.5 Guidelines for intravenous fluid administration in maintenance and replacement of losses

For maintenance fluid balance:
Each day 2500 ml fluid containing about 140 mmol sodium and 60 mmol potassium are required to maintain balance in 75-kg man. A good regimen is 2 litres 5% dextrose and 1 litre physiological saline every 24 hours

For hypovolaemic patients:
An estimate of the losses is made (e.g. in hospital patients from a review of the input/output charts) and these must be given in addition to the normal daily requirements

DISORDERS OF SODIUM REGULATION

Hyponatraemia

Hyponatraemia (serum sodium < than 135 mmol/l) may be the result of the following:

- Relative water excess (dilutional hyponatremia); this is the most common cause
- Salt loss in excess of water, e.g. diarrhoea and renal diseases as described above
- Pseudohyponatraemia, in which hyperlipidaemia or hyperproteinaemia results in a spuriously low measured sodium concentration. The sodium is confined to the aqueous phase but its concentration is expressed in terms of the total volume of plasma (i.e. water plus lipid). In this situation plasma osmolality is normal and therefore treatment of 'hyponatraemia' is unnecessary.

True hyponatraemia must be differentiated from artefactual 'hyponatraemia' caused by taking blood from the drip arm into which a fluid of low sodium is being infused.

Hyponatraemia resulting from water excess (dilutional hyponatraemia)

An excess of body water relative to sodium is differentiated from hyponatraemia caused by sodium loss, because there are none of the clinical features of extracellular volume depletion.

Aetiology

Hyponatraemia is often seen in patients with severe cardiac failure, hepatic cirrhosis or the nephrotic syndrome in which there is an inability of the kidney to excrete 'free water'. This is compounded by the use of diuretics. There is evidence of volume overload and the patient is usually oedematous. Where there is no evidence of extracellular volume overload causes include the syndrome of inappropriate ADH secretion (SIADH), Addison's disease and hypothyroidism.

Clinical features

Symptoms rarely occur until the serum sodium is less than 120 mmol/l. They result from the movement of water into the brain cells in response to the fall in extracellular osmolality, and include headache, confusion, convulsions and coma.

Investigation

Hyponatraemia in association with cardiac failure, cirrhosis or nephrotic syndrome is usually clinically obvious and no further investigation is necessary. If there is no evidence of volume overload the most probable cause is SIADH or diuretic therapy (page 416).

Management

The underlying cause must be corrected where possible. Most cases are simply managed by water restriction (to 1000 ml or even 500 ml/day) with a review of diuretic treatment. Hypertonic saline is restricted to patients with very severe symptomatic hyponatraemia who are not fluid overloaded. It must be given slowly (not more than 70 mmol/h), the aim being to increase the serum sodium to more than 125 mmol/l. A rapid rise in extracellular osmolality, particularly if there is 'overshoot' to high serum sodium and osmolality, will then result in severe shrinking of brain cells and the syndrome of 'central pontine myelinolysis' which can be fatal.

Hypernatraemia

Hypernatraemia (serum sodium > 145 mmol/l) is almost always the result of reduced water intake or water loss in excess of sodium. More rarely it is caused by excessive administration of sodium.

Aetiology
Insufficient intake is most often found in elderly people, neonates or unconscious patients when access to water is denied or confusion or coma eliminates the normal response to thirst. The situation is exacerbated by increased losses of fluid, e.g. sweating, diarrhoea.

Water loss relative to sodium occurs in pituitary diabetes insipidus, nephrogenic diabetes insipidus, osmotic diuresis and water loss from the lungs or skin.

Clinical features
Symptoms are non-specific and include nausea, vomiting, fever and confusion.

Investigations
Simultaneous urine and plasma osmolality and sodium should be measured.

Passage of urine with an osmolality lower than that of plasma in this situation is clearly abnormal and indicates diabetes insipidus (page 417). If urine osmolality is high this suggests an osmotic diuresis or excessive extrarenal losses of water (e.g. heat stroke).

Management
Treatment is that of the underlying cause and replacement of water, either orally if possible or intravenously with 5% dextrose. The aim is to correct over 48 hours, as over-rapid correction may lead to cerebral oedema. If there is clinical evidence of volume depletion this implies that there is a sodium deficit as a well as a water deficit, and intravenous 0.9% saline should be used.

DISORDERS OF POTASSIUM REGULATION

Dietary intake of potassium varies between 80 and 150 mmol daily. Potassium is predominantly an intracellular ion, only

2% of total body potassium being extracellular. Serum levels are mainly controlled by renal excretion under the influence of aldosterone in the renal tubules. In addition levels are influenced by extrarenal losses (e.g. gastrointestinal) and uptake of K^+ into cells. Alkalosis associated with a fall in intracellular H^+ concentration results in a net flux of potassium into cells, with a fall in plasma potassium; acidosis has the reverse effect.

Hypokalaemia

This is a serum potassium concentration of < 3.5 mmol/l.

Aetiology
The most common causes of hypokalaemia (Table 6.6) are diuretic treatment and hyperaldosteronism.

Table 6.6 Causes of hypokalaemia

Increased renal excretion	Diuretics, e.g. thiazides, loop diuretics
	Solute diuresis, e.g. glucosuria
	Primary hyperaldosteronism
	Secondary hyperaldosteronism
	Liver failure
	Heart failure
	Nephrotic syndrome
	Ingestion of mineralocorticoids
	Corticosteroids
	Carbenoxolone
	Liquorice
	Renal tubular acidosis: types 1 and 2
	Renal tubular damage, e.g. drugs
	Rare syndromes: Bartter's, Liddle's
Gastrointestinal losses	Vomiting, diarrhoea, villus adenoma, fistulae, ileostomies
Severe dietary deficiency	
Redistribution into cells	Alkalosis, β-agonists, insulin

Clinical features
Hypokalaemia is usually asymptomatic, although muscle weakness may occur if severe. There is an increased risk of cardiac arrhythmias, particularly in patients with cardiac disease. Hypokalaemia also predisposes to digoxin toxicity.

Management
The underlying cause should be identified and treated where possible. Usually withdrawal of diuretics or purgatives, and replacement with oral potassium supplements, is all that is required. Indications for intravenous infusion of potassium are hypokalaemic diabetic ketoacidosis and severe cases

(< 2.5 mmol/l) are associated with hypokalaemic cardiac arrhythmias. This should be performed slowly, and replacement at rates of greater than 20 mmol/h should only be done with ECG monitoring and hourly measurement of serum potassium.

Hyperkalaemia

This is defined as a serum potassium concentration of > 5.0 mmol/l. True hyperkalaemia must be differentiated from artefactual hyperkalaemia which results from lysis of red cells during vigorous phlebotomy.

Aetiology

The most common causes (Table 6.7) are acute renal failure, drug interference with potassium excretion, and hyporeninaemic hypoaldosteronism (page 213).

Table 6.7 Causes of hyperkalaemia

Excessive intake	
Impaired renal excretion	Renal failure
	Potassium-sparing diuretics (amiloride)
	Hypoaldosteronism:
	Addison's disease
	Hyporeninaemic hypoaldosteronism
	Angiotensin-converting enzyme (ACE) inhibitors
Release from cells	Acidosis
	Crush injury
	Suxamethonium

Clinical features

Hyperkalaemia usually produces few symptoms or signs until high enough to cause cardiac arrest. It is often associated with metabolic acidosis causing Kussmaul's respiration.

Management

A serum potassium of more than 7 mmol/l is a medical emergency and may be associated with typical ECG changes (reduced P wave, widened QRS complex and tented T waves).

If ECG changes are present, 10 ml of 10% calcium gluconate should be given to protect the myocardium from hyperkalaemia. Intravenous glucose (50 ml 50% dextrose with 10 units insulin) will drive K^+ intracellularly and reduce serum K^+ temporarily. Severe acidosis should be treated with intravenous bicarbonate (1.26%).

Definitive treatment requires removal of K^+ from the body either by cation-exchange resins (Calcium Resonium) or haemodialysis.

DISORDERS OF MAGNESIUM REGULATION

Disturbance of magnesium balance is uncommon and usually associated with more obvious fluid and electrolyte disturbance. Like potassium, magnesium is mainly an intracellular cation and balance is maintained mainly via the kidney.

Hypomagnesaemia

Aetiology

A low magnesium (plasma magnesium < 0.7 mmol/l) may arise from deficient intake, defective absorption (malabsorption, small gut resection), excessive gut loss (diarrhoea, fistulae) or through excessive urinary losses (excessive diuresis, renal tubular acidosis, hyper-aldosteronism).

Clinical features

Symptoms and signs include irritability, tremor, ataxia, carpopedal spasm, seizures, and confusional and hallucinatory states. ECG may show a prolonged QT interval, and flattened T waves.

Management

The underlying cause must be corrected where possible and oral supplements given. Intravenous replacement may be needed with severe cases.

Hypermagnesaemia

Aetiology

Hypermagnesaemia (plasma magnesium > 1.1 mmol/l) primarily occurs in patients with renal failure who have been given magnesium-containing laxatives or antacids.

Clinical features

Symptoms develop when plasma magnesium exceeds 2 mmol/l, and include neurological and cardiovascular depression with narcosis, respiratory depression and cardiac conduction defects.

Management

The only treatment usually necessary is withdrawal of magnesium therapy. In severe cases intravenous calcium gluconate may be necessary to reverse the cellular toxic effects of magnesium.

DISORDERS OF ACID–BASE BALANCE

The concentration of hydrogen ions is extremely important to cell metabolism and is normally controlled very tightly. The pH (the negative logarithm of $[H^+]$) is maintained at 7.4 (range 7.35–7.45). The major source of H^+ is tissue respiration ($H_2O + CO_2 = H^+ + HCO_3^-$) with organic acid production and free fatty acid production contributing to lesser degrees. The kidney and lungs constantly regulate acid–base balance through excretion of H^+ and reabsorption of HCO_3^- in the kidneys and CO_2 in the lungs. In addition, the liver contributes to acid–base balance through metabolism of ammonia. Between production and excretion there is an extremely effective buffering system maintaining a constant H^+ inside and outside the cell. Buffers include haemoglobin proteins, bicarbonate and phosphate.

Acid–base disturbances may be caused by:

- Abnormal carbon dioxide removal in the lungs ('respiratory' acidosis and alkalosis).
- Abnormalities in the regulation of bicarbonate and other buffers in the blood ('metabolic' acidosis and alkalosis).

Respiratory acidosis

This is usually associated with ventilatory failure with retention of carbon dioxide. The $P_a\text{CO}_2$ and $[H^+]$ rise (see page 369).

Respiratory alkalosis

Hyperventilation results in increased removal of carbon dioxide resulting in a fall of $P_a\text{CO}_2$ and $[H^+]$.

Metabolic acidosis

This is the result of accumulation of any acid other than carbonic acid. The most common cause is lactic acidosis following shock or cardiac arrest.

Clinical features

These include hyperventilation, hypotension caused by arteriolar vasodilatation and the negative inotropic effect of acidosis, and cerebral dysfunction associated with confusion and fits.

Differential diagnosis (the anion gap)

The first step is to identify whether the acidosis is the result of retention of HCl or of another acid. This is achieved by measurement of the anion gap. The main electrolytes measured in plasma are sodium, potassium, chloride and bicarbonate. The sum of the cations, sodium and potassium, normally exceeds that of chloride and bicarbonate by 10–18 mmol/l. This anion gap is usually made up of negatively charged proteins, phosphate and organic acids. If the anion gap is normal in the presence of acidosis, it can be concluded that HCl is being retained or $NaHCO_3$ is being lost. Causes of a normal anion gap acidosis are given in Table 6.8.

Table 6.8 Causes of metabolic acidosis with a normal anion gap

Increased gastrointestinal HCO_3^- loss	Diarrhoea
	Ileostomy
	Ureterosigmoidostomy
Increased renal HCO_3^- loss	Acetazolamide ingestion
	Proximal (type 2) renal tubular acidosis
	Hyperparathyroidism
	Tubular damage, e.g. drugs, heavy metals
Decreased renal H^+ excretion	Distal (type 1) renal tubular acidosis
	Type 4 renal tubular acidosis
Increased HCl production	Ammonium chloride ingestion
	Increased catabolism of lysine, arginine

If the anion gap is *increased* (i.e. > 18 mmol/l), the acidosis is the result of an exogenous acid, e.g. salicylates or one of the acids normally present in small unmeasured quantities, such as lactate. Causes of a high anion gap acidosis are given in Table 6.9.

Table 6.9 Causes of a high anion gap metabolic acidosis

Renal failure	
Ketoacidosis	Diabetes
	Starvation
	Alcohol poisoning
Drug poisoning	Salicylates
	Methanol
	Ethylene glycol
Lactic acidosis	Type A
	Strenuous exercise
	Shock
	Severe hypoxia
	Type B
	Metformin accumulation
	Leukaemia, lymphoma
	Poisoning, ethanol, paracetamol
	Acute liver failure

Lactic acidosis

Increased production of lactic acid occurs when cellular respiration is abnormal, resulting from either lack of oxygen (type A) or a metabolic abnormality (type B). The most common form in clinical practice is type A lactic acidosis occurring in septicaemic or cardiogenic shock.

Diabetic ketoacidosis

This is a high anion gap acidosis caused by accumulation of organic acids, acetoacetic acid and hydroxybutyric acid (see page 428).

Renal tubular acidosis

Renal tubular acidosis refers to systemic acidosis caused by impairment of the ability of the renal tubules to maintain acid–base balance. This group of disorders is uncommon and only rarely a cause of significant clinical disease.

TYPE 4 RENAL TUBULAR ACIDOSIS

This is the most common of these disorders and is also known as *hyporeninaemic hypoaldosteronism*. Typical features are acidosis and hyperkalaemia occurring in the setting of mild chronic renal failure, usually caused by tubulointerstitial disease or diabetes. Plasma aldosterone and renin are low and do not respond to stimulation. Treatment is with fludrocortisone, diuretics, sodium bicarbonate and ion exchange resins for reduction of serum potassium.

TYPE 3 RENAL TUBULAR ACIDOSIS

Extremely rare, representing a combination of type 1 and type 2.

TYPE 2 RENAL TUBULAR ACIDOSIS

This is the result of failure of H^+ secretion in the distal tubule. Typical features are hypokalaemia, and inability to produce an acid urine in spite of systemic acidosis. Hypercalciuria results in renal stone formation, recurrent urinary tract infection and osteomalacia. The disorder is associated with many diseases, including autoimmune disease, drugs and any cause of nephrocalcinosis. Treatment is with oral sodium bicarbonate, citrate and potassium supplements.

TYPE 1 RENAL TUBULAR ACIDOSIS

This is very rare in adults and caused by failure of sodium bicarbonate reabsorption in the proximal tubule. Typical features include acidosis, hypokalaemia, an inability to produce an acid urine in spite of systemic acidosis and the appearance of bicarbonate in the urine. Treatment is with sodium bicarbonate, which may be required in large doses.

Uraemic acidosis

Reduction of the capacity to secrete H^+ and NH_4^+ in addition to bicarbonate wasting contribute to the acidosis of chronic renal failure. Acidosis occurs particularly when there is tubular damage such as reflux and chronic obstructive nephropathy. It is associated with hypercalciuria and renal osteodystrophy because H^+ ions are buffered by bone in exchange for calcium. Treatment is with sodium or calcium carbonate although acidosis in end-stage renal failure is only usually fully corrected by adequate dialysis.

Metabolic alkalosis

This is much less common than acidosis and is often associated with potassium or volume depletion. The main causes are persistent vomiting, diuretic therapy or hyperaldosteronism. Vomiting causes alkalosis both by causing volume depletion and through loss of gastric acid.

Clinical features
Cerebral dysfunction is an early feature of alkalosis. Respiration may be depressed.

Management
This includes fluid replacement, if necessary, with replacement of sodium, potassium and chloride. The bicarbonate excess will correct itself.

FINAL MEDICINE EXAMINATION: WATER AND ELECTROLYTES

1. A 39-year-old woman is admitted to a hospital with a 3-week history of nausea and vomiting and weakness following a chest infection. She has a past history of depression and hypothyroidism for which she was taking thyroxine. On examination she is dehydrated, drowsy and pigmented with a blood pressure of 70/40 mmHg. She is oliguric and investigation shows: haemoglobin 14.9 g/dl, white blood cells 7.4×10^9/l, urea 22.8 mmol/l, creatinine 290 μmol/l, sodium 118 μmol/l potassium 5.7 mmol/l, bicarbonate 23 mmol/l, thyroxine 29.6 nmol/l, free T_4 4.5 pmol/l, TSH > 50 mU/l.

   (a) What are the probable diagnoses and their cause?

   (b) What further investigations are indicated?

   (c) What is your initial treatment?

2. Write short notes on potassium deficiency.

3. What are the possible causes of a low plasma sodium concentration and how may they be distinguished? What clinical effects may be attributable to this abnormality?

ANSWERS

1. (a) This presentation is typical of an Addisonian crisis precipitated by the chest infection. The patient is

markedly hypotensive and dehydrated on clinical examination. The raised urea and creatinine are compatible with dehydration and prerenal acute renal failure (page 240). The serum sodium is very low and, in combination with the clinical findings, suggest that this is caused by salt and water loss (page 206) either from the kidney or the gastrointestinal tract. The combination of pigmented skin, a history of probable autoimmune disease (most common cause of hypothyroidism is autoimmune) and hyperkalaemia suggest Addison's disease (page 411) resulting from autoimmune adrenal destruction. The thyroid function tests show evidence of hypothyroidism (low thyroxine, low T_4 and raised TSH).

(b) Blood glucose (to look for hypoglycaemia), random plasma cortisol and ACTH, chest radiograph, blood cultures, serum adrenal autoantibodies.

(c) The immediate management is intravenous physiological saline (1 litre over 30 min), 100 mg intravenous hydrocortisone, intravenous dextrose if hypoglycaemic, antibiotics if evidence of infection.

2. Potassium deficiency (which implies total body depletion) is not the same as hypokalaemia (which means a low serum concentration and may be caused by deficiency or redistribution into cells). Depletion occurs with excess losses or inadequate intake (rare) and the causes are listed in Table 6.6.

3. The causes, investigation and symptoms of hyponatraemia are discussed on page 206.

CHAPTER 7

Renal Disease

Presenting features of renal disease

The most common diseases of the kidney and urinary tract are benign prostatic hypertrophy in men and urinary tract infection (UTI) in women. The symptoms suggesting renal tract disease are frequency of micturition, dysuria, haematuria, urinary retention and alteration of urine volume (either polyuria or oliguria). In addition there may be pain situated anywhere along the renal tract from loin to groin. Non-specific symptoms may be the presenting features, e.g. lethargy, anorexia and pruritus, which occur in chronic renal failure.

Renal disease may be asymptomatic and discovered by the incidental finding of hypertension, a raised serum urea or proteinuria and haematuria on stix testing.

Urine stix testing

Commercial reagent stix detect the presence of protein, glucose, ketones, bilirubin, urobilinogen and blood in the urine. They also measure urine pH which is useful in the investigation and management of renal tubular acidosis (page 213). Each test is based on a colour change in a strip of absorbent cellulose impregnated with the appropriate reagent. The stix is dipped briefly into a fresh specimen of urine collected in a clean container and the colour changes compared with the manufacturer's colour charts on the reagent strip container. The degree of colour change is a semi-quantitative assessment of the amount of substance present. Haematuria or proteinuria suggests renal tract disease.

PROTEINURIA

The glomerular ultrafiltrate normally contains a small amount of protein most of which is absorbed in the proximal renal tubule and only small amounts (up to 200 mg per 24 hours) appear in the urine. Most reagent stix can detect a protein concentration of 150 mg/l or more in the urine. Pyrexia, exercise and adoption of the upright posture may all produce a mild increase in urinary protein output. 'Postural proteinuria' is the term used when proteinuria occurs in the upright posture but not when supine. It may be diagnosed by testing for protein in several early morning urine samples passed after overnight recumbency, and then testing several samples after being up and about. The condition is usually benign and the amount of protein excreted is small.

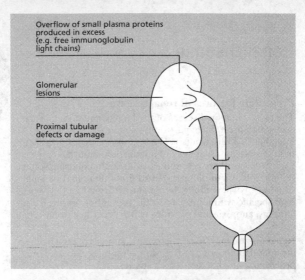

Figure 7.1 Sources of urinary protein. (Adapted from Mallick, 1991, Presenting features of renal disease. *Medicine International*, vol. 85, p. 3512.)

Persistent proteinuria (Figure 7.1) detected on stix testing requires full investigation. The first step is to quantitate protein excretion by a 24-hour urine collection. Proteinuria greater than 2 g/24 hours is usually the result of glomerular disease (page 220) and greater than 3–5 g/24 hours may result in the nephrotic syndrome (page 226). Proteinuria caused by failure of proximal tubular reabsorption is uncommon and this is seldom an isolated defect; there are usually multiple proximal tubular defects causing glycosuria, aminoaciduria, phosphaturia and renal tubular acidosis (*Fanconi's syndrome*). Bence-Jones proteins (immunoglobulin light chains in patients with myeloma) are not detected by stix and are identified by immunoelectrophoresis of urine.

HAEMATURIA

Haematuria may arise from any site in the kidney or urinary tract (Figure 7.2) and may be macroscopic, with bloody urine, or microscopic and found only on stix testing. A positive stix test must always be followed by careful microscopy of fresh urine to confirm the presence of red cells, to look for red cell casts and to exclude haemoglobinuria (page 115) which is uncommon but also results in a positive test. The presence of red cell casts on urine microscopy indicates bleeding of glomerular origin (see later). In the absence of red cell casts,

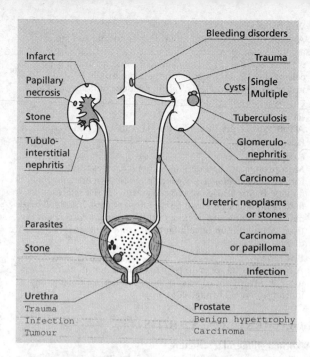

Figure 7.2 Sites and causes of bleeding from the urinary tract.

further investigations, such as urine cytology, intravenous urography and cystoscopy, are required to define the site of bleeding.

With macroscopic haematuria the source of bleeding may be suggested by a careful history. Haematuria that is only apparent at the start of micturition is usually associated with urethral disease. Haematuria that occurs at the end of micturition suggests bleeding from the prostate or bladder base whereas blood seen as an even discoloration throughout the urine suggests bleeding from a source in the bladder or above.

Urine microscopy

Microscopy of urine is performed on all patients suspected of having renal disease. A fresh clean-catch mid-stream specimen of urine is essential to make a valid interpretation of the results.

WHITE CELLS

A value of > 10 per mm^3 of urine is abnormal and indicates an inflammatory reaction within the urinary tract. Usually it is the result of a UTI. The causes of sterile pyuria (i.e. pus cells without bacterial infection) are a partially treated UTI, urinary tract tuberculosis, calculi, bladder tumour, papillary necrosis and interstitial nephritis.

RED CELLS

A value of > 1 per mm^3 is abnormal and must be investigated (see above).

CASTS

Mucoprotein precipitated in the renal tubules results in the formation of *hyaline casts* which on their own are a normal finding. Incorporation of red cells results in *red cell casts,* a finding pathognomonic of glomerulonephritis. *White cell casts* may be seen in acute pyelonephritis. *Granular casts* result from disintegration of cellular debris and indicate renal disease.

BACTERIA

A bacterial count over 100 000 organisms per millilitre of urine in a fresh mid-stream urine specimen is a reliable indicator of a UTI (page 228).

GLOMERULONEPHRITIS

Normal glomerular structure

A renal glomerulus (there are about 1 million glomeruli in each kidney) consists of a capillary plexus invaginating the blind end of the proximal renal tubule (Figure 7.3). The glomerular capillaries are lined by a *fenestrated endothelium* which rests on the *glomerular basement membrane* (GBM). External to the GBM are the *visceral epithelial* cells (podocytes). These cells only make contact with the GBM by finger-like projections called *foot processes,* which are separated from one another by 'slit pores' (Figure 7.3). This unique structure of the glomerular membrane accounts for the tremendous permeability allowing 125–200 ml of glomerular filtrate to be formed every minute (this is the glomerular filtration rate or GFR). The composition of the glomerular filtrate is similar to plasma but contains only small amounts of protein (all of low molecular weight), most of which is reabsorbed in the proximal tubule. The water and electrolyte composition of the glomerular filtrate are normally substantially altered by tubular reabsorption and secretion until it reaches the renal pelvis as urine.

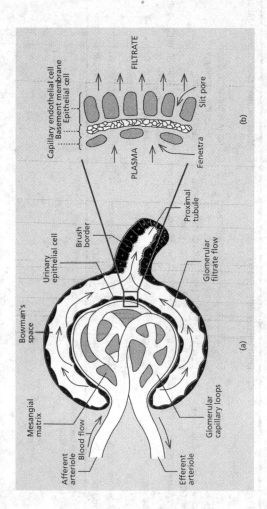

Figure 7.3 (a) Diagrammatic representation of the normal glomerulus; (b) the components of the glomerular membrane. (Adapted from Read et al., 1993, *Essential Medicine*, Edinburgh, Churchill Livingstone; Guyton, 1987, *Human Physiology and Mechanisms of Disease*, 4th edn, London, W B Saunders.)

Table 7.1 Categories of glomerulonephritis (GN) and associated clinical conditions*

Histological type	Light microscopic appearances	Most common clinical presentation
Proliferative glomerulonephritis		
Diffuse	Endothelial and mesangial cell proliferation	Acute nephritic syndrome
Focal segmental	As above but changes are focal	Haematuria, proteinuria
With crescent formation (rapidly progressive GN)	Crescent formation (aggregates of macrophages and epithelial cells in Bowman's space)	Acute renal failure
Mesangiocapillary (mesangioproliferative)	Thickening of GBM, mesangial cell proliferation	Haematuria, proteinuria, nephritic and nephrotic syndrome
IgA nephropathy	Mesangial cell proliferation	Haematuria in young men
Membranous GN	Thickening of GBM	Nephrotic syndrome in adults
Minimal change nephropathy	Normal (fusion of epithelial cell foot processes on EM)	Nephrotic syndrome in children
Focal glomerulosclerosis	Segmental scarring of glomeruli	Proteinuria or nephrotic syndrome

* There is not a complete correlation between the histopathological types and the clinical features.
GBM, Glomerular basement membrane.

Glomerulonephritis is a general term for a group of disorders in which there is immunologically mediated injury to the glomerulus. Two chief pathogenic mechanisms are recognized:

- *Deposition or* in situ *formation of immune complexes* (most human glomerulonephritides). Circulating antigen–antibody complexes are deposited in the kidney or complexes are formed locally when antigen becomes trapped in the glomerulus. The antigen may be exogenous, e.g. β-*haemolytic streptococci*, or endogenous, e.g. DNA in systemic lupus erythematosus.

- *Deposition of antiglomerular basement membrane antibody* (anti-GBM, < 5%). Anti-GBM antibody reacts with an antigen in the GBM producing glomerular damage. The antibody may also react with alveolar capillary basement membrane and can cause both lung haemorrhage and glomerulonephritis (Goodpasture's syndrome).

In some glomerulonephritides, e.g. associated with Wegener's granulomatosis and microscopic polyarteritis, there is no evidence of immune complex deposition. Injury is mediated by a vasculitis causing a focal segmental necrotizing glomerulonephritis with haematuria, proteinuria and deteriorating renal function.

Pathogenesis
Deposition of immune complexes in the glomerulus leads to an inflammatory response which triggers secondary mechanisms of glomerular injury. These include complement activation, fibrin deposition, platelet aggregation and activation of kinin systems. The histological response to immune complex deposition is very variable.

Glomerulonephritis is classified on the basis of light microscopic appearances supplemented by information gained from immunohistochemical techniques and electron microscopy (EM). The main forms of histopathologically identified glomerulonephritis and the clinical features most often associated with each are listed in Table 7.1. The terms 'focal' and 'diffuse' refer to the kidney as a whole and 'segmental' and 'global' refer to the glomeruli. Thus in focal segmental glomerulonephritis only some glomeruli are affected and only a part of the glomerulus.

Aetiology
In most patients with immune complex-mediated glomerulonephritis the cause is unknown, i.e. the nature of the antigen is not determined. In a minority of cases antigens derived from viruses, bacteria, parasites, drugs and from the host may be involved (Table 7.2).

Table 7.2 Some causes of immune complex mediated glomerulonephritis

Infections
Lancefield group A β-haemolytic streptococci
Streptococcus viridans (infective endocarditis)
Mumps virus
Hepatitis B virus
Tropical infections: schistosomiasis, *Plasmodium malariae*, filariasis

Systemic disease
Systemic lupus erythematosus (SLE)

Malignant tumours

Drugs, e.g. penicillamine

Clinical features
Glomerulonephritis presents in one of four ways:

● Asymptomatic proteinuria/haematuria (page 218)

● Acute nephritic syndrome

● Nephrotic syndrome

● Renal failure, acute and chronic (page 240)

Acute nephritic syndrome

Diffuse proliferative glomerulonephritis underlies many of the cases of acute nephritic syndrome in adults and children. The prototype *exogenous* pattern is poststreptococcal glomerulonephritis whereas that produced by an *endogenous* antigen is lupus nephritis seen in SLE. The typical case of poststreptococcal glomerulonephritis develops in a child 1–3 weeks after a streptococcal infection (pharyngitis or cellulitis) with a Lancefield group A β-haemolytic streptococcus. The bacterial antigen becomes trapped in the glomerulus leading to an acute diffuse proliferative glomerulonephritis.

Clinical features
The syndrome comprises:

● Haematuria (macroscopic or microscopic)

● Proteinuria (usually <2g /day)

● Hypertension caused by salt and water retention

● Oedema (periorbital, leg or sacral)

● Oliguria

● Uraemia

Investigations
A thorough history and examination are essential to assess the severity of the illness and to determine any associated underlying conditions. The investigations to consider in

Table 7.3 Investigations indicated in glomerular disease

Investigations	Significance
Baseline measurements	To determine current status, monitor progress and response to treatment
• Measurement of creatinine clearance	
• 24-hour urinary protein excretion	
• Serum urea and electrolytes	
• Serum albumin	
Diagnostically useful tests	
Urine microscopy	Red cell casts indicate glomerulonephritis
Culture (swab from throat or infected skin)	Diagnosis of recent streptococcal infection
Serum antistreptolysin-O titre	
Blood glucose	Diagnosis of diabetes mellitus
Antinuclear and anti-DNA antibodies	Positive in SLE
cANCA (page 196)	Positive in Wegener's granulomatosis
pANCA (page 196)	Positive in microscopic polyarteritis
Antiglomerular basement membrane antibody	Goodpasture's disease
Hepatitis B surface antigen	Negative result excludes HBV infection
Chest radiograph	Cavities in Wegener's granulomatosis, malignancy?
Renal biopsy	Indicated in some adults with nephrotic or nephritic syndrome

nephritic syndrome are listed in Table 7.3. If the clinical diagnosis of a nephritic illness is clear-cut, e.g. in poststreptococcal glomerulonephritis, renal ultrasonography and renal biopsy are usually unnecessary.

Management
Poststreptococcal glomerulonephritis usually has a good prognosis and supportive measures are often all that is required until spontaneous recovery takes place. Hypertension is treated with salt restriction, loop diuretics (page 314) and vasodilators. Fluid balance is monitored by daily weighing and daily recording of fluid input and output charts. In oliguric patients with evidence of fluid overload (e.g. oedema, pulmonary congestion and severe hypertension) fluid restriction is necessary. Life-threatening complications such as hypertensive encephalopathy (see page 313), pulmonary oedema (see page 284) and severe uraemia (see page 244) are treated in the usual ways.

In glomerulonephritis complicating SLE or the systemic vasculitides (see below), immunosuppression with prednisolone, cyclophosphamide or azathioprine improves renal function.

Nephrotic syndrome

Nephrotic syndrome consists of heavy proteinuria (> 3–5 g/24 h), hypoalbuminaemia and oedema. Structural damage to the glomerular basement membrane leads to loss of electrostatic and physical barriers which normally prevents passage of large-molecular-weight proteins into the glomerular filtrate. Increased protein loss, in addition to increased catabolism of protein in the kidney, leads to hypoalbuminaemia. The pathogenesis of oedema in the nephrotic syndrome is poorly understood. The classic explanation is that intravascular hypovolaemia (hypoalbuminaemia reduces plasma oncotic pressure, salt and water move into extravascular compartment) results in activation of the renin–angiotensin–aldosterone system which promotes sodium and water reabsorption in the distal nephron. However, it now seems probable that there is also a primary intrarenal defect in sodium excretion.

Aetiology
All types of glomerulonephritis can cause the nephrotic syndrome, although in Europe and the USA membranous disease is the most common cause in adults and minimal change glomerulonephritis in children. Membranous glomerulonephritis is usually idiopathic but may occur in association with drugs, neoplasms or infections (Table 7.2).

Minimal change glomerulonephritis occurs most commonly in boys under 5 years of age. It accounts for 90% of cases of nephrotic syndrome in children and 20–25% in adults; however, it is rare in black African populations. The pathogenesis of this condition is not known; immune complexes are absent on immunofluorescence but the increase in glomerular permeability is thought to be immunologically mediated in some way.

Amyloid (page 442) involving the kidneys and diabetes mellitus (page 433) are also important causes of the nephrotic syndrome but, unlike minimal change and membranous glomerulonephritis, the mechanism is not immune mediated.

Other renal diseases, e.g. polycystic kidneys, chronic pyelonephritis, may cause proteinuria, but rarely severe enough to cause the nephrotic syndrome.

Clinical features
Oedema of the ankles, genitals and abdomen is the principal finding. The face (periorbital oedema) and arms may also be involved in severe cases.

Differential diagnoses
Nephrotic syndrome must be differentiated from other causes of oedema and hypoalbuminaemia. In congestive cardiac failure (page 275) there is oedema and a raised jugular venous pressure (JVP). In nephrotic syndrome the JVP is normal or low unless there is concomitant renal failure and oliguria. Hypoalbuminaemia and oedema occur in cirrhosis but there are usually signs of chronic liver disease on examination (page 79).

Investigations
The diagnosis is established by demonstrating:

- Heavy proteinuria (> 3–5 g daily in adults)

- Hypoalbuminaemia (< 30 g/l)

Hyperlipidaemia is common in the nephrotic syndrome and is the result of increased hepatic synthesis of cholesterol and triglycerides which accompanies hepatic albumin synthesis. Further investigations to be considered are listed in Table 7.3.

In the UK most cases of childhood nephrotic syndrome are caused by minimal change glomerulonephritis and therefore treatment is usually started with corticosteroids without recourse to a renal biopsy. In adults a renal biopsy is performed unless the diagnosis is clear-cut, e.g. nephrotic syndrome in a patient with long-standing diabetes mellitus must be advanced diabetic glomerulopathy. If a drug is implicated, e.g. penicillamine, the correct management is to stop the drug.

Management
GENERAL
Oedema is treated with bed rest, dietary salt restriction and diuretic therapy. Intravenous diuretics and occasionally

intravenous salt-poor albumin may be required to initiate a diuresis. Diuresis, once established, can usually be maintained with oral diuretics alone. If diuresis is too vigorous it may precipitate circulatory collapse and acute renal failure.

SPECIFIC TREATMENT

Minimal change disease is almost always steroid-responsive in children although less commonly in adults. High-dose prednisolone therapy (40–60 mg daily) should be given over a period of 8 weeks and then reduced slowly. Of patients who enter remission 30–50% will have a relapse within 3 years and this is treated with a further course of steroids. In patients with frequent relapses and in steroid-unresponsive patients, immunosuppressive therapy with cyclophosphamide or cylcosporin may be employed.

The benefits of immunosuppressive therapy in membranous glomerulonephritis remain contentious. In other types of glomerulonephritis remission may occur if the underlying disease can be treated, e.g. in patients with SLE, treatment with steroids or cyclophosphamide may induce long-term remission.

Complications

- VENOUS THROMBOSIS. Hypovolaemia and a hypercoagulable state predispose to thrombus formation in both renal (seen on ultrasonography) and peripheral veins. Prolonged bed rest should be avoided but, if necessary, patients should receive prophylactic anticoagulation with subcutaneous heparin (page 142).

- SEPSIS. Loss of immunoglobulin in the urine increases the susceptibility to infection which is an important cause of death in these patients.

- ACUTE RENAL FAILURE is rarely the result of progression of the underlying renal disease. However, acute renal failure may occur as a result of hypovolaemia particularly after diuretic therapy or with renal vein thrombosis.

URINARY TRACT INFECTION

Urinary tract infection is common in women with about 35% having symptoms of a UTI at some time in their lives. It is relatively uncommon in children and in men where it usually indicates underlying disease.

Pathogenesis

Infection of the urinary tract is most often via the ascending transurethral route and this is facilitated by sexual intercourse and urethral catheterization. Women are more susceptible to infection because the short urethra and proximity to the anus facilitates transfer of bowel organisms to the bladder. Infection is most often caused by bacteria from the patient's own bowel flora (Table 7.4) but in 20–30% of young women it is caused by skin organisms: *Staphylococcus saprophyticus* or *Staph. epidermidis*.

Table 7.4 Organisms causing urinary tract infection in domicilliary practice

Organism	Approximate frequency (%)
Escherichia coli and other 'coliforms'	68+
Proteus mirabilis	12
*Klebsiella aerogenes**	4
*Enterococci**	6
Staphylococcus saprophyticus or *Staph. epidermidis*†	10

* More common in hospital practice.
† More common in women.

Common abnormalities that encourage bladder infection (*cystitis*) include the following:

● Urinary obstruction or stasis

● Previous damage to the bladder epithelium

● Bladder stones

● Poor bladder emptying

Ascending infection of the ureters results in renal parenchymal infection (*acute pyelonephritis*). This is facilitated by vesicoureteric reflux and dilated hypotonic ureters. *Chronic pyelonephritis* (also called atrophic pyelonephritis or reflux nephropathy) arises from childhood UTIs in combination with vesicoureteric reflux leading to progressive renal scarring. It presents as hypertension or chronic renal failure in childhood and adult life.

Clinical features

The most common symptoms of lower urinary tract infection are frequency of micturition, dysuria (painful voiding), suprapubic pain, and tenderness, haematuria and smelly urine.

In acute pyelonephritis, there may also be loin pain and tenderness with fever and systemic upset. However, localization of infection on the basis of symptoms alone is unreliable.

In elderly people, symptoms may be atypical, with incontinence, nocturia or just a vague change in well-being.

Investigations

URINE MICROSCOPY AND CULTURE. The diagnosis depends on

finding more than 100 000 of the same organism per millilitre of urine in a clean-catch mid-specimen urine (MSU). Lower counts or mixed growths are of uncertain significance and the test should be repeated. If in doubt, urine must be obtained by suprapubic bladder aspiration where any growth of a uropathogenic organism is evidence of infection.

EXCRETION UROGRAPHY is performed to look for physiological and anatomical abnormalities of the urinary tract which may predispose to UTI. It is indicated in women with repeated infections and after a single infection in children and men.

Management

A 5-day course of oral amoxycillin, nitrofurantoin or trimethoprim is usually effective. A high fluid intake should be encouraged during treatment and for some weeks after. In women with relapsing infection, low-dose prophylactic antibiotics may be required for a period of 6–12 months. Patients with acute pyelonephritis may be acutely ill and usually require initial treatment with parenteral antibiotics such as amoxycillin or an aminoglycoside (e.g. gentamicin).

Complications

In fit patients with normal urinary tracts, UTIs rarely result in serious kidney damage. In patients with abnormal urinary tracts (e.g. stones) or systemic disease involving the kidney (e.g. diabetes mellitus), the complications are renal papillary necrosis (page 232) and development of a renal or perinephric abscess. Abscesses can be seen on ultrasonography and usually require surgical drainage in addition to antibiotic therapy.

Urinary tract infection in pregnancy

Approximately 6% of pregnant women have significant bacteriuria in pregnancy and, if untreated, 20% of these will develop acute pyelonephritis. Early detection and treatment of bacteriuria is thus indicated.

Abacteriuric frequency or dysuria ('urethral syndrome')

The urethral syndrome occurs in women and presents with dysuria and frequency but in the absence of bacteriuria. It may be associated with vaginitis in postmenopausal women, irritant chemicals (e.g. soaps) and sexual intercourse.

Tuberculosis of the urinary tract

Tuberculosis (TB) of the urinary tract may present with all the symptoms of a UTI, i.e. dysuria, frequency or haematuria, and should be considered particularly in the Asian immigrant population of the UK. Classically, there is sterile pyuria (page 220). Diagnosis depends on culture of mycobacteria from early morning urine samples. Treatment is as for pulmonary tuberculosis (page 344).

TUBULOINTERSTITIAL NEPHRITIS

Interstitial inflammation with tubular damage is a regular feature of bacterial pyelonephritis but, contrary to former belief, it rarely, if ever, leads to chronic renal damage in the absence of reflux, obstruction or other complicating factors. The importance of other factors, particularly drugs, in the causation of this disorder has now been realized.

Acute tubulointerstitial nephritis

Acute tubulointerstitial nephritis is most often the result of a hypersensitivity reaction to drugs (Table 7.5), most commonly drugs of the penicillin family and non-steroidal anti-inflammatory drugs (NSAIDs).

Table 7.5 Common causes of acute tubulointerstitial nephritis

Penicillins
NSAIDs
Sulphonamides
Phenindione
Allopurinol
Cephalosporins
Rifampicin
Diuretics – frusemide, thiazides
Cimetidine
Phenytoin

Patients present with acute renal failure and the features of a hypersensitivity reaction: fever, arthralgia, skin rashes and blood eosinophilia. Renal biopsy shows an intense interstitial cellular infiltrate, predominantly eosinophils, and variable tubular necrosis. Management involves withdrawal of the offending drug and treatment of acute renal failure (page 244). High-dose prednisolone therapy is often used, although its value has not been proven. The prognosis is generally good; patients should avoid further exposure to the offending drug.

Chronic tubulointerstitial nephritis

The most common cause of chronic tubulointerstitial nephritis is prolonged consumption of large amounts of analgesic drugs, particularly NSAIDs and drugs containing phenacetin (now withdrawn) ('analgesic nephropathy'). Some causes are show in Table 7.6.

Table 7.6 Causes of chronic tubulointerstitial nephritis

Chronic pyelonephritis
Non-steroidal anti-inflammatory drugs
Diabetes mellitus
Sickle-cell disease
Sjögren's syndrome
Hyperuricaemic nephropathy

Presentation is usually with polyuria, proteinuria (usually < 1 g/day) or uraemia. Polyuria and nocturia are the result of tubular damage in the medullary area of the kidney, leading to defects in the renal concentrating ability. Necrosis of the papillae, which may subsequently slough off and be passed in the urine, sometimes causes ureteric colic or acute ureteral obstruction. Management is largely supportive. In cases of analgesic nephropathy, the drug should be stopped and replaced if necessary with paracetamol or dihydrocodeine.

HYPERTENSION AND THE KIDNEY

Hypertension may be the cause or the result of renal disease, and it may be difficult to differentiate between the two on clinical grounds. Investigations, as described on page 313, should be performed on all patients although intravenous urography (IVU) is usually unnecessary.

Essential hypertension

Hypertension leads to characteristic histological changes in the renal vessels and intrarenal vasculature over time. These changes include intimal thickening with reduplication of the elastic lamina, reduction in kidney size and an increase in the proportion of sclerotic glomeruli. These changes are usually accompanied by some deterioration in renal function.

Accelerated or *malignant phase hypertension* is marked by the development of fibrinoid necrosis in afferent glomerular arterioles and fibrin deposition in arteriolar walls. A rapid rise in blood pressure may trigger these arteriolar lesions and a vicious circle is then established whereby fibrin deposition leads to renal damage, increased renin release and hence a further increase in blood pressure.

Treatment of hypertension is described on page 313. The outlook is good if treatment is started before renal impairment has occurred.

Renal hypertension
Bilateral renal disease

Hypertension commonly complicates bilateral renal disease such as chronic glomerulonephritis, bilateral reflux

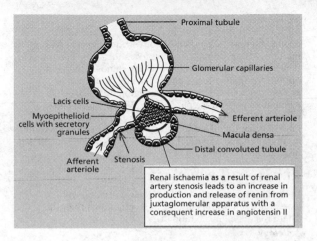

Figure 7.4 The mechanism of hypertension in unilateral renal artery stenosis. (Adapted from Davidson, 1991, *Principles and Practice of Medicine*, Edinburgh, Churchill Livingstone.)

nephropathy or analgesic nephropathy. Two main mechanisms are responsible:

● Activation of the renin–angiotensin–aldosterone system
● Retention of salt and water, leading to an increase in blood volume and hence blood pressure

Unilateral renal disease

Hypertension may arise as a result of unilateral renal artery stenosis (caused by fibromuscular hyperplasia in young women, atheroma in elderly people) or unilateral reflux nephropathy. The mechanism of hypertension is illustrated in Figure 7.4.

SCREENING FOR UNILATERAL RENAL DISEASE

● Rapid sequence excretion urography is widely employed. Injected contrast medium is filtered more slowly and concentrated to a greater extent within the nephron on the side of the stenosis
● Radionucleotide studies using diethylenetriamine pentaacetate (DTPA) (page 257) can demonstrate decreased renal perfusion on the affected side
● Renal arteriography remains the gold standard for the diagnosis of renal artery disease

Management

Most patients do well with hypotensive therapy without the need for surgery. Angiotensin-converting enzyme (ACE) inhibitors are avoided because they can lead to acute renal failure in the presence of renal artery stenosis. Surgical options for renal artery stenosis include transluminal angioplasty to dilate the stenotic region, reconstructive vascular surgery and nephrectomy. With good selection of patients, more than 50% are cured or improved by intervention. In unilateral reflux nephropathy, nephrectomy is advocated, particularly if the abnormal kidney is making an insignificant contribution to overall excretion function.

RENAL STONE DISEASE

In the UK approximately 2% of the population will experience renal stone disease at some time in their life. There is a male:female ratio of 2:1.

Aetiology

Calcium-containing stones are the most common (Table 7.7).

Table 7.7 Types and frequency of renal stones

Types of renal stone	Approximate frequency (%)

Calcium-containing:
    Calcium oxalate (65%)
    Calcium phosphate (15%)
	80

Magnesium ammonium phosphate	10–15
Uric acid	3–5
Cystine	1–2

CALCIUM STONES

More than half of all patients with calcium oxalate stones have *idiopathic hypercalciuria*. People with this condition both absorb from the gut and excrete in the urine a higher fraction of dietary calcium than normal people. Serum calcium levels are normal. Less common causes of hypercalciuria are the following:

- Hypercalcaemia (page 193): most patients with hypercalcaemia who form stones have primary hyperparathyroidism

- Excessive dietary intake of calcium

- Excessive resorption of calcium from the skeleton as occurs with prolonged immobilization or weightlessness

Increased oxalate excretion favours the formation of calcium oxalate, even if calcium excretion is normal:

- Primary hyperoxaluria is a rare autosomal recessive enzyme deficiency leading to increased oxalate production and corresponding oxalate excretion. There is widespread calcium oxalate crystal deposition in the kidneys and later in other tissues (myocardium, tissues and bone). Renal failure typically develops in the late teens or early twenties. More frequent causes of mild hyperoxaluria are dietary or enteric hyperoxaluria.

- Dietary hyperoxaluria from excessive ingestion of high oxalate-containing foods (e.g. spinach, rhubarb and tea) or from dietary calcium restriction with compensatory increased absorption of oxalate

- Enteric hyperoxaluria: small bowel disease, e.g. Crohn's disease or resection is associated with increased absorption of oxalate from the colon. Dehydration secondary to fluid loss from the gut also plays a part in stone formation

Primary renal disease may lead to calcium stone formation. Medullary sponge kidney is associated with hypercalciuria and a tendency to develop stones (page 252). The alkaline urine seen in the renal tubular acidoses favours the precipitation of calcium phosphate.

INFECTION-INDUCED STONES

Urinary tract infection with organisms that produce urease (*Proteus*, *Klebsiella* and *Pseudomonas* spp.) is associated with stones containing ammonium, magnesium and calcium. Urease hydrolyses urea to ammonia and thus raises the urine pH. An alkaline urine and high ammonia concentration favour stone formation. These stones are often large and fill the pelvicalyceal system, producing the typical radio-opaque staghorn calculus.

URIC ACID STONES

Uric acid stones are sometimes associated with hyperuricaemia with or without clinical gout (page 180). Patients with ileostomies are also at risk of developing urate stones because urine acidity is reduced (as a result of gut bicarbonate loss), and uric acid becomes less soluble in the more alkaline urine.

CYSTINE STONES

These may occur with cystinuria, an autosomal recessive condition affecting cystine and dibasic amino acid transport (lysine, ornithine and arginine) in the epithelial cells of renal tubules and the gastrointestinal tract. The excessive urinary excretion of cystine, which is the least soluble of the naturally occurring amino acids, leads to the formation of crystals and calculi.

Clinical features (Table 7.8)

Table 7.8 Clinical features of urinary tract calculi

Asymptomatic
Pain
Haematuria
Urinary tract infection
Urinary tract obstruction

Most people with urinary tract calculi are asymptomatic; pain is the most common symptom. Large staghorn renal calculi may cause loin pain. *Ureteric stones* cause renal colic, a severe intermittent pain lasting for hours. The pain is felt anywhere between the loin and the groin, and may radiate into the scrotum or labium or into the tip of the penis. Nausea and vomiting are common. Microscopic haematuria is almost always present. The patient will be pyrexial only if there is a UTI associated with the stone. *Bladder stones* present with urinary frequency and haematuria. *Urethral stones* may cause bladder outflow obstruction, resulting in anuria and painful bladder distension.

Investigations

In a patient presenting with renal colic the clinical diagnosis is confirmed by plain abdominal radiograph ('KUB' – kidney, ureters and bladder) and emergency intravenous urography. Ninety per cent of renal stones are radio-opaque and calcification may be seen in the line of the renal tract. Intravenous urography (IVU) shows a delayed nephrogram on the side of the stone.

Table 7.9 Investigations in a patient with urinary calculi

First line	Second line, in recurrent stone formers

Urine
  Chemical analysis of any stone passed
  MSU for culture and sensitivity
	Two 24-hour urine collections for calcium, oxalate and uric acid output

Blood
  Serum urea and electrolytes
  Serum calcium
  Serum uric acid
  Serum bicarbonate
	Random urine for cystine screening

Radiography
  Plain film
  Excretion urography	

A detailed history may reveal possible aetiological factors for stone formation, e.g. vitamin D consumption, gouty arthritis, recurrent UTIs, intestinal resection. The subsequent work-up for a renal calculus is indicated in Table 7.9.

Management

INITIAL TREATMENT

In the case of renal colic, a strong analgesic (e.g. an opiate or an NSAID) should be given to relieve the pain. Most ureteric stones that are 5 mm or less in diameter will pass spontaneously. Indications for surgical intervention include persistent pain, infection above the site of obstruction and failure of the stone to pass down the ureter. The options for stone removal include the following:

- Percutaneous nephrolithotomy for stones in the renal pelvis and calyces
- Extracorporeal shock wave lithotripsy for renal stones
- Cystoscopic removal of ureteric and bladder stones
- Open surgery for very large stones

PREVENTION OF RECURRENCE

Further therapy depends on the type of stone and any underlying condition identified during screening investigations. For prevention of all stones, whatever the cause, it is important to maintain a high intake of fluid (to produce a urine volume of 2–2.5 l/day), particularly during the summer months. When no metabolic or renal abnormality has been identified ('idiopathic stone formers') adequate hydration is the mainstay of treatment.

Idiopathic hypercalciuria. Dietary intake of calcium should be reduced by avoiding milk, cheese and white bread. A water softener may be helpful for patients who live in hard water areas. If hypercalciuria persists, a thiazide diuretic, e.g. bendrofluazide, will reduce urinary calcium excretion.

Mixed infective stones. Recurrent stones should be prevented by maintenance of a high fluid intake and measures to stop bacteriuria. This will require long-term follow-up and may demand the use of long-term, low-dose, prophylactic antibiotics.

Uric acid stones may be prevented by maintaining an alkaline urine (with oral sodium bicarbonate) and by use of the xanthine oxidase inhibitor allopurinol, which allows the excretion of the soluble precursor compound, hypoxanthine, in preference to uric acid.

Cystine stones. Patients may be unable to tolerate the very high fluid intake (5 litres of water in 24 hours) needed to maintain solubility of cystine in the urine. An alternative is

D-penicillamine which chelates cystine forming a more soluble complex.

Nephrocalcinosis (Table 7.10)

The term 'nephrocalcinosis' means diffuse renal parenchymal calcification that is detectable radiologically. The condition is typically painless. Hypertension and renal impairment commonly occur. The treatment is of the underlying cause.

Table 7.10 Common causes of nephrocalcinosis

Mainly medullary
Hypercalcaemia
Renal tubular acidosis
Primary hyperoxaluria
Medullary sponge kidney
Tuberculosis

Mainly cortical (rare)
Renal cortical necrosis

URINARY TRACT OBSTRUCTION

The urinary tract may be obstructed at any point along its length between the kidney and the urethral meatus. This results in dilatation of the tract above the obstruction. Dilatation of the renal pelvis is known as *hydronephrosis*.

Aetiology

The causes of obstruction may be classified into four groups, listed in Table 7.11. In adults the most common causes are prostatic obstruction, gynaecological cancer and calculi.

Table 7.11 Causes of urinary tract obstruction

Within the lumen
Calculi
Blood clots
Sloughed renal papillae
Tumour

Within the wall
Stricture: ureteric or urethral
Neuropathic bladder
Pelviureteric junction obstruction
Obstructive megaureter

Pressure from outside
Prostatic hypertrophy/tumour
Pelvic tumours
Phimosis
Retroperitoneal fibrosis

Clinical features

The symptoms of urinary tract obstruction are the following.

PAIN is usually a dull ache in the flank or back.

ALTERATION OF URINE VOLUME: complete anuria is strongly suggestive of complete bilateral obstruction or complete obstruction of a single functioning kidney. Partial obstruction causes polyuria as a result of tubular damage and impairment of concentrating mechanisms.

With bladder outlet obstruction, hesitancy, poor stream, terminal dribbling and a sense of incomplete emptying occur. Retention with overflow is characterized by the frequent passage of small quantities of urine.

Depending on the site of obstruction an enlarged bladder or hydronephrotic kidney may be felt on examination. Pelvic and rectal examination are essential in determining the cause of obstruction.

Investigations

Imaging studies are performed to identify the site and nature of the obstruction and, together with serum biochemistry, to assess function of the affected kidney.

ULTRASONOGRAPHY AND EXCRETION UROGRAPHY are the initial investigations. Ultrasonography confirms the diagnosis of obstruction and may show hydronephrosis. Excretion urography identifies the site of obstruction and shows a characteristic appearance (a delayed nephrogram which eventually becomes denser than the non-obstructed side).

RADIONUCLIDE STUDIES (page 257) contribute to the management of obstruction by quantifying the degree of obstruction and function of the kidney. In general, absence of uptake of the radiopharmaceutical indicates renal damage that is sufficiently severe to render correction of the obstruction unprofitable.

Subsequent investigations may include CT, retrograde and anterograde urography, cystoscopy and pressure–flow studies during bladder filling and voiding. Anterograde urography is particularly useful in both the diagnosis and therapy of patients with urinary obstruction. A fine catheter is introduced into the renal pelvis under ultrasonic guidance. This allows the introduction of dye to determine the site and cause of obstruction; in addition, urine may be temporarily drained from an obstructed system while definitive treatment is planned.

Management

Surgery is the usual treatment for persistent urinary tract obstruction. Elimination of obstruction may be associated with a massive postobstructive diuresis, resulting partly from a solute diuresis from salt and urea retained during obstruction and partly from the renal concentrating defect. In some cases definitive relief of obstruction is not possible and urinary diversion may be required. This may be simply an indwelling urethral catheter, a stent placed across the obstructing lesion or by formation of an ileal conduit.

RENAL FAILURE

The term 'renal failure' means failure of renal excretory function as a result of the depression of the glomerular filtration rate (GFR). This is accompanied to a variable extent by failure of erythropoietin production, vitamin D hydroxylation, regulation of acid–base balance, and regulation of salt and water balance and blood pressure.

- *Acute renal failure* (ARF) is a sudden and rapid decline in renal function which lasts days to weeks. It is usually reversible or self-limiting.

- *Chronic renal failure* (CRF) develops over months or years. It is usually not reversible but treatment may slow progression.

Acute renal failure

Aetiology
Acute renal failure (ARF) may be

- Prerenal
- Renal
- Postrenal

It may also result from a combination of these factors, e.g. in postsurgical ARF fluid depletion (prerenal), systemic infection and nephrotoxic drugs (renal) may all play a role. ARF may also complicate chronic renal failure (*'acute-on-chronic'*).

PRERENAL. Failure of perfusion of the kidneys with blood occurs in prerenal failure. The kidney is able to maintain glomerular filtration close to normal in spite of wide variations in the renal perfusion pressure and volume status – so-called 'autoregulation'. Maintenance of a normal GFR in the face of decreased systemic pressure depends on the intrarenal production of prostaglandins and angiotensin II. With severe or prolonged hypovolaemia, there is eventually a drop in glomerular filtration termed 'prerenal failure'. Drugs that impair renal autoregulation, such as ACE inhibitors and NSAIDs, increase the risk of prerenal failure in hypovolaemia.

Table 7.12 Prerenal causes of acute renal failure

Hypovolaemia
Haemorrhage
Burns
Diarrhoea
Pancreatitis
Diabetic ketoacidosis
Diuretics
Sepsis

Decreased cardiac output
Myocardial infarction
Massive pulmonary embolism
Congestive cardiac failure

Severe liver failure (hepatorenal syndrome)

Renal artery obstruction

Prerenal failure is most commonly the result of hypovolaemia, and is characterized in the early stages by lack of structural damage and rapid reversibility once normal renal perfusion has been restored. Hypovolaemia is identified from the clinical history and, on physical examination, by the presence of hypotension, a postural drop in blood pressure, a low jugular venous pressure (JVP) and reduced tissue turgor. Measurement of urinary electrolytes (Table 7.13) can help in distinguishing between prerenal failure and intrinsic renal failure but these are no substitute for a proper clinical assessment.

If, on the basis of the history and clinical examination, prerenal (hypovolaemia) failure is diagnosed or strongly suspected, the effect of volume repletion on renal function must be tested. Volume repletion should be with an appropriate fluid: blood in the case of posthaemorrhagic shock and physiological saline if fluid depletion is caused by vomiting, diarrhoea or polyuria. In some cases, e.g. with a very sick patient, volume replacement is guided by measurement of the central venous pressure. With pure prerenal failure, urine output should increase with volume replacement. If hypovolaemia is corrected (i.e. the JVP or CVP is normal) and urine output does not increase, the kidneys may respond to a strong diuretic stimulus (e.g. frusemide 120 mg i.v. over 10 minutes which may be repeated once if there is no response). If urine output does not increase with these measures, then the patient has progressed to acute tubular necrosis (ATN) and the management is that of established intrinsic renal failure (see later).

Table 7.13 Criteria for distinction between prerenal and intrinsic cause of renal dysfunction

	Prerenal	Intrinsic
Urine specific gravity	> 1.020	< 1.010
Urine osmolality (mosmol/l)	> 500	< 350
Urine sodium (mmol/l)	< 20	> 40
Fractional excretion of sodium (Na$^+$)	< 1%	> 1%

$$\text{Fractional excretion of Na}^+ = \frac{[\text{Urine Na}^+/\text{Plasma Cr}]}{[\text{Plasma Na}^+/\text{Urine Cr}]} \times 100\%$$

where Cr is creatinine.

POSTRENAL. Postrenal ARF is caused by obstruction to the flow of urine anywhere along the renal tract (page 238) and is usually quickly reversed if the obstruction is relieved. All patients with ARF must be examined for evidence of obstruction (enlarged palpable kidneys or bladder, large prostate on rectal examination, pelvic masses on vaginal examination in women) and undergo renal ultrasonography to look for hydronephrosis and dilated ureters. Treatment is usually by a temporary measure, e.g. urethral/suprapubic catheterization or percutaneous nephrostomy until definitive treatment of the obstructing lesion can be undertaken.

INTRINSIC RENAL FAILURE. Failure to restore the circulation and to re-establish adequate renal blood flow, in prerenal failure, leads to structural changes referred to as ATN which may also result from exposure to nephrotoxins. The other causes of intrinsic renal failure are glomerulonephritis, interstitial nephritis and vasculitis (Table 7.14). In established renal failure the kidney loses its ability to concentrate the urine and conserve sodium. This may, in addition to clinical examination, be useful in differentiating renal from prerenal failure where the kidney is able to concentrate the urine and conserve sodium (see Table 7.13).

Table 7.14 Causes of intrinsic renal failure

Vascular
Vasculitis
Malignant hypertension

Acute glomerulonephritis

Acute interstitial nephritis
Drug hypersensitivity
Infections

Acute tubular necrosis
Ischaemia
Exogenous nephrotoxins: gentamicin, cephaloridine, intravenous contrast agents
Endogenous nephrotoxins: Bence-Jones protein, uric acid, myoglobin

Clinical features of established ARF

The early stages of renal failure are often completely asymptomatic. Symptoms are common when the blood urea concentration is over 40 mmol/l but many patients develop uraemic symptoms at lower levels of blood urea. It is not the accumulation of urea itself that causes symptoms, but a combination of many different metabolic abnormalities.

ALTERATION OF URINE VOLUME. Oliguria usually occurs with acute renal failure but there may be polyuria with passage of large quantities of dilute urine.

NEUROLOGICAL. Weakness, fatigue and lassitude occur. Mental confusion, seizures and coma may also occur with severe uraemia, but this is less commonly seen since the introduction of effective renal replacement therapy.

SKIN. Symptoms include pallor, pruritus, pigmentation and bruising.

CARDIOPULMONARY. Breathlessness occurs from a combination of anaemia and pulmonary oedema secondary to volume overload.

There may be deep sighing respiration (Kussmaul's respiration) resulting from systemic metabolic acidosis. Pericarditis occurs with severe untreated uraemia and may be complicated by a pericardial effusion and tamponade.

GASTROINTESTINAL. Nausea, anorexia and vomiting are common.

HAEMATOLOGICAL. Anaemia is most commonly seen in chronic renal failure but may occur in ARF. Impaired platelet function causes bruising and exacerbates gastrointestinal bleeding.

Investigations

The purpose of investigation is two-fold:

1. To document the degree of renal impairment and obtain baseline values so that the response to treatment can be monitored. This is accomplished by measurement of serum urea and electrolytes, and a 24-hour creatinine clearance.
2. To establish the underlying cause of ARF so that specific treatment (e.g. intensive immunosuppression in Wegener's granulomatosis) may be instituted as early as possible and thus prevent progression to irreversible renal failure.

BLOOD COUNT. Anaemia and a very high ESR may suggest myeloma or a vasculitis.

URINE STIX TESTING AND MICROSCOPY. Glomerulonephritis is suggested by haematuria and proteinuria on urine stix testing and the presence of red cell casts on urine microscopy (page 218).

URINARY ELECTROLYTES. Measurement of urinary electrolytes (see Table 7.13) excludes a significant prerenal element to ARF.

RADIOLOGY. Every patient should undergo renal ultrasonography (for renal size and to exclude obstruction). CT is useful for the diagnosis of retroperitoneal fibrosis and some other causes of urinary obstruction, and may also indicate cortical scarring.

HISTOLOGICAL INVESTIGATIONS. Renal biopsy should be considered in every patient with unexplained renal failure and normal sized kidneys.

OPTIONAL INVESTIGATIONS (depending on the case)

- Serum protein electrophoresis
- Immunological: serum autoantibodies, ANCAs (page 196) and complement
- Infectious screen: antibodies to hepatitis B and C and HIV
- Blood cultures

Management

The principles of management of established ARF are summarized in Table 7.15. In all patients with intrinsic renal failure hypovolaemia and obstruction must be excluded as contributing factors.

Table 7.15 Principles of management of a patient with acute renal failure

1 Emergency resuscitation
   To prevent death from hyperkalaemia (page 209) or pulmonary oedema (page 284)

2 Establish the aetiology and treat the underlying cause
   - History including family history, systemic disease, use of nephrotoxic drugs
   - Examination includes assessment of haemodynamic status, pelvic and rectal examination
   - Investigations

3 Prevention of further renal damage
   Avoid sepsis, hypovolaemia and nephrotoxic drugs

4 Management of established renal failure
   - Once fluid balance has been corrected the daily fluid intake should equal fluid lost on the previous day plus insensible losses (approximately 500 ml)
   - Adequate nutrition – enteral or parenteral
   - Nursing care, e.g. prevention of pressure sores
   - Monitor daily: urine volume, serum biochemistry, body weight
   - Frequent review regarding the need for dialysis

5 Careful fluid and electrolyte balance during recovery phase
   The patient may pass large volumes of dilute urine until the kidney recovers concentrating ability

Indications for dialysis include severe hyperkalaemia (> 6.5 mmol/l), severe metabolic acidosis, pulmonary oedema and progressive uraemia with encephalopathy or pericarditis. Whether haemodialysis, haemofiltration or peritoneal dialysis is used depends on the facilities available and the clinical circumstances, e.g. haemodialysis requires anticoagulation and thus would be inappropriate in a patient with recent haemorrhage from peptic ulceration.

Prognosis
The prognosis depends on the underlying cause. In those who survive, renal function usually recovers over 2–3 weeks.

Chronic renal failure

Aetiology
The causes of chronic renal failure (CRF) are listed in Table 7.16. In European countries glomerulonephritis is the single most common cause of end-stage renal failure. In some cases the kidneys are so scarred that it is difficult to determine the underlying cause.

Table 7.16 The causes of end-stage renal failure

Glomerulonephritis	
Chronic pyelonephritis	accounting for approximately 50% of cases
Diabetes mellitus	
Renal vascular disease	
Polycystic kidneys	
Multisystem disease, e.g. SLE	
Drugs	
Amyloidosis	
Hereditary disease	

Clinical features and investigations
Clinical features and investigations are similar to those in ARF (page 243). In CRF there is nocturia and polyuria as a result of the impaired concentrating ability of the kidney. In addition there may be symptoms and signs resulting from the long-term complications of CRF:

ANAEMIA. This is present in the great majority of patients with CRF. The pathogenesis is multifactorial:

● Decreased erythropoietin production by the diseased kidney
● Depressed bone marrow activity
● Shortened red cell survival
● Increased blood loss (from the gut, during haemodialysis and as a result of repeated sampling)

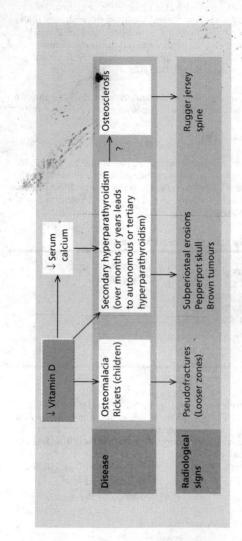

Figure 7.5 Pathogenesis and radiological features of renal osteodystrophy.

- Dietary deficiency of haematinics (iron, vitamin B_{12} and folate)

BONE DISEASE. The term 'renal osteodystrophy' embraces the various forms of bone disease that develop in CRF, i.e. osteomalacia, osteoporosis, secondary and tertiary hyperparathyroidism, and osteosclerosis. Renal phosphate retention and impaired production of 1,25-dihydroxyvitamin D (the active hormonal form of vitamin D) lead to a fall in serum calcium concentration and hence to a compensatory increase in parathyroid hormone (PTH) secretion. A sustained excess of PTH results in skeletal decalcification with the classic radiological features described in Figure 7.5. Osteosclerosis (hardening of bone) may be a result of hyperparathyroidism. Alternate bands of sclerotic and porotic bone in the vertebra produce the characteristic 'rugger jersey spine' radiographic appearance.

NEUROLOGICAL. A motor and sensory neuropathy may occur in uraemia. Most commonly the sensory neuropathy may manifest as peripheral paraesthesiae. Median nerve compression in the carpal tunnel is common and usually caused by β_2-microglobulin-related amyloidosis (see later). Autonomic dysfunction may present as postural hypotension and disturbed gastrointestinal motility. Dialysis produces an improvement in neuropathy.

CARDIOVASCULAR DISEASE. The highest mortality in CRF is from cardiovascular disease which is increased as a result of the presence of hypertension, abnormalities of lipid metabolism and vascular calcification. Renal disease also results in a form of cardiomyopathy with both systolic and diastolic dysfunction.

OTHER COMPLICATIONS. These include an increased risk of peptic ulceration, acute pancreatitis, hyperuricaemia, sexual dysfunction and failure to thrive in children.

Differentiating ARF from CRF
Distinction between ARF and CRF depends on the history, duration of symptoms and previous urinalysis or measurement of renal function. A normochromic anaemia, small kidneys on ultrasonography and the presence of renal osteodystrophy (see below) favour a chronic process.

Management
The underlying cause of renal disease should be treated aggressively wherever possible, e.g. tight metabolic control in diabetes. A low protein diet (40 g/day) and good blood pressure control may slow the decline in renal function. Of the antihypertensive agents, ACE inhibitors have particular protective effects on the glomeruli but must be used with caution in the presence of coexistent renal vascular disease.

CALCIUM AND PHOSPHATE. Hyperphosphataemia is treated by dietary restriction and oral calcium carbonate (a phosphate-binding agent). The serum calcium should be maintained in the normal range through the use of synthetic vitamin D analogues such as 1α-cholecalciferol or the vitamin D metabolite 1,25-dihydroxyvitamin D_3 (1,25-$(OH)_2D_3$).

ANAEMIA. Recombinant human erythropoietin is a very effective but expensive treatment for the anaemia of CRF and has largely replaced repeated blood transfusions. It is administered subcutaneously or intravenously three times weekly. Failure to respond may be the result of haematinic deficiency, bleeding, malignancy or infection. The disadvantages of treatment are that erythropoietin may accelerate hypertension and lead to convulsions.

ACIDOSIS. Systemic acidosis accompanies the decline in renal function and may contribute to increased serum potassium levels as well as dyspnoea and lethargy. Treatment is with oral sodium bicarbonate; the increased sodium load may exacerbate oedema and reduce blood pressure control.

PREPARATION FOR DIALYSIS AND TRANSPLANTATION. In most patients with CRF there is a progressive loss of renal function which proceeds at a constant rate for that patient (Figure 7.6). The graph of the reciprocal creatinine concentration plotted against time may be used to predict when the patient is likely to develop end-stage renal failure and so require a form of renal replacement therapy. This may be haemodialysis, chronic ambulatory peritoneal dialysis or renal transplantation.

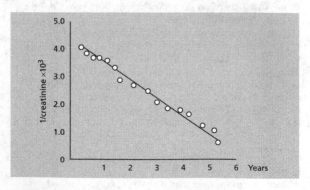

Figure 7.6 A reciprocal plot of serum creatinine against time. Such a slope is particular to an individual patient. It may be used to predict the time of onset of end-stage renal failure and thus prepare the patient for dialysis, e.g. formation of an arteriovenous fistula.

RENAL REPLACEMENT THERAPY

Dialysis

'Uraemic toxins' can be efficiently removed from the blood by the process of diffusion across a semipermeable membrane towards the low concentrations present in dialysis fluid (Figure 7.7). The gradient is maintained by replacing used dialysis fluid with fresh solution. In *haemodialysis,* blood in an extracorporeal circulation is exposed to dialysis fluid separated by an artificial semipermeable membrane. In *peritoneal dialysis* the peritoneum is used as the semipermeable membrane and dialysis fluid is instilled into the peritoneal cavity.

Haemodialysis

Adequate dialysis requires a blood flow of at least 200 ml/min and the most reliable way of achieving this is by surgical construction of an *arteriovenous fistula,* usually in the forearm. This provides a permanent and easily accessible site for insertion of needles. An adult of average size usually requires 4–5 hours of haemodialysis three times a week which may be performed in hospital or, in the UK, many patients have self-supervised home haemodialysis. All patients are anticoagulated (usually with heparin) because contact of blood with foreign surfaces activates the clotting cascade. The most common acute complication of haemodialysis is hypotension caused, in part, by excessive removal of extracellular fluid.

Peritoneal dialysis

CONTINUOUS AMBULATORY PERITONEAL DIALYSIS
Continuous ambulatory peritoneal dialysis (CAPD) requires insertion of a permanent catheter (Tenkoff catheter) into the

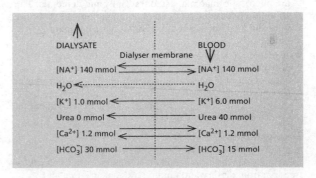

Figure 7.7 The principle of haemodialysis.

peritoneum via a subcutaneous tunnel. Up to 3 litres of dialysate are introduced and exchanged three to five times a day.

INTERMITTENT PERITONEAL DIALYSIS

Dialysate is introduced into the peritoneal cavity via a catheter and exchanged every 60–120 minutes, requiring the patient to remain in bed during treatment. It is mainly used in ARF.

Peritonitis is the most common serious complication of peritoneal dialysis. Infection with *Staph. epidermidis* accounts for 50% of cases. Treatment is with appropriate antibiotics which are often given intraperitoneally.

Haemofiltration

Haemofiltration is a form of haemodialysis used most commonly in the treatment of ARF. The procedure employs a highly permeable membrane which allows large amounts of fluid and solute to be removed from the patient. It is readily performed in intensive care units on very sick patients in whom haemodialysis or peritoneal dialysis would be very difficult.

Long-term complications of dialysis

Cardiovascular disease (as a result of atheroma) and sepsis are the leading causes of death in long-term dialysis patients. Causes of fatal sepsis include peritonitis complicating peritoneal dialysis and *Staph. aureus* infection (including endocarditis) complicating the use of indwelling access devices for haemodialysis.

- Aluminium intoxication occurs as a result of accumulation from dialysis solution and from intestinal absorption of aluminium-containing phosphate binders. Clinical features are microcytic anaemia, osteodystrophy and dementia. The condition is avoided by the use of aluminium-free dialysis fluid and avoiding aluminium-containing phosphate binders.

- Amyloidosis is the result of the accumulation and polymerization of β_2-microglobulin. This molecule (a component of HLA proteins on most cell membranes) is normally excreted by the kidneys, but is not removed by dialysis membranes. Deposition results in the carpal tunnel syndrome and joint pains, particularly of the shoulders.

Transplantation

Successful renal transplantation offers the potential for complete rehabilitation in end-stage renal failure. It allows freedom from dietary and fluid restriction, anaemia and infertility are corrected and the need for parathyroidectomy reduced. In the best centres graft survival is 80% at 10 years.

Kidneys are obtained from cadavers or, less frequently, from healthy first-degree relatives. The donor must be ABO compatible and good HLA matching increases the chances of successful transplantation. The donor kidney is placed in the iliac fossa and anastomosed to the iliac vessels of the recipient; the donor ureter is placed into the recipient's bladder. Graft rejection is reduced by giving long-term immunosuppressive treatment (unless the donor is an identical twin, i.e. genetically identical) which comprises corticosteroids, azathioprine and cyclosporin A. Antilymphocyte globulin is a potent immunosuppressive and is increasingly used in both the treatment and prevention of rejection. The complications of renal transplantation and immunosuppression include opportunistic infection (e.g. *Pneumocystis carinii*), hypertension, development of tumours (skin malignancies and lymphomas) and, occasionally, recurrence of the renal disease (e.g. Goodpasture's syndrome).

CYSTIC RENAL DISEASE

Solitary and multiple renal cysts

Renal cysts are common, particularly with advancing age. They are usually asymptomatic and discovered incidentally on ultrasonography or excretion urography performed for some other reason. Occasionally they may cause pain and/or haematuria.

Adult polycystic disease

Adult polycystic disease (APCD) is an autosomal dominantly inherited condition (gene on the short arm of chromosome 16) in which multiple cysts develop throughout both kidneys. Cysts increase in size at a variable rate with advancing age. There is progressive asymmetrical renal enlargement with compression of intervening renal tissue and progressive loss of excretory function.

Clinical features
The disease presents at any age after the second decade. Presenting symptoms include the following:

- Acute loin pain and/or haematuria as a result of haemorrhage into a cyst
- Abdominal discomfort caused by renal enlargement
- Development of hypertension or symptoms of uraemia

About 30% of patients will develop hepatic cysts which are usually clinically insignificant. More rarely cysts develop in the pancreas, spleen, ovary and other organs. Berry aneurysms of the cerebral vessels are found in 10–30% of patients; this may result in subarachnoid haemorrhage

Diagnosis
Clinical examination commonly reveals large irregular
kidneys, hypertension and possibly hepatomegaly. Definitive
diagnosis is established by ultrasonography.

Management
Treatment involves careful control of blood pressure and salt
replacement if necessary. As the disease is always
progressive, many patients will require renal replacement by
dialysis and/or transplanation. Children and siblings of
patients with the disease should be offered ultrasonographic
screening. This is carried out in the second decade because
diagnosis before this age is difficult and hypertension is rare
in the very young.

Medullary sponge kidney

Medullary sponge kidney is an uncommon condition
characterized by dilatation of the collecting ducts in the
papillae with associated stasis of urine. In severe cases there
are numerous cysts and the medullary area has a sponge-like
appearance. In 20% of patients there is hypercalciuria or
renal tubular acidosis (see page 213). The diagnosis is made
by excretion urography. Most patients have intermittent colic
with the passage of small stones or haematuria with well-
preserved renal function.

TUMOURS OF THE KIDNEY AND GENITOURINARY TRACT

Renal cell carcinoma

Renal cell carcinoma (previously called hypernephroma or
Grawitz's tumours) are the most common renal tumours in
adults, presenting most commonly in the fifth decade, with a
male to female ratio of 2:1. They arise from the proximal
tubular epithelium and may be solitary, multiple and
occasionally bilateral.

Clinical features
Haematuria, loin pain and a mass in the flank are the most
common presenting features. Other features include malaise,
weight loss, fever and occasionally polycythaemia (page 125).
Twenty-five per cent have metastases at presentation to bone,
liver and the lung, where they are often solitary and large
('cannon-ball' metastases).

Investigations
EXCRETION UROGRAPHY will reveal a space-occupying lesion
in the kidney.

ULTRASONOGRAPHY will demonstrate a solid lesion and can
assess patency of the renal vein and inferior vena cava.

CT AND MRI are useful for tumour staging.

Management
Surgery forms the mainstay of treatment. Nephrectomy is carried out unless there is bilateral involvement or the contralateral kidney functions poorly. Medroxyprogesterone may be of value in controlling metastatic disease.

Prognosis
The 5-year survival rate is 60–70% when the tumour is confined to the renal parenchyma, but less than 5% in those with distant metastases.

Urothelial tumours

The calyces, renal pelvis, ureter, bladder and urethra are lined by transitional cell epithelium. Bladder tumours are the most common form of transitional cell malignancy. These tumours occur most commonly after the age of 40 years and are four times more common in males. Predisposing factors include the following:

- Cigarette smoking
- Industrial chemicals, e.g. β-naphthylamine, benzidine
- Drugs, e.g. phenacetin, cyclophosphamide
- Chronic inflammation, e.g. schistosomiasis

Clinical features
Painless haematuria is the most common symptom of bladder cancer although pain may occur from clot retention. Transitional cell cancers of the kidney and ureters may cause haematuria and flank pain.

Investigations
CYTOLOGY of the urine may show malignant cells.

EXCRETION UROGRAPHY may show filling defects but small tumours may not be seen.

CYSTOSCOPY if no evidence of upper urinary tract pathology has been found.

Management
Pelvic and ureteric tumours are treated with surgical resection. Treatment of bladder tumours depends on the stage but options include local diathermy or cystoscopic resection, bladder resection, radiotherapy, and local and systemic chemotherapy.

DISEASES OF THE PROSTATE GLAND

Benign enlargement of the prostate gland

Benign prostatic enlargement is extremely common, occurring most commonly after the age of 60 years. There is hyperplasia of both glandular and connective tissue elements of the gland, although the aetiology of the condition remains unknown.

Clinical features

Frequency of micturition, delay in initiation of micturition and postvoiding dribbling are common symptoms. Acute urinary retention or retention with overflow incontinence may occur. An enlarged smooth prostate may be felt on rectal examination.

Investigations

Serum electrolytes and renal ultrasonography are performed to exclude renal damage resulting from obstruction. Serum prostate-specific antigen (PSA) is markedly raised in prostate cancer which may present similarly (see below).

Management

Patients with moderate symptoms can be treated medically. α-Adrenergic antagonists are most commonly used. Finasteride is an inhibitor of α-reductase (the enzyme converting testosterone to dihydrotestosterone) and may be of value in decreasing prostatic volume and increasing urine flow. Patients with severe symptoms or with dilatation of the upper urinary tract require surgery, most commonly with transurethral resection.

Prostatic carcinoma

Prostatic carcinoma is common, accounting for 7% of all cancers in men. Malignant change within the prostate is increasingly common with increasing age, being present in 80% of men aged 80 years and over. In most cases these malignant foci remain dormant.

Clinical features

Most patients present with symptoms of bladder outflow obstruction identical to those of benign prostatic hypertrophy. Patients may also present with metastases, particularly to bone. In some cases malignancy is unsuspected until histological investigation is carried out on the resected specimen after prostatectomy. Rectal examination may reveal a hard irregular gland.

Investigation

Investigation is as for benign prostatic enlargement with measurement of serum PSA. Supplemental tests include transrectal ultrasonography which helps in tumour staging and transrectal biopsy for histological confirmation.

Management

Microscopic tumour is usually managed by watchful waiting. Treatment of disease confined to the gland is radical prostatectomy or radiotherapy, both resulting in 80–90% 5-year survival. The treatment of metastatic disease depends on removing androgenic drive to the tumour. This is achieved by bilateral orchidectomy, synthetic luteinizing hormone-releasing hormone analogues, e.g. goserelin, or antiandrogens, e.g. cyproterone acetate.

URINARY INCONTINENCE

Normal bladder physiology

As the bladder fills with urine two factors act to ensure continence until the bladder is next emptied:

1. Intravesical pressure remains low as a result of stretching of the bladder wall and the stability of the bladder muscle (detrusor) which does not contract involuntarily
2. The sphincter mechanisms of the bladder neck and urethral muscles

At the onset of voiding the sphincters relax (mediated by decreased sympathetic activity) and the detrusor muscle contracts (mediated by increased parasympathetic activity). Overall control and coordination of micturition is by higher brain centres which include the cerebral cortex and the pons.

STRESS INCONTINENCE

Stress incontinence occurs as a result of sphincter weakness which may be iatrogenic in men (post-prostactectomy) or the result of childbirth in women. There is a small leak of urine when intra-abdominal pressure rises, e.g. with coughing, laughing or standing up. In young women pelvic floor exercises may help the problem. In postmenopausal women the contributing factor of urethral atrophy may be helped by oestrogen creams.

URGE INCONTINENCE

In urge incontinence there is a strong desire to void and the patient may be unable to hold his or her urine. The usual cause is detrusor instability which occurs most often in women and the aetiology is not known. Mild cases may respond to bladder retraining (gradually increasing the time interval between voiding). More severe cases are treated with anticholinergic agents which decrease detrusor excitability. Less commonly, urge incontinence is caused by bladder hypersensitivity from local pathology (e.g. UTI, bladder stones, tumours) and treatment is then of the underlying cause.

OVERFLOW INCONTINENCE

Overflow incontinence is most often seen in men with prostatic hypertrophy causing outflow obstruction. There is leakage of small amounts of urine and, on abdominal examination, the distended bladder is felt rising out of the pelvis. If the obstruction is not relieved then renal damage will develop.

NEUROLOGICAL CAUSES

These are usually apparent from the history and examination which reveal accompanying neurological deficits. Brain-stem damage, e.g. trauma, may lead to incoordination of detrusor muscle activity and sphincter relaxation so that the two contract together during voiding. This results in a high-pressure system with the risk of obstructive uropathy. The aim of treatment is to reduce outflow pressure either with α-adrenergic blockers or by sphincterotomy. Autonomic neuropathy, e.g. in diabetic individuals, decreases detrusor excitability and results in a distended atonic bladder with a large residual urine which is liable to infection. Permanent catheterization may be necessary.

In elderly people incontinence may be the result of a combination of factors: diuretic treatment, dementia (antisocial incontinence) and difficulty in getting to the toilet because of immobility.

A DICTIONARY OF TERMS: RENAL MEDICINE

OLIGURIA is the excretion of less than 300 ml of urine per day. Causes are extreme dehydration, hypotension, obstruction and acute renal failure.

ANURIA is a condition in which no urine is voided. It suggests complete urinary tract obstruction.

POLYURIA is a persistent large increase in urine output, usually associated with nocturia. The causes are polydipsia, solute diuresis (e.g. hyperglycaemia with glycosuria), diabetes insipidus and chronic renal failure.

GLOMERULAR FILTRATION RATE (GFR). This is the most widely used test of renal function. In routine clinical practice the most reliable index of GFR is measurement of endogenous creatinine clearance which is calculated from a 24-hour urine collection and measurement of a single serum creatinine value during the 24 hours.

EXCRETION UROGRAPHY (INTRAVENOUS UROGRAPHY [IVU] OR INTRAVENOUS PYELOGRAPHY [IVP]). Serial radiographs are taken of the kidney and the full length of the abdomen, following intravenous injection of contrast, usually an organic iodine-containing medium.

ANTEROGRADE PYELOGRAPHY. A catheter is passed percutaneously into a renal calyx. This allows injection of contrast medium to demonstrate upper urinary tract obstruction and drainage of an obstructed system.

MICTURATING CYSTOSCOPY is used mainly for the evaluation of vesicoureteric reflux in children. Contrast medium is instilled into the bladder via a catheter, and the ureters and kidneys are then screened during micturition.

- Static scanning is performed after an intravenous injection of technetium-99m-labelled dimercaptosuccinic acid (^{99m}Tc-DMSA) which is taken up by the kidneys. It allows an assessment of the *function* of each kidney
- Dynamic scanning is performed after an intravenous injection of technetium-99m-labelled diethylenetriamine pentaacetate (^{99m}Tc-DTPA) which is taken up by the kidneys and excreted into the collecting systems, ureter and bladder. It allows assessment of *renal blood flow*, *estimation of GFR* and *assessment of obstructive uropathy*

FINAL MEDICINE EXAMINATION: RENAL MEDICINE

Three topics occur commonly and with almost equal frequency. These are chronic renal failure, the causes and management of acute renal failure, and the causes of proteinuria and the nephrotic syndrome.

1. What are the clinical features of 'end-stage' renal failure, and how may it be treated?

2. What clinical and other evidence would lead you to suspect the diagnosis of chronic renal failure in a 50-year-old man? How would you determine the cause of renal failure?

3. In a patient presenting with a plasma creatinine of 500 mmol/l which features would suggest that the renal failure is chronic, rather than acute?

   (a) Reduced renal size detected by ultrasonography.

   (b) A urine sodium concentration of less than 10 mmol/l.

   (c) Elevated serum alkaline phosphatase and subperiosteal erosions on radiograph of the hands.

   (d) A haemoglobin of 14 g/l.

   (e) The presence of ureteric obstruction on renal ultrasonography.

   (f) Evidence of polyneuropathy.

4. List the causes of renal failure resulting from poor perfusion of the kidneys. What are the clinical and laboratory features?

5. What factors contribute to the development of acute renal failure in a patient with multiple injuries following a road traffic accident? Outline your management during the first 24–48 hours.

6. Write short notes on the causes and differential diagnosis of acute renal failure.

7. A 50-year-old man presents with bilateral ankle swelling and is found to have a serum albumin of 28 g/l. Discuss the differential diagnosis in terms of history, possible physical findings and further helpful investigations.

Other questions are:

8. Describe how patients with glomerulonephritis may present.

9. Discuss the presentation and management of recurrent urinary tract infection in women.

ANSWERS

1. The clinical features and treatment of end-stage renal failure are discussed on page 245.

2. A patient presenting with any of the complications discussed on page 245 would lead you to suspect chronic renal failure (CRF), but the usual ways in which patients present are with hypertension, nocturia and polyuria or with symptoms of anaemia. The investigations for renal failure are discussed on page 243. A renal biopsy is performed in patients with normal sized kidneys. Small kidneys are technically difficult to biopsy, histological investigations are hard to interpret and at this late stage the prognosis would not be influenced by treatment of the underlying condition.

3. (a), (c) and (f) suggest chronic renal failure. The urine sodium concentration is very low and this may occur with prerenal acute renal failure (when the kidney is conserving sodium) and with chronic renal failure when the concentrating ability of the kidney is lost and large amounts of dilute urine are produced. The normal Hb is in favour of acute renal failure.

4. This is discussed on page 241. Poor perfusion of the kidneys is usually caused by hypovolaemia; other causes include pump failure (cardiogenic shock) or shock resulting from a pulmonary embolism. The clinical and laboratory features are described on pages 241 and 242.

5. The most probable cause is poor renal perfusion secondary to hypovolaemia from blood loss. Other causes include rhabdomyolysis (extensive crush injury to muscle leads to release of myoglobin which is directly toxic to renal tubular cells), ruptured urethra (suspect with severe pelvic fractures and anuria) and

later septicaemia and drugs (e.g. gentamicin). Initial management is to correct hypovolaemia with whole blood (measurement of central venous pressure will guide replacement) followed by a bolus of frusemide (page 241) if the patient remains oliguric. If urine output does not increase and urethral rupture is excluded as the cause of oliguria, then treatment is of established acute tubular necrosis (page 244). The investigations must include measurement of the muscle enzyme creatinine phosphokinase.

6. This is discussed on page 240.

7. Hypoalbuminaemia is caused by decreased synthesis (liver disease) or increased loss from the kidneys or rarely the gut (protein-losing enteropathy). The main differential is between liver disease and nephrotic syndrome. Important points in the history are risk factors for chronic liver disease (e.g. alcohol, intravenous drug abuse) and diseases that may be associated with nephrotic syndrome (e.g. diabetes, chronic infections and amyloidosis, drugs). Signs of chronic liver disease must be looked for on physical examination. Initial investigations are liver biochemistry and stix test of the urine for protein.

8. This is discussed on page 224.

9. This is discussed on pages 229–230.

CHAPTER 8

Cardiovascular Disease

Common presenting symptoms of heart disease

The common symptoms of heart disease are chest pain, breathlessness, palpitations and syncope.

Chest pain

Acute chest pain or discomfort is a common presenting symptom of cardiovascular disease and must be differentiated from non-cardiac causes. The site of pain, its character, radiation and associated symptoms will often point to the cause (Table 8.1).

Dyspnoea

Dyspnoea is an abnormal awareness of breathing. The causes are discussed on page 323. Left heart failure is the most common cardiac cause of exertional dyspnoea which may be accompanied by orthopnoea (breathlessness on lying flat).

Palpitations

A palpitation is an awareness of the heart beat. The normal heart beat is sensed when the patients is anxious, excited, exercising or lying on the left side. In other circumstances it usually indicates a cardiac arrhythmia, commonly ectopic beats or a paroxysmal tachycardia (page 269).

Syncope and dizziness

Syncope means a temporary impairment of consciousness as a result of cerebral ischaemia. There are many causes (page 478) but the most common is a simple faint. The cardiac causes of syncope are the result of either very fast (e.g. ventricular tachycardia) or very slow heart rates (e.g. complete heart block) which are unable to maintain an adequate cardiac output. Attacks occur suddenly and without warning. They last only 1 or 2 minutes with complete recovery in seconds (compare epilepsy where complete recovery may be delayed for some hours). Obstruction to ventricular outflow also causes syncope (e.g. aortic stenosis, hypertrophic cardiomyopathy) which typically occurs on exercise when the requirements for increased cardiac output cannot be met.

Other symptoms

Tiredness, lethargy and exertional fatigue occur with cardiac failure and result from poor perfusion of brain and skeletal muscle. Heart failure also causes salt and water retention

Table 8.1 Common causes of chest pain

Usually retrosternal

Angina pectoris	Crushing pain on exercise, relieved by rest. May radiate to jaw or arms
Myocardial infarction	Similar in character to angina but more severe, occurs at rest, lasts longer
Pericarditis	Sharp pain aggravated by movement, respiration and changes in posture
Aortic dissection	Severe tearing chest pain which radiates to the back
Reflux oesophagitis	Occurs at night and when bending or lying down. Pain may radiate into the neck

Other sites

Pulmonary infarct	Typically pleuritic in nature, i.e. sharp, well-localized pain aggravated by inspiration, coughing and
Pneumonia	movement
Pneumothorax	
Costochondritis	Musculoskeletal pain is usually a sharp, well-localized pain and with a tender area on palpation
Fractured rib	

leading to oedema, which in ambulant patients is most prominent over the ankles. In severe cases it may involve the genitalia and thighs.

The electrocardiogram

The electrocardiogram (ECG) is a recording from the body surface of the electrical activity of the heart. The standard ECG has 12 leads:

- Chest leads, V1–V6, which look at the heart in a *horizontal plane* (Figure 8.1)
- Limb leads which look at the heart in a *vertical plane* (Figure 8.2). Limb leads are unipolar (AVR, AVL and AVF) or bipolar (I, II, III)

The ECG machine is arranged so that when a depolarization wave spreads towards a lead the needle moves upwards, and when it spreads away from the lead the needle moves downwards.

The ECG wave form and definitions (Figure 8.3)

The P wave is the first deflection and caused by atrial depolarization. When abnormal it may be:

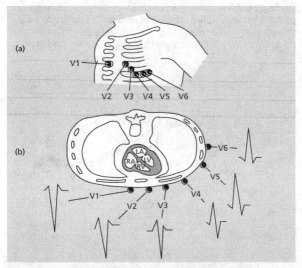

Figure 8.1 (a) The V leads are attached to the chest wall overlying the intercostal spaces as shown: V4 in the midclavicular line, V5 in the anterior axillary line, V6 in the midaxillary line. (b) Leads V1 and V2 look at the right ventricle, V3 and V4 look at the interventricular septum, V5 and V6 look at the left ventricle. The normal QRS complex in each lead is shown.

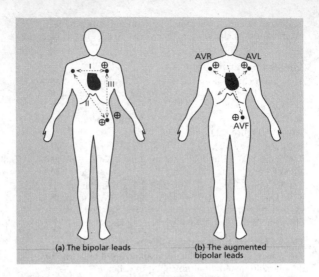

Figure 8.2 Lead I is derived from electrodes on the right arm (negative pole) and left arm (positive pole), lead II is derived from electrodes on the right arm (negative pole) and left leg (positive pole) and lead III from electrodes on the left arm (negative pole) and the left leg (positive pole).

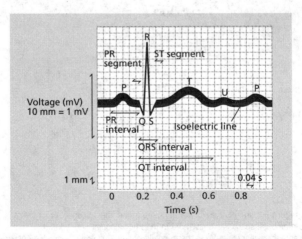

Figure 8.3 The waves and elaboration of the normal ECG. (Modified from Goldman, M J, 1976, *Principles of Clinical Electrocardiography*, 3rd edn, Los Alto, Longman.)

- Broad and notched (> 0.12 s) in left atrial enlargement ('P mitrale', e.g. mitral stenosis)
- Tall and peaked (> 2.5 mm) in right atrial enlargement ('P pulmonale', e.g. pulmonary hypertension)
- Replaced by flutter or fibrillation waves (page 272)
- Absent in sinoatrial block (page 268)

The QRS complex represents ventricular depolarization:

- A negative (downward) deflection preceding an R wave is called a Q wave. Normal Q waves are small and narrow; deep, wide Q waves (except in AVR and V1) indicate myocardial infarction (page 289)
- A deflection upwards is called an R wave whether or not it is preceded by a Q wave
- A negative deflection following an R wave is termed an S wave

Ventricular depolarization starts in the septum and spreads from left to right (Figure 8.4). Subsequently the main free walls of the ventricles are depolarized. Thus, in the right ventricular leads (V1 and V2), the first deflection is upwards (R wave) as the septal depolarization wave spreads towards those leads. The second deflection is downwards (S wave) as the bigger left ventricle (in which depolarization is spreading away) outweighs the effect of the right ventricle (Figure 8.1).

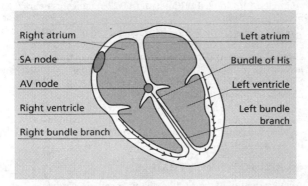

Figure 8.4 In normal circumstances only the specialized conducting tissues of the heart undergo spontaneous depolarization (*automaticity*) which initiates an action potential. The sinus node discharges more rapidly than the other cells and is the normal pacemaker of the heart. The impulse generated by the sinus node spreads first through the atria producing atrial systole and then through the atrioventricular node to the His–Purkinje system producing ventricular systole.

The opposite pattern is seen in the left ventricular leads (V5 and V6) with an initial downwards deflection (small Q wave reflecting septal depolarization) followed by a large R wave caused by left ventricular depolarization.

Left ventricular hypertrophy (e.g. with systemic hypertension) causes a tall R wave (> 25 mm) in the left ventricular leads and deep S waves in the right ventricular leads. There may also be ST segment depression and T wave inversion.

Right ventricular hypertrophy (e.g. in pulmonary hypertension) causes tall R waves in the right ventricular leads.

The QRS duration reflects the time that excitation takes to spread through the ventricle. A wide QRS complex (> 0.10 s) occurs if conduction is delayed, e.g. with right or left bundle-branch block, or if conduction is through abnormal pathways, e.g. ventricular ectopic.

T waves result from ventricular repolarization. In general the direction of the T wave is the same as that of the QRS complex. Inverted T waves occur in many conditions and although usually abnormal they are a non-specific finding.

The PR interval is measured from the start of the P wave to the start of the QRS complex. It is the time taken for excitation to pass from the sinus node, through the atrium, atrioventricular node and His–Purkinje system to the ventricle. A prolonged PR interval (> 0.22 s) indicates heart block (page 268).

The ST segment is the period between the end of the QRS complex and the start of the T wave. ST elevation (> 1 mm above the isoelectric line) occurs in the early stages of myocardial infarction (page 289) and with acute pericarditis. ST segment depression (> 0.5 mm below the isoelectric line) indicates myocardial ischaemia.

The heart rate. At normal paper speed (25 mm/s in the UK) each 'big square' is 0.2 s. The heart rate (if the rhythm is regular) is calculated by counting the number of big squares between consecutive R waves and dividing into 300.

CARDIAC ARRHYTHMIAS

An abnormality of the cardiac rhythm is called a cardiac arrhythmia. Such a disturbance of rhythm may cause sudden death, syncope, dizziness, palpitations or no symptoms at all. Paroxysmal arrhythmias may not be detected on a single ECG recording. Twenty-four-hour ambulatory ECG monitoring (continuous recording for 24 hours) and event recorders (portable device activated by the patient to record the ECG when symptoms occur) are outpatient investigations often used to detect arrhythmias causing intermittent symptoms.

There are two main types of arrhythmia:

- *Bradycardia* where the heart rate is slow (< 60 beats/min). The slower the heart rate the more probable that the arrhythmia will be symptomatic
- *Tachycardia,* where the heart rate is fast (> 100 beats/min). Tachycardias are more likely to be symptomatic when the arrhythmia is fast and sustained. They are subdivided into *supraventricular tachycardias*, which arise from the atrium or the atrioventricular junction, and *ventricular tachycardias*, which arise from the ventricles

Arrhythmias and conduction disturbances complicating acute myocardial infarction are discussed on page 293.

Sinus rhythms
Sinus arrhythmia

Fluctuations of autonomic tone result in phasic changes in the sinus discharge rate. Thus, during inspiration, para-sympathetic tone falls and the heart rate quickens, and on expiration the heart rate falls. This variation is normal, particularly in children and young adults.

Sinus bradycardia

Sinus bradycardia is normal during sleep and in well-trained athletes. During the acute phase of a myocardial infarction it often reflects ischaemia of the sinus node. Other causes include hypothermia, hypothyroidism, cholestatic jaundice, raised intracranial pressure, and drug therapy with β-blockers, digitalis and other antiarrhythmic drugs. Patients with symptomatic bradycardia are treated with a permanent cardiac pacemaker. Intravenous atropine is used in the acute situation.

Sinus tachycardia

Sinus tachycardia is a physiological response during exercise and excitement. It may also occur with fever, anaemia, cardiac failure, thyrotoxicosis and drugs (e.g. catecholamines and atropine). Treatment is aimed at correction of the underlying cause. If necessary, β-blockers may be used to slow the sinus rate, but not in heart failure.

Pathological bradycardias

There are two main forms of severe bradycardia: sinus node disease and atrioventricular block.

Sinus node disease (sick sinus syndrome)

Most cases of chronic sinus node disease are the result of idiopathic fibrosis occurring in elderly people. Bradycardia is caused by intermittent failure of sinus node depolarization or failure of the sinus impulse to propagate through the perinodal tissue to the atria. This is seen on the ECG as a long pause between consecutive P waves (> 2 s). The slow heart rate predisposes to ectopic pacemaker activity and tachyarrhythmias are common (tachybrady syndrome).

Insertion of a permanent pacemaker is only indicated in symptomatic patients to prevent dizzy spells and blackouts. Antiarrhythmic drugs are used to treat tachycardias. Thromboembolism is common in sick sinus syndrome and patients should receive anticoagulation treatment unless there is a contraindication.

Atrioventricular block

There are three forms: first-degree heart block, second-degree (partial) block and third-degree (complete) block. The common causes are ischaemic heart disease, cardiomyopathy and, particularly in elderly people, fibrosis of the conducting tissue.

● *First-degree atrioventricular (AV) block* is the result of delayed atrioventricular conduction and reflected by a prolonged PR interval on the ECG. No change in heart rate occurs and treatment is unnecessary

● *Second-degree (partial AV) block* occurs when some atrial impulses fail to reach the ventricles. Asymptomatic patients require no treatment other than careful follow-up because there may be progression to complete heart block. Symptomatic patients are treated with insertion of a permanent pacemaker. There are three forms (Figure 8.5):
  – MOBITZ I BLOCK (Wenckebach's phenomenon) in which the PR interval gradually increases, culminating in a dropped beat
  – MOBITZ II BLOCK occurs when a dropped QRS complex is not preceded by progressive PR prolongation
  – A 2:1 or 3:1 block occurs when every second or third P wave conducts to the ventricles. A 4:1 or 5:1 block can also occur

● *Third-degree (complete) AV block*. There is no association between atrial and ventricular activity and ventricular contractions are maintained by a spontaneous escape rhythm (usually about 40/min) from an automatic centre below the site of block. The ECG shows regular P waves and QRS complexes which occur independently of one another. The usual symptoms are dizziness and blackouts (Stokes–Adams attacks). If the ventricular rate is very slow, cardiac failure may occur. Insertion of a permanent pacemaker is usually required for complete heart block. In

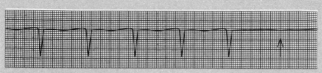

(a) Wenckebach (Mobitz type I)

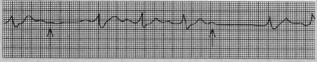

(b) Mobitz type II

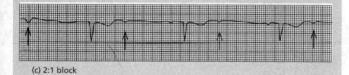

(c) 2:1 block

Figure 8.5 Three varieties of second-degree atrioventricular (AV) block. Arrows indicate non-conducting P waves.

the acute situation, e.g. myocardial infarction, recovery may be expected and intravenous atropine or a temporary pacemaker may be all that is necessary

Intraventricular conduction disturbances

The intraventricular conduction system consists of the His bundle, the right and left bundle branches and the anterosuperior and posteroinferior divisions of the left bundle-branch block. Complete block of a bundle branch is associated with a wider QRS complex (0.12 s or more). The shape of the QRS depends on whether the right or the left bundle is blocked.

Pathological tachycardias

Mechanisms of arrhythmia production

The mechanisms responsible for most tachyarrhythmias are *abnormal automaticity* and *re-entry mechanisms*.

ABNORMAL AUTOMATICITY

Arrhythmias arise if there is enhanced automaticity of the normal conducting tissue or automaticity is acquired by damaged cells of the atria or ventricles; this causes ectopic beats and, if sustained, tachyarrhythmias.

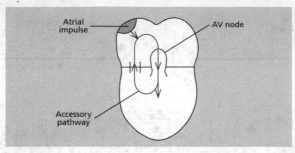

Figure 8.6 A re-entry circuit. The impulse is conducted normally through the AV node and initiates ventricular depolarization. In certain circumstances the accessory pathway is able to transmit the impulse *retrogradely* back into the atria, thus completing a circuit and initiating a self-sustaining re-entry tachycardia.

RE-ENTRY

Re-entry may occur if there are two separate pathways for impulse conduction (Figure 8.6).

Atrial tachyarrhythmias

Ectopic beats, tachycardia, flutter and fibrillation may all arise from the atrial myocardium. They share common aetiologies, which are listed in Table 8.2.

Table 8.2 Causes of atrial arrhythmias

Ischaemic heart disease
Rheumatic heart disease
Thyrotoxicosis
Cardiomyopathy
Lone atrial fibrillation (i.e. no cause discovered)
Wolff–Parkinson–White syndrome
Pneumonia
Atrial septal defect
Carcinoma of the bronchus
Pericarditis
Pulmonary embolus
Acute and chronic alcohol abuse

ATRIAL ECTOPIC BEATS

These are caused by premature discharge of an ectopic atrial focus. On the ECG this produces an early and abnormal P wave, usually followed by a normal QRS complex. Treatment is not usually required unless they cause troublesome palpitations or are responsible for provoking more significant arrhythmias.

ATRIAL FLUTTER

Atrial flutter is almost always associated with organic disease of the heart. The atrial rate is usually about 300 beats/min. The AV node usually conducts every second flutter beat giving a ventricular rate of 150 beats/min. The ECG (Figure 8.7(a)) characteristically shows 'saw tooth' flutter waves (F waves) which are most clearly seen when AV conduction is transiently impaired by carotid sinus massage or drugs. Treatment of an acute paroxysm is electrical cardioversion. Prophylaxis is achieved with class 1a, 1c or III drugs (Table 8.3). Rate control of a chronic arrhythmia is with AV nodal blocking drugs, e.g. digoxin.

ATRIAL FIBRILLATION

This is a common arrhythmia, occurring in between 5% and 10% of patients over 65 years of age. It also occurs, particularly in a paroxysmal form, in younger patients. Atrial activity is chaotic and mechanically ineffective. The AV node conducts a proportion of the atrial impulses to produce an irregular ventricular response. There are no clear P waves on the ECG (Figure 8.7(b)), only a fine oscillation of the baseline (so-called fibrillation or f waves). When atrial fibrillation arises in an apparently normal heart it is sometimes possible to convert to sinus rhythm either electrically (by cardioversion) or chemically (with class 1a, 1c or III drugs). When atrial fibrillation is caused by an acute precipitating event such as alcohol toxicity, chest infection or thyrotoxicosis, the underlying cause should be treated initially. Chronic atrial fibrillation occurring in a diseased heart will usually not respond to cardioversion, and treatment is by control of the ventricular rate, usually with digoxin. Most patients receive anticoagulation treatment because of the risk of atrial thrombosis and embolism.

Junctional tachycardia

Junctional tachycardias are paroxysmal in nature and usually occur in the absence of structural heart disease. They are re-entrant arrhythmias caused by an abnormal pathway in the AV node or by an accessory pathway (bundle of Kent) as in the Wolff–Parkinson–White syndrome (Figure 8.8). The usual history is of a sudden onset of fast (140–280/min) regular palpitations. On the ECG the P waves may be seen very close to the QRS complex or are not seen at all. The QRS complex is usually of normal shape because, as with other supraventricular arrhythmias, the ventricles are activated in the normal way, down the bundle of His. Occasionally the QRS complex is wide, because of a rate-related bundle branch block, and it may be difficult to distinguish from ventricular tachycardia.

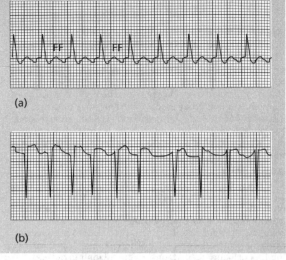

Figure 8.7 (a) Atrial flutter. The flutter waves are marked with an F, only half of which are transmitted to the ventricles. (b) Atrial fibrillation. There are no P waves, the ventricular response is fast and irregular.

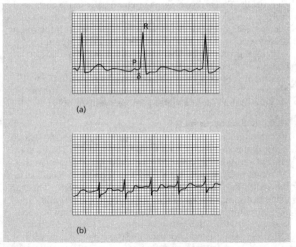

Figure 8.8 (a) An ECG showing Wolff–Parkinson–White syndrome. During sinus rhythm electrical impulses are conducted quickly through the abnormal pathway resulting in a short PR interval and a slurred proximal limb of the QRS complex (δ wave). (b) A trace demonstrating the paroxysmal tachycardia which may result from this syndrome.

Table 8.3 Vaughan Williams classification of antiarrhythmic drug therapy

Class	Mechanism of action	Individual drugs
Ia	Membrane-stabilizing action	Quinidine, procainamide, disopyramide
Ib		Lignocaine, mexiletine
1c		Flecainide, propafenone
II	β-Adrenergic blockers	Metoprolol, atenolol, propranolol
III	Increases refractory period of conducting system	Amiodarone, sotalol, bretyllium
IV	Calcium channel blocking agents	Verapamil, diltiazem

Adenosine and digoxin are other antiarrhythmic drugs which do not fit into this classification.
These drugs all have proarrhythmic side effects (among others) and should be used with caution.
All except amiodarone are negatively inotropic and may exacerbate heart failure.

Termination of an attack:

● Manoeuvres that increase vagal stimulation of the sinus node: carotid sinus massage, ocular pressure or the Valsalva manoeuvre

● Drug treatment: adenosine is a very short-acting, AV nodal blocking drug given as a bolus dose intravenously. It will terminate most junctional tachycardias. Transient side effects include complete heart block, hypotension, nausea and bronchospasm. An alternative treatment is intravenous verapamil (contraindicated if the QRS complex is wide and thus differentiation from ventricular tachycardia is difficult)

● DC cardioversion

Prophylaxis:

● Radiofrequency ablation of the accessory pathway via a cardiac catheter

● Flecainide, disopyramide, amiodarone and β-blockers are the drugs most commonly used

Ventricular arrhythmias

Ventricular ectopic beats, (extrasystoles, premature beats)

Ventricular ectopic beats may be asymptomatic or patients may complain of extra beats, missed beats or heavy beats. The ectopic electrical activity is not conducted to the ventricles through the normal conducting tissue, and thus the QRS complex on the ECG is widened with a bizarre configuration (Figure 8.9). In normal individuals ectopic beats are of no significance but treatment is sometimes given for symptoms. In patients with heart disease they are associated with a worse prognosis but it has not been shown that suppression alters this.

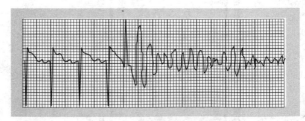

Figure 8.9 A rhythm strip demonstrating four beats of sinus rhythm followed by a ventricular ectopic beat that initiates ventricular fibrillation. The ST segment is elevated owing to acute myocardial infarction.

Ventricular tachycardia

Ventricular tachycardia and ventricular fibrillation are usually associated with underlying heart disease, e.g. ischaemia, cardiomyopathy and hypertensive heart disease. Ventricular tachycardia is defined as three or more consecutive ventricular beats occurring at a rate of 120/min or more. The ECG shows a rapid ventricular rhythm with broad abnormal QRS complexes which can sometimes be confused with a broad complex junctional tachycardia. Ventricular tachycardia may produce severe hypotension when urgent DC cardioversion is necessary. If there is no haemodynamic compromise, treatment is usually with intravenous lignocaine. Prophylaxis is usually with mexiletine, disopyramide, flecainide or amiodarone. Patients who are refractory to all medical treatment may need an implantable defibrillator (a small device implanted behind rectus abdominus and connected to the heart; it recognizes ventricular tachycardia or ventricular fibrillation and automatically delivers a defibrillation shock to the heart).

Ventricular fibrillation

This is a very rapid and irregular ventricular activation (Figure 8.9) with no mechanical effect and hence no cardiac output. Ventricular fibrillation rarely reverts spontaneously and management is immediate cardioversion (see Cardiac arrest).

Cardiac arrest

In cardiac arrest there is no effective cardiac output. The patient is unconscious, apnoeic with absent arterial pulses (best felt in the carotid artery in the neck). Irreversible brain damage occurs within 3 minutes if an adequate circulation is not established.

Prognosis of cardiac arrest

In many patients resuscitation is unsuccessful, particularly in those who collapse out of hospital and are brought into hospital in an arrested state. In patients who are successfully resuscitated the prognosis is often poor because they have severe underlying heart disease. The exception is those patients who are successfully resuscitated from a ventricular fibrillation arrest in the early stages of myocardial infarction, when the prognosis is much the same as for other patients with an infarct.

CARDIAC FAILURE

Cardiac failure occurs when, in spite of normal venous pressures, the heart is unable to maintain sufficient cardiac output to meet the demands of the body. It is a common

Basic life support (ABC)

Call for help

Thump the chest firmly over the sternum; occasionally reverts VT/VF to sinus rhythm

AIRWAY

• Place patient on his or her back on a firm surface
• Remove obstructing material, e.g. blood and vomit
• Open the airway by flexing the neck and extending the head

BREATHING

• Give four breaths in quick succession of mouth-to-mouth resuscitation. Watch for the rise and fall of the patient's chest indicating adequate ventilation

CIRCULATION

• Circulation is achieved by external chest compression
• The heel of one hand is placed over the lower half of the victim's sternum and the heel of the second hand is placed over the first with straight arms the sternum is depressed by 1–2 inches

Compressions: respiration   = 5:1 if two rescuers, 60 compressions per minute
                              = 15:2 if one rescuer, 80 compressions per minute

Advanced life support

• Institute as soon as help arrives, continue cardiac massage throughout except during defibrillation
• Defibrillate immediately (ventricular fibrillation is the most common arrhythmia in cardiac arrest)
• Give 100% O_2 via Ambu-Bag, intubate as soon as possible and initiate positive pressure ventilation
• Establish intravenous access and connect ECG leads
• If intravenous access not possible give drugs via endotracheal tube (3 × intravenous dose)

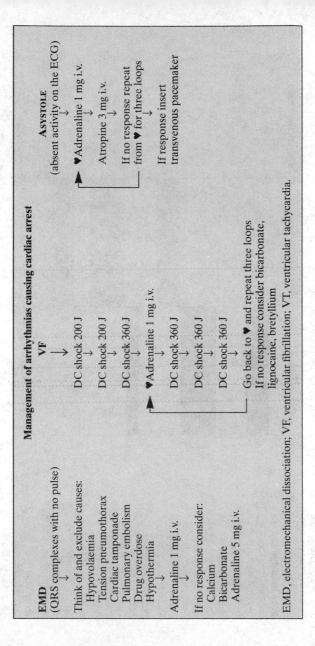

Management of arrhythmias causing cardiac arrest

EMD
(QRS complexes with no pulse)

Think of and exclude causes:
Hypovolaemia
Tension pneumothorax
Cardiac tamponade
Pulmonary embolism
Drug overdose
Hypothermia
↓
♥Adrenaline 1 mg i.v.
↓
If no response consider:
Calcium
Bicarbonate
Adrenaline 5 mg i.v.

VF
→ DC shock 200 J
→ DC shock 200 J
→ DC shock 360 J
→ ♥Adrenaline 1 mg i.v.
→ DC shock 360 J
→ DC shock 360 J
→ DC shock 360 J
→ Go back to ♥ and repeat three loops
If no response consider bicarbonate, lignocaine, bretyllium

ASYSTOLE
(absent activity on the ECG)
→ ♥Adrenaline 1 mg i.v.
→ Atropine 3 mg i.v.
→ If no response repeat from ♥ for three loops
→ If response insert transvenous pacemaker

EMD, electromechanical dissociation; VF, ventricular fibrillation; VT, ventricular tachycardia.

Table 8.4 Causes of heart failure: the predominant clinical picture is indicated

	Left heart failure	Right heart failure	Biventricular failure
Myocardial dysfunction			
Ischaemic heart disease	■		
Systemic hypertension	■		
Dilated cardiomyopathy			▨
Volume overload			
Ventricular septal defect	■		
Mitral regurgitation	■		
Aortic regurgitation	■		
Pulmonary regurgitation		▨	
Tricuspid regurgitation		▨	
Outflow obstruction			
Aortic stenosis	■		
Pulmonary hypertension		▨	
Pulmonary embolism		▨	
Pulmonary stenosis		▨	
Compromised ventricular filling			
Constrictive pericarditis		▨	
Pericardial tamponade		▨	
Restrictive cardiomyopathy			▨
Arrhythmia			
Severe bradycardia			▨
Severe tachycardia			▨

condition with an estimated incidence of 10 per 1000 in those over the age of 65 years.

Aetiology

Low-output failure develops when the heart is unable to generate adequate output.

High-output failure is uncommon and occurs when the heart is unable to meet the perfusion requirements of tissue metabolism in spite of an increased cardiac output. Causes include anaemia, systemic to pulmonary shunts, thyrotoxicosis, Paget's disease and beri-beri (page 502).

Pathophysiology

When the heart fails, compensatory mechanisms attempt to maintain cardiac output and peripheral perfusion. However, as heart failure progresses the mechanisms are overwhelmed and become pathophysiological.

NEUROHUMORAL ACTIVATION

Sympathetic nervous system. Activation of the sympathetic nervous system improves ventricular function by increasing heart rate and myocardial contractility. Constriction of venous capacitance vessels redistributes flow centrally and the increased venous return to the heart (preload) further augments ventricular function by the Starling mechanism (Figure 8.10). Sympathetic stimulation, however, also leads to arteriolar constriction, thus increasing the afterload and reducing cardiac output.

Renin–angiotensin system. The fall in cardiac output and increased sympathetic tone lead to diminished renal perfusion, activation of the renin–angiotensin system and hence increased fluid retention. Salt and water retention further increases venous pressure and maintains stroke volume by the Starling mechanism (Figure 8.10). As salt and water retention increases, however, peripheral and pulmonary congestion cause oedema and contribute to dyspnoea. Angiotensin II also causes arteriolar constriction, thus increasing the afterload and the work of the heart.

Atrial natriuretic peptides (ANPs). Distension of the atria leads to release of these peptides which have vasodilator and natriuretic properties. The effect of their action may represent a beneficial, albeit inadequate, compensatory response leading to reduced cardiac load (preload and afterload).

VENTRICULAR DILATATION

Myocardial failure leads to a reduction of the volume of blood ejected with each heart beat, and thus an increase in the volume of blood remaining after systole. The increased diastolic volume stretches the myocardial fibres and, as Starling's law would suggest, myocardial contraction is

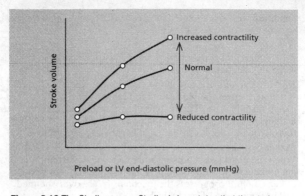

Figure 8.10 The Starling curve. Starling's law states that the stroke volume is directly proportional to the diastolic filling (i.e. the preload or ventricular end-diastolic pressure). Changes in contractility (e.g. increased with sympathetic stimulation) and afterload have an independent effect on ventricular function. In heart failure (bottom line) the ventricular function curve is relatively flat so that increasing the preload has only a small effect on cardiac output.

restored. Once cardiac failure is established, however, the compensatory effects of cardiac dilatation become limited by the flattened contour of Starling's curve. Eventually the increased venous pressure contributes to the development of pulmonary and peripheral oedema. In addition, as ventricular diameter increases greater tension is required in the myocardium to expel a given volume of blood, and oxygen requirements increase.

Clinical features
It is clinically useful to divide heart failure into the syndromes of right, left and biventricular (congestive) cardiac failure but, it is rare for any one part of the heart to fail in isolation.

RIGHT HEART FAILURE
The most frequent cause of chronic right heart failure is secondary to left heart failure. Other causes are indicated in Table 8.4. There is jugular venous distension, hepatomegaly and dependent pitting oedema (over the ankles and calves in ambulant patients, over the sacrum in bed-bound patients). Less frequently ascites occurs. Non-specific features are fatigue, anorexia and nausea.

LEFT HEART FAILURE
The most common cause of left heart failure is ischaemic heart disease. Other causes are listed in Table 8.4. The

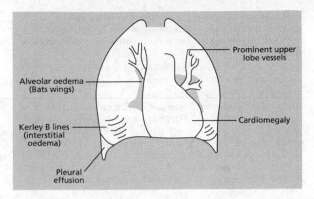

Figure 8.11 The chest radiograph in left ventricular failure.

clinical features are largely the result of pulmonary congestion with symptoms of fatigue, exertional dyspnoea, orthopnoea and paroxysmal nocturnal dyspnoea (page 323). The signs are tachypnoea, tachycardia, a displaced apex beat and basal lung crackles. A third heart sound occurs and is the result of rapid filling of the ventricles. In severe failure dilatation of the mitral annulus results in functional mitral regurgitation.

BIVENTRICULAR FAILURE (CONGESTIVE)
This term is used variously but is best restricted to cases where right heart failure is a result of pre-existing left heart failure. The physical signs are thus a combination of the above syndromes.

ACUTE HEART FAILURE
This is a medical emergency with left or right heart failure developing over minutes or hours.

Investigations
Heart failure is usually a clinical diagnosis and investigations are performed to confirm this and identify the underlying cause.

RADIOLOGY. The chest radiograph is usually unhelpful in determining the cause of heart failure but shows cardiac enlargement (cardiothoracic ratio > 50% on a postero-anterior chest film) and characteristic appearances in left heart failure (Figure 8.11).

ECG may show evidence of underlying causes, e.g. arrhythmias, ischaemia, left ventricular hypertrophy in hypertension.

ECHOCARDIOGRAPHY is the most useful diagnostic investigation. It allows an assessment of left ventricular function, identifies valvular abnormalities and pericardial effusion.

BLOOD TESTS. These include full blood count, urea and electrolytes, and sometimes thyroid function tests.

OTHER INVESTIGATIONS. Radionuclide ventriculography (technetium-99m scan) is sometimes performed to quantitate ejection fraction (page 317), and identify sections of the left ventricular wall that contract abnormally. Cardiac catheterization is usually reserved for the small proportion of patients with a surgically correctable lesion, e.g. aortic or mitral valve abnormalities. In such cases the surgeon requires precise definition of the lesion and demonstration of the coronary anatomy.

Treatment of chronic heart failure
Treatment is aimed at relieving symptoms, retarding disease progression and improving survival (Table 8.5).

Table 8.5 The management of chronic heart failure

General measures
Reduction of physical activity, thus reducing the work of the heart
Bed rest in severe cases
Reduction of salt intake – no added salt at meals
Avoid alcohol which has negative inotropic effects

Correct aggravating factors
Arrhythmias, anaemia, hypertension, pulmonary infections

Specific therapy

Drugs	Diuretics
	Vasodilators
	Inotropic agents
	Antiarrhythmic drugs
Surgery	Replacement of diseased valves
	Cardiac transplantation
	Repair of ventricular septal defect

DRUG TREATMENT
Diuretics
Diuretics are the first line of treatment in patients with heart failure. They act by promoting renal sodium excretion with enhanced water excretion as a secondary effect. The resulting loss of fluid reduces ventricular filling pressures (preload) and thus decreases pulmonary and systemic congestion.

● The thiazide diuretics, e.g. bendrofluazide, are mild diuretics which inhibit sodium reabsorption in the distal renal tubule. The exception is metolazone which causes a profound diuresis and is used in severe heart failure unresponsive to large doses of loop diuretics. The major side effects of the thiazides are hypokalaemia, hyperglycaemia and hyperuricaemia.

- Loop diuretics, e.g. frusemide and bumetanide, inhibit sodium reabsorption in the ascending limb of the loop of Henle. They are potent diuretics used in moderate/severe heart failure. These drugs produce marked renal potassium loss and promote hyperuricaemia.

- Potassium-sparing diuretics are relatively ineffective when given alone and are usually prescribed in combination with a loop diuretic. Spironolactone, an aldosterone antagonist, is the most effective but causes gynaecomastia. Amiloride and triamterene have a direct action on ion transport in the distal renal tubule. They increase sodium loss and reduce potassium loss.

VASODILATOR THERAPY

Vasodilators have a beneficial effect in heart failure by reducing venous constriction (reduction of preload) and arteriolar constriction (reduction of afterload).

- Angiotensin-converting enzyme (ACE) inhibitors, e.g. captopril and enalapril, enhance renal salt and water excretion and increase cardiac output by reducing afterload. They not only improve symptoms, but also limit the development of progressive heart failure and prolong survival, and should be prescribed to all patients with heart failure in addition to diuretic therapy. The major side effect is first-dose hypotension. Patients at greatest risk are those with severe heart failure receiving large doses of diuretics. These patients should omit the preceding dose of diuretic and begin therapy in hospital with the first dose given at bedtime. Other side effects are prerenal renal failure (page 240), hyperkalaemia, persistent cough and rash.

- Other vasodilators: the combination of isosorbide mononitrate (a venodilator) and hydralazine (arteriolar vasodilator) improves symptoms and survival and is used when ACE inhibitors are not tolerated or their use is contraindicated. Other vasodilators, used less commonly, include prazosin, nitroprusside and the calcium channel antagonists.

INOTROPIC AGENTS

- Digoxin is of undoubted benefit in patients with congestive heart failure and atrial fibrillation. Studies are continuing to assess the role of digoxin in patients with heart failure and sinus rhythm.

- β-Adrenergic agonists: dopamine and dobutamine are only effective intravenously and are used in the treatment of cardiogenic shock (page 285) or occasionally as a temporary measure in a patient with severe intractable heart failure. Xamoterol is a β-blocking drug with high intrinsic sympathomimetic activity. It is effective in improving cardiac performance but its use is limited because it may precipitate an acute deterioration in patients with severe heart failure.

ANTIARRHYTHMIC DRUGS

Arrhythmias are frequent in heart failure and are implicated in sudden death. There is conflicting evidence that prophylactic antiarrhythmic drugs improve survival and treatment should be restricted to those who are symptomatic from arrhythmias. Most antiarrhythmic drugs, with the exception of amiodarone, are negatively inotropic and may cause worsening heart failure.

Prognosis

There is usually a gradual deterioration necessitating increased doses of diuretics and sometimes admission to hospital. The prognosis is poor in those with severe heart failure (i.e. breathless at rest or on minimal exertion) with a 1-year survival rate of 50%. Younger patients with severe intractable heart failure are usually referred to a specialist cardiothoracic centre for consideration of cardiac transplantation. Eighty per cent of patients survive 1 year; early deaths are the result of operative mortality, organ rejection and overwhelming infection secondary to immunosuppressive treatment. After this time the greatest threat to health is accelerated coronary atherosclerosis the cause of which is unknown.

Pulmonary oedema

This is a very frightening life-threatening emergency characterized by rapid onset of extreme breathlessness. Causes include acute, severe left ventricular failure (e.g. myocardial infarction, acute mitral and aortic regurgitation), mitral stenosis and arrhythmias. An acute elevation of left atrial pressure produces corresponding elevation of the pulmonary capillary pressure and increased transudation of fluid into the pulmonary interstitium and alveoli (*cardiogenic pulmonary oedema*). *Non-cardiogenic pulmonary oedema* is seen in very ill patients and is discussed on pages 372–373.

Clinical features

The patient is acutely breathless, wheezing and anxious. There is usually a cough productive of frothy blood-tinged (pink) sputum. Increased sympathoadrenal activity leads to profuse sweating, tachycardia and peripheral circulatory shutdown. On auscultation there is a gallop rhythm, and wheezes and crackles are heard throughout the chest.

Investigations

RADIOLOGY. The chest radiograph shows distension of the upper lobe veins (indicating a raised pulmonary venous pressure) and bilateral perihilar shadowing in a 'butterfly' or 'bat's wing' distribution caused by alveolar fluid. Interstitial pulmonary oedema produces Kerley B lines (Figure 8.11).

ECG AND CARDIAC ENZYMES may show evidence of a myocardial infarction as the precipitating event.

ARTERIAL BLOOD GASES show hypoxaemia. Initially the $P_a\text{CO}_2$ falls because of overbreathing but later increases because of impaired gas exchange.

Management

In many cases the patient is so unwell that treatment (Table 8.6) must begin before investigations are completed. Intravenous opiates, e.g. morphine, and diuretics are the first-line agents. Morphine relieves dyspnoea by a combination of vasodilatation and relief of anxiety. Respiratory depression occurs with large doses (> 10 mg). Diuretics produce immediate vasodilatation in addition to the more delayed diuretic response. If the patient does not improve, intravenous nitrates may be used to reduce the preload. Occasionally, in severe cases which do not respond to treatment, ventilation is necessary.

Table 8.6 Management of pulmonary oedema

Sit the patient up
60% oxygen by face mask
Frusemide 40–80 mg i.v.
Morphine 2.5–10 mg i.v. + an antiemetic, e.g. metoclopramide 10 mg i.v.

Treat exacerbating and precipitating factors
   Hypertension
   Pulmonary infection
   Arrhythmias

Consider
   Intravenous nitrate infusion
   Intravenous aminophylline (250 mg over 10 min) to relieve bronchospasm

Cardiogenic shock

Cardiogenic shock (pump failure) is an extreme type of cardiac failure characterized by hypotension, a low cardiac output and signs of poor tissue perfusion, such as oliguria, cold extremities and poor cerebral function. Its most common cause is massive myocardial infarction and management is discussed on page 366.

ISCHAEMIC HEART DISEASE

Myocardial ischaemia results from an imbalance between the supply of oxygen to cardiac muscle and myocardial demand. The most common cause is coronary artery atheroma which results in a fixed obstruction to coronary blood flow. Other causes of ischaemia include anaemia, aortic stenosis and coronary artery thrombosis, spasm or rarely arteritis (e.g. polyarteritis).

Atheroma consists of atherosclerotic plaques (seen *post mortem* as raised yellow–white areas covering the intimal surface of the artery) rich in cholesterol and other lipids, surrounded by smooth muscle cells and fibrous tissue. A number of risk factors have been identified for coronary atherosclerosis, some of which are irreversible and some which can be modified.

Irreversible risk factors

AGE
Atherosclerosis is progressively more common as age increases. It rarely presents in the young except in familial hyperlipidaemia (page 439).

SEX
Men are more often affected than women, although the incidence in women after the menopause is similar to men. The cause for this difference is poorly understood.

FAMILY HISTORY
Coronary artery disease is often present in several members of the same family. It is unclear, however, whether family history is an independent risk factor as so many other factors are familial. Recently, it has been shown that a specific genotype associated with higher circulating ACE levels may be significantly more common in patients who have had a myocardial infarction than in age-matched controls.

Potentially reversible risk factors

HYPERLIPIDAEMIA
Elevated cholesterol levels increase the risk of premature atherosclerosis, particularly when associated with low levels of high-density lipoproteins (HDLs). High triglyceride levels are less definitely linked with coronary atheroma.

SMOKING
The risk of developing coronary artery disease is directly related to the number of cigarettes smoked in men. This relationship, although still important, is less clear in women. Stopping smoking reduces the risk but does not eliminate it.

HYPERTENSION
Both elevated systolic and diastolic hypertension are linked to an increased incidence of coronary artery disease.

OTHER FACTORS
Diabetes mellitus, lack of exercise and obesity have all been linked to an increased incidence of atheroma.

Angina
Angina pectoris is a descriptive term for chest pain arising from the heart as a result of myocardial ischaemia.

Clinical features
Angina is usually described as central crushing chest pain, coming on with exertion and relieved by rest within a few minutes. It is often exacerbated by cold weather, anger and excitement, and it frequently radiates to the arms and neck. Variants of classic angina include *decubitus angina* (occurs on lying down) and *Prinzmetal's angina* (caused by coronary artery spasm). Angina which is increasing rapidly in severity, occurs at rest or is of recent onset is known as *unstable angina* (crescendo angina or preinfarction angina). Physical examination in patients with angina is often normal but must include a search for risk factors (e.g. hypertension and xanthelasma occurring in hyperlipidaemia).

Diagnosis
The primary diagnosis is clinical because investigations may be normal. Occasionally chest wall pain or oesophageal reflux causes diagnostic confusion (page 31).

Investigations
RESTING ECG typically shows ST segment depression and T-wave flattening or inversion during an attack. The ECG is normal in up to 80% of people between attacks.

EXERCISE ECG testing is positive in about 75% of people with severe coronary artery disease; a normal test does not exclude the diagnosis. ST segment depression (> 1 mm) at a low workload or a paradoxical fall in blood pressure with exercise usually indicates severe coronary artery disease, and these patients should be considered for coronary angiography.

RADIO-ISOTOPE STUDIES (thallium-201 perfusion scan, page 317) are particularly useful in those with equivocal exercise tests. Ischaemic areas show as 'cold spots' during exercise.

CORONARY ANGIOGRAPHY is occasionally used when the cause of pain is unclear. More commonly the test is performed to delineate the exact coronary anatomy before consideration of coronary artery surgery.

Management
GENERAL
Underlying problems such as obesity, thyrotoxicosis, anaemia

or aortic valve disease should be treated. Smoking should be discouraged, other risk factors evaluated and steps made to correct them.

MEDICAL

Acute attacks are treated with sublingual glyceryl trinitrate. Patients should be encouraged to use glyceryl trinitrate before exertion rather than waiting for the pain to develop. The main side effect is a severe bursting headache which is relieved by inactivating the tablet either by swallowing or spitting it out.

When angina occurs frequently or with only modest exertion, regular prophylactic therapy should be employed. Nitrates or β-blockers are usually used as first-line agents and calcium antagonists added if necessary. Aspirin is also given to reduce the risk of subsequent myocardial infarction.

● Nitrates reduce venous and intracardiac diastolic pressure, reduce impedance to the emptying of the left ventricle and dilate coronary arteries. They are available in a variety of slow-release preparations, including infiltrated skin plasters, buccal pellets and long-acting oral nitrate preparations, e.g. isosorbide mononitrate, isosorbide dinitrate. The major side effect is headache which tends to diminish with continued use

● β-Adrenergic blocking drugs, e.g. metoprolol and atenolol, reduce heart rate and the force of ventricular contraction, both of which reduce the myocardial oxygen demand. They are contraindicated in heart failure and asthma, and relatively contraindicated in peripheral vascular disease

● Calcium antagonists, e.g. nifedipine, diltiazem and verapamil, block calcium influx into the cell and the utilization of calcium within the cell. They relax the coronary arteries and reduce the force of left ventricular contraction, thus reducing oxygen demand. The side effects (postural dizziness, headache, ankle oedema) are the result of systemic vasodilatation

When angina persists or worsens in spite of general measures and optimal medical treatment, patients should be considered for coronary artery bypass grafting (CABG) or angioplasty.

CORONARY ANGIOPLASTY: localized atheromatous lesions are dilated at cardiac catheterization using small inflatable balloons. This technique is widely applied for angina resulting from isolated, proximal, non-calcified, atheromatous plaques. Complications include acute occlusion in 2–4% of cases (necessitating full surgical back-up) and restenosis (30% in the first 6 months).

SURGERY: the saphenous vein from the leg, or the internal mammary artery from the chest, is anastomosed to the proximal aorta and coronary artery distal to the obstruction. Surgery successfully relieves angina in about 90% of cases and, when performed for left main stem obstruction or three-vessel disease, an improved lifespan and quality of life can be expected. Operative mortality rate is less than 1%. Most patients eventually develop recurrence of angina because of accelerated atherosclerosis in the graft (particularly vein grafts) which can be treated by stenting.

MANAGEMENT OF UNSTABLE ANGINA

This is a medical emergency with a risk of myocardial infarction if treatment is inadequate. Management involves admission to hospital, bed rest, intravenous heparin, aspirin and a combination of all three antianginal drugs. Early coronary angiography with a view to surgery or angioplasty is recommended, particularly when symptoms continue in spite of optimum medical treatment.

Prognosis

The average annual mortality rate for patients with stable angina is 4% a year, with the worst prognosis in those with extensive coronary artery disease.

Myocardial infarction

Myocardial infarction is now the most common cause of death in developed countries. It is almost always the result of rupture of an atherosclerotic plaque with development of thrombosis and total occlusion of the artery.

Clinical features

Central chest pain similar to that occurring in angina is the most common presenting symptom. Unlike angina it usually occurs at rest, is more severe and lasts for some hours. The pain is often associated with restlessness, sweating, nausea and vomiting. There are usually few signs unless complications develop (see later) although the patient often appears pale, sweaty and grey. About 20% of patients have no pain, and such 'silent' infarctions either go unnoticed or present with hypotension, arrhythmias or pulmonary oedema. This occurs most commonly in elderly patients or those with diabetes or hypertension.

Investigations

In most cases the diagnosis is made on the basis of the clinical history and early ECG appearances. Serial changes (over 3 days) in the ECG and cardiac enzymes confirm the diagnosis and allow an assessment of infarct size (on the magnitude of the enzyme rise and extent of ECG changes). A normal ECG in the early stages does not exclude the diagnosis.

ECG usually shows a characteristic pattern. Within hours there is ST segment elevation followed by T-wave flattening or inversion (Figure 8.12). Pathological Q waves are broad

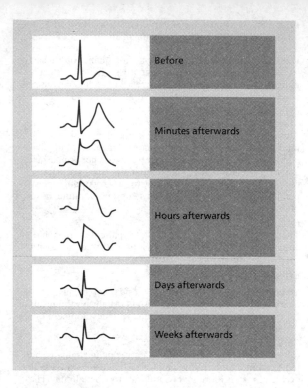

Figure 8.12 ECG evolution of myocardial infarction. After the first few minutes the T waves become tall, pointed and upright, and there is ST segment elevation. After the first few hours the T waves invert, the R wave voltage is decreased and Q waves develop. After a few days the ST segment returns to normal. After weeks or months the T wave may return to upright but the Q wave remains.

(>1 mm) and deep (>2 mm, or >25% of the amplitude of the following R wave) negative deflections that start the QRS complex. They are seen once full-thickness infarction (as opposed to non-Q-wave or subendocardial infarction) has occurred. They develop because the infarcted muscle is electrically silent so the recording leads 'look through' the infarcted area. This means that the electrical activity being recorded (on the opposite ventricular wall) is moving away from the electrode and is therefore negative.

Typically ECG changes are confined to the leads that 'face' the infarct. Leads II, III and AVF are involved in inferior

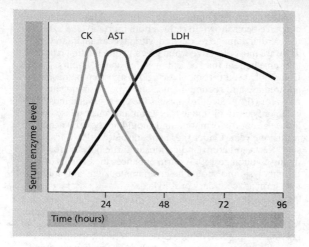

Figure 8.13 The enzyme profile in acute myocardial infarction. CK, creatinine kinase; AST, aspartate aminotransferase; LDH, lactate dehydrogenase.

infarcts, I, II and AVL in lateral infarcts, and V2–V6 in anterior infarcts. As there are no posterior leads, a posterior wall infarct is diagnosed by the appearance of reciprocal changes in V1 and V2 (i.e. the development of tall initial R waves, ST segment depression and tall upright T waves).

CARDIAC ENZYMES: necrotic cardiac muscle releases enzymes into the systemic circulation. The most commonly measured are creatinine kinase (CK), aspartate aminotransferase (AST) and lactic dehydrogenase (LDH), although none is specific for cardiac muscle damage. There is a characteristic time course for the release of the enzymes into the blood, and thus they are usually measured for 3 days following suspected myocardial infarction (Figure 8.13).

OTHER INVESTIGATIONS

These include a chest radiograph, full blood count, serum urea and electrolytes, blood glucose and lipids (lipids taken within the first 12 hours reflect preinfarction levels, but after this time they are altered for up to 6 weeks).

Management

The aims of treatment are relief of pain, limitation of infarct size and treatment of complications.

FIBRINOLYTIC THERAPY should be given immediately. These agents can achieve early reperfusion in 50–70% of patients (compared to a spontaneous reperfusion of less than 30%) and have been shown to reduce both mortality and extent of myocardial damage associated with myocardial infarction. They are most effective when given within the first 6 hours but some benefit may be achieved for up to 24 hours. Commonly used thrombolytic agents are streptokinase, anistreplase and recombinant tissue-type plasminogen activator (tPA). Streptokinase is the cheapest and most commonly used, although this agent and anistreplase both induce antibody formation and should not be used again within one year. Under these circumstances, tPA is used. The side effects and contraindications to thrombolysis are discussed on page 140. Aspirin enhances the benefits of thrombolysis and should be given immediately and continued long term as secondary prophylaxis.

TRANSFER TO CORONARY CARE UNIT (CCU). Fatal cardiac arrhythmias occur most commonly in the period immediately following the infarct. Patients should be admitted as soon as possible to the CCU where close ECG monitoring and immediate resuscitation are possible. The management of myocardial infarction is summarized in Table 8.7.

Table 8.7 Management of myocardial infarction

Immediate management
- Pain relief
  Diamorphine (5–10 mg i.v. or s.c.) + an antiemetic, e.g. metoclopramide 10 mg i.v.
- Streptokinase: 1.5 million units over 1 hour by intravenous infusion pump
- 60% oxygen by face mask
- Aspirin: 150 mg orally stat, 150 mg daily thereafter
- Heparin: 5000 units 8-hourly s.c. until mobile to prevent deep venous thrombosis
- Treat complications (pp. 293–294)

Subsequent management of uncomplicated infarction
- Mobilize gradually after 24–48 hours if pain-free
- Initiate secondary prevention therapy
  Aspirin 150 mg daily
  β-Blockers, e.g. atenolol, metoprolol orally
  Stop smoking
  Treat hyperlipidaemia and other risk factors
- Consider ACE inhibitors: they reduce mortality and prevent development of heart failure where echocardiography shows reduced ejection fraction (< 35%)
- Submaximal exercise test just before hospital discharge
  Consider angiography if ischaemic ECG changes or chest pain in early stages
- Discharge from hospital after 7 days

Complications
The common complications are listed in Table 8.8.

Table 8.8 Complications associated with myocardial infarction

Early (within 2–3 days)	Late
Arrhythmias	Dressler's syndrome
Heart block	Shoulder–hand syndrome
Heart failure	Ventricular aneurysm
Myocardial rupture (usually fatal)	Recurrent arrhythmias
Pericarditis	Thromboembolism
Thromboembolism	

DISTURBANCE OF RATE, RHYTHM AND CONDUCTION
Atrial arrhythmias
Sinus tachycardia is common; treatment is that of the underlying cause, particularly pain, anxiety and heart failure. Sinus bradycardia is especially associated with inferior myocardial infarction and treatment with intravenous atropine is given if there are associated symptoms. Atrial fibrillation occurs in about 10% of patients and is usually a transient rhythm disturbance which can be treated with digoxin until return to sinus rhythm.

Ventricular arrhythmias
Ventricular ectopic beats are very common and may precede the development of ventricular tachycardia or fibrillation. Anti-arrhythmic drug treatment has not, however, been shown to affect progression to these more serious arrhythmias. Ventricular tachycardia may degenerate into ventricular fibrillation or may itself produce shock or cardiac failure. Treatment of VT is with intravenous lignocaine or direct current cardioversion if there is severe hypotension. Ventricular fibrillation may be primary (occurring in the first 24–48 hours) or secondary (occurring late after infarction and associated with large infarcts and heart failure). Treatment is with immediate DC cardioversion. Late ventricular fibrillation is associated with a poor prognosis and a high incidence of sudden death.

Heart block occurring with inferior infarction is common and usually resolves spontaneously. Some patients respond to intravenous atropine but a temporary pacemaker may be necessary if the rhythm is very slow or producing symptoms.

Complete heart block occurring with anterior wall infarction indicates involvement of both bundle branches by extensive myocardial necrosis and hence a very poor prognosis.

CARDIAC FAILURE in a mild form occurs in up to 40% of patients following myocardial infarction and may be prevented by administration of ACE inhibitors, e.g. captopril. Extensive infarction may cause pulmonary oedema (page 284), which may also occur following rupture of the ventricular septum or mitral valve papillary muscle. Both conditions present with worsening heart failure, a systolic thrill and a loud pansystolic murmur. Mortality is high and urgent surgical correction is often needed.

THROMBOEMBOLISM occurs most commonly following prolonged bed rest and with cardiac failure. Pulmonary embolism may result from a deep vein thrombosis or a ventricular mural thrombus.

PERICARDITIS is characterized by sharp chest pain and a pericardial rub. Treatment is with non-steroidal anti-inflammatory drugs (NSAIDs) until spontaneous resolution occurs within 1–2 days. Late pericarditis (Dressler's syndrome) is rare; usually it occurs weeks to months after infarction and corticosteroids may be necessary in some patients.

SHOULDER–HAND SYNDROME consists of pain and immobility of the left arm in the weeks and months following an acute myocardial infarction. Treatment is with early mobilization and physiotherapy.

Rehabilitation
If possible full mobilization should be achieved within 1 week to 10 days, and strong reassurance and encouragement supplied. At 6 weeks patients may resume driving and consider return to work at 3 months.

Mortality from myocardial infarction
Approximately 75% of deaths occur within the first 24 hours, many before reaching hospital. Of those who leave hospital alive, about 15–25% die in the first year, and thereafter the annual mortality rate is 5–10%.

Rheumatic fever

Rheumatic fever is an inflammatory disease that occurs in children and young adults (the first attack usually occurs between 5 and 15 years of age) as a result of infection with group A streptococci. It is a complication of less than 1% of streptococcal pharyngitis, developing 2–3 weeks after the onset of sore throat. It is thought to develop because of an autoimmune reaction triggered by the streptococci and is not the result of direct infection of the heart.

Epidemiology
The incidence in developed countries has decreased dramatically since the 1920s. This is thought to be the result of improved sanitation, a change in the virulence of the organism and use of antibiotics.

Clinical features

The disease presents suddenly with fever, joint pains and loss of appetite. The major clinical features are as follows:

- Carditis affects all three layers of the heart and presents with changing heart murmurs, mitral and aortic regurgitation, cardiac failure and chest pain caused by pericarditis
- Polyarthritis is classically a fleeting polyarthritis affecting the large joints, e.g. knees, ankles and elbows
- Sydenham's chorea (or St Vitus' dance) is involvement of the central nervous system that develops late after a streptococcal infection. Sufferers are noticeably 'fidgety' and display spasmodic, unintentional movements
- Skin manifestations include erythema marginatum (transient pink coalescent rings develop on the trunk) and small non-tender subcutaneous nodules which occur over tendons, joints and bony prominences

Investigations

BLOOD COUNT shows a leukocytosis and a raised ESR.

The diagnosis is based on the *revised Duckett Jones criteria* [CM p. 591] which depends on the combination of certain clinical features and evidence of recent streptococcal infection.

Treatment

Treatment is with complete bed rest, high-dose aspirin and penicillin to eradicate residual streptococcal infection.

Chronic rheumatic heart disease

More than 50% of those who suffer acute rheumatic fever *with carditis* will later (after 10–20 years) develop chronic rheumatic valvular disease, predominantly affecting the mitral and aortic valves (see below).

VALVULAR HEART DISEASE

Cardiac valves may be incompetent (regurgitant) or stenotic or both. Abnormal valves produce turbulent blood flow which is heard as a murmur on auscultation. Murmurs may sometimes be heard with normal hearts ('innocent murmurs') often reflecting a hyperdynamic circulation, e.g. in pregnancy, anaemia and thyrotoxicosis. Benign murmurs are soft, midsystolic, may vary with posture and are not associated with signs of organic heart disease.

Diagnosis of valve dysfunction is made clinically and by echocardiography and cardiac catheterization. Treatment is both medical and surgical; this may be valve replacement, valve repair (some incompetent valves) or valvotomy (the fused cusps of a stenotic valve are separated along the commissures). The timing of surgery is critical and must not be delayed until there is irreversible ventricular dysfunction or pulmonary hypertension.

Prosthetic heart valves

Prosthetic heart valves may be pig valves (a porcine xenograft) which tend to degenerate within about 10 years but patients do not need anticoagulation. These valves are often used in elderly patients. Mechanical valves last much longer but patients need lifelong anticoagulation. There are several types: a ball-and-cage design (Starr–Edwards valve), a tilting disc (Björk–Shiley valve) or a double tilting disc (St Jude valve). Valves are susceptible to infection and thrombosis and may produce haemolysis or systemic emboli.

The individual valve lesions are considered separately below but disease may affect more than one valve (particularly in rheumatic heart disease and endocarditis) when a combination of clinical features are produced. Damaged and prosthetic valves are at risk of infection during an episode of bacteraemia (e.g. after tooth extraction, endoscopy and surgery) and patients should always receive prophylactic antibiotics to cover the procedure (page 305).

Mitral stenosis

Aetiology

Almost all mitral stenosis is the result of rheumatic heart disease, although a history of rheumatic fever is not always obtained.

Pathophysiology

Reduction in the area of the normal valve orifice impairs left ventricular filling which results in a reduced cardiac output particularly during exercise. To maintain left ventricular filling there is a progressive increase in left atrial pressure resulting in left atrial hypertrophy and dilatation. The dilated atrium is prone to fibrillate which further compromises ventricular filling. Thrombus may form in the dilated fibrillating atrium and give rise to systemic emboli (e.g. to the brain resulting in a stroke). Chronically elevated left atrial pressure leads to an increase in pulmonary capillary pressure and pulmonary oedema. An increase in tone in the pulmonary arterioles leads to pulmonary hypertension may eventually lead to right ventricular hypertrophy and failure.

Symptoms

Usually symptoms do not occur until the valve orifice is moderately stenosed (area of < 2 cm). Exertional dyspnoea which becomes progressively more severe is usually the first symptom. Cough productive of blood-tinged sputum is common and, occasionally, frank haemoptysis may occur. The onset of atrial fibrillation may produce an abrupt deterioration and precipitate pulmonary oedema.

Signs

- Cyanotic or dusky-pink discoloration on the upper cheeks produces the so-called mitral facies or malar flush
- The pulse is often irregular as a result of atrial fibrillation
- The apex beat is 'tapping' in quality as a result of a combination of a palpable first heart sound and left ventricular backward displacement produced by an enlarging right ventricle
- Auscultation at the apex reveals a loud first heart sound, an opening snap (when the mitral valve opens) in early diastole, followed by a rumbling middiastolic murmur. If the patient is in sinus rhythm the murmur becomes louder when atrial systole occurs (presystolic accentuation) caused by increased flow across the narrowed valve

There may be features of pulmonary hypertension and right ventricular hypertrophy (loud second heart sound, parasternal heave) and eventually in severe mitral stenosis the signs of right heart failure develop (page 280).

Investigations

Investigations are performed to confirm the diagnosis, to estimate the severity of valve stenosis and to look for pulmonary hypertension.

CHEST X-RAY appearances of mitral stenosis are indicated diagramatically in Figure 8.14.

ECG usually shows atrial fibrillation. In patients in sinus rhythm atrial hypertrophy results in a bifid P wave ('P mitrale').

ECHOCARDIOGRAPHY is the most useful investigation to confirm the diagnosis. Doppler studies will assess the severity of stenosis by estimating the valve area and the pressure gradient across it.

CARDIAC CATHETERIZATION is required only if echo-cardiography is inadequate or if there is coexisting heart disease (e.g. coronary heart disease). The typical finding is a diastolic pressure that is higher in the left atrium than in the left ventricle.

Management

GENERAL: treatment is often not required for mild mitral stenosis. Complications are treated medically, e.g. digoxin for atrial fibrillation, diuretics for heart failure and anti-coagulation (in patients in atrial fibrillation) to prevent clot formation and embolization.

SPECIFIC: if pulmonary congestion persists, in spite of medical therapy, then surgical relief of mitral stenosis is indicated.

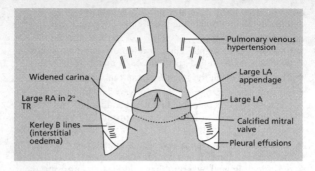

Figure 8.14 The chest radiograph in mitral stenosis. LA, left atrium; RA, right atrium; TR, tricuspid regurgitation.

The techniques used include valvotomy or mitral valve replacement. A new technique, trans-septal balloon valvotomy, involves dilatation of the valve with a balloon passed into the left atrium via the femoral vein and right atrium, and puncture of the interatrial septum.

Valvotomy is only suitable for non-calcified competent valves.

Mitral regurgitation

Aetiology
Rheumatic heart disease and a prolapsing mitral valve are the most common causes of mitral regurgitation (Table 8.9).

Table 8.9 Causes of mitral regurgitation

Rheumatic heart disease
Mitral valve prolapse
Infective endocarditis*
Ruptured chordae tendinae*
Rupture of the papillary muscle* complicating myocardial infarction
Papillary muscle dysfunction
Dilating left ventricular disease causing 'functional' mitral regurgitation
Hypertrophic cardiomyopathy
Rarely: systemic lupus erythematosus, Marfan's syndrome,
Ehlers–Danlos syndrome

* These disorders may produce acute regurgitation.

Pathophysiology
The circulatory changes depend on the speed of onset and severity of regurgitation. Long-standing regurgitation produces little increase in the left atrial pressure because flow is accommodated by an enlarged left atrium. With acute

mitral regurgitation, there is a rise in left atrial pressure resulting in an increase in pulmonary venous pressure and pulmonary oedema.

Symptoms
Acute regurgitation presents as pulmonary oedema. Chronic regurgitation causes progressive exertional dyspnoea, fatigue and lethargy (resulting from reduced cardiac output). Thromboembolism is less common than with mitral stenosis although infective endocarditis is much more common.

Signs
- The apex is displaced laterally with a diffuse thrusting character
- The first heart sound is soft
- There is a pansystolic murmur loudest at the apex radiating widely over the precordium and into the axillae
- A third heart sound is often present, caused by rapid filling of the dilated left ventricle in early diastole

Investigations
CHEST RADIOGRAPHY shows signs of left atrial enlargement and an increased heart size resulting from left ventricular dilatation.

ECG shows P mitrale before the onset of atrial fibrillation. There may be evidence of left ventricular hypertrophy (page 265).

ECHOCARDIOGRAPHY confirms the diagnosis and will usually indicate the cause. Doppler studies allow an assessment of the severity of the lesion.

CARDIAC CATHETERIZATION is necessary only when there is uncertainty about the haemodynamic significance of the lesion.

Management
In mild cases, treatment with diuretics or ACE inhibitors is employed as symptoms dictate. Progress is monitored with serial echocardiograms; progressive ventricular enlargement is usually an indication for surgical intervention with either valve repair or replacement.

Prolapsing mitral valve (floppy mitral valve, Barlow's syndrome)

This is a common condition often seen in young women. One or more of the mitral valve's leaflets prolapses back into the left atrium during ventricular systole, producing mitral regurgitation in a few cases.

Aetiology
The cause is unknown but it may be associated with Marfan's syndrome, thyrotoxicosis, rheumatic or ischaemic heart disease.

Clinical features

Most patients are asymptomatic. Atypical chest pain is the most common symptom. Some patients complain of palpitations caused by atrial and ventricular arrhythmias. The typical finding on examination is a midsystolic click which may be followed by a murmur. Occasionally there are features of mitral regurgitation.

Investigation

Echocardiography is diagnostic and shows the prolapsing valve cusps.

Management

Chest pain and palpitations are treated with β-blockers. Anticoagulation to prevent thromboembolism is indicated if there is significant mitral regurgitation and atrial fibrillation.

Aortic stenosis

Aetiology

There are three causes of aortic valve stenosis:

- Calcification of a congenital bicuspid valve
- Rheumatic heart disease
- Senile degeneration and calcification

Pathophysiology

Obstruction to left ventricular emptying results in left ventricular hypertrophy. In turn this results in relative ischaemia of the myocardium and consequent angina, arrhythmias and eventually left ventricular failure.

Symptoms

There are usually no symptoms until the stenosis is moderately severe (when the aortic orifice is reduced to a third of its normal size). Angina, dyspnoea and exercise-induced syncope are the main symptoms. Ventricular arrhythmias may cause sudden death.

Signs

Typical signs of aortic stenosis are:

- A slow rising pulse, best felt in the carotid arteries in the neck
- A thrusting non-displaced apex beat
- A harsh ejection systolic murmur (palpated as a thrill) loudest in the aortic area and radiating into the neck. The murmur may be preceded by an ejection click which is the result of the sudden opening of a deformed but mobile valve

Investigations

CHEST RADIOGRAPH shows a normal heart size, prominence of the ascending aorta (poststenotic dilatation) and there may be valvular calcification.

ECG may show evidence of left ventricular hypertrophy.

ECHOCARDIOGRAPHY is diagnostic in most cases. The aortic valve is thickened, calcified and immobile. Doppler studies allow an assessment of the pressure gradient across the valve during systole.

CARDIAC CATHETERIZATION is used primarily to exclude coexisting coronary artery disease (which may also cause the angina).

Management

The treatment of symptomatic aortic stenosis is with aortic valve replacement. Untreated, the prognosis is poor with a life expectancy of less than 3 years. Asymptomatic severe aortic stenosis (pressure gradient across the valve > 50 mmHg during systole) is also usually treated by valve replacement. Otherwise asymptomatic patients are advised to avoid strenuous exercise and are followed up carefully. Antibiotic prophylaxis against infective endocarditis is essential.

Aortic regurgitation

Aetiology

Aortic regurgitation is the result of disease of the valve cusps or dilatation of the aortic root and valve ring. The most common causes are rheumatic fever and infective endocarditis complicating an already damaged valve (Table 8.10).

Table 8.10 Causes and associations of aortic regurgitation

Damage to the aortic valve cusps	Bicuspid aortic valve
	Acute rheumatic fever*
	Chronic rheumatic heart disease
	Infective endocarditis*
Dilatation of aorta and valve ring	Syphilis
	Arthritides
	Reiter's syndrome
	Ankylosing spondylitis
	Rheumatoid arthritis
	Severe hypertension
	Dissection of the aorta*
	Aortic endocarditis
	Marfan's syndrome
	Osteogenesis imperfecta

* These conditions may produce acute aortic regurgitation.

Pathophysiology

Chronic regurgitation volume loads the left ventricle and results in ventricular hypertrophy and dilatation. Eventually contraction of the ventricle deteriorates, resulting in left ventricular failure. These adaptations do not occur with acute regurgitation and patients may present with pulmonary oedema.

Symptoms
In chronic regurgitation patients remain asymptomatic for many years before developing exertional dyspnoea and fatigue as a result of left ventricular failure.

Signs
- A 'collapsing' (water-hammer) pulse with wide pulse pressure is pathognomic. Rare manifestations of this sign are:
    - visible capillary pulsation in the nail bed (Quincke's sign)
    - head nodding with each heartbeat (de Musset's sign)
    - femoral artery sounds heard as a pistol shot
    - systolic bruit heard on compression of the femoral artery (Durozier's sign)
- The apex is displaced laterally and is thrusting in quality.
- An early diastolic murmur is heard at the left sternal edge and is accentuated when the patient sits forward with the breath held in expiration. Increased stroke volume produces turbulent flow across the aortic valve heard as a midsystolic murmur.
- A middiastolic murmur (Austin Flint murmur) is heard in severe disease and is the result of the regurgitant jet producing premature closure of the anterior mitral valve leaflet.

Investigations
CHEST RADIOGRAPH shows a large heart and dilatation of the ascending aorta.

ECG shows evidence of left ventricular hypertrophy.

ECHOCARDIOGRAPHY shows vigorous cardiac contraction and a dilated left ventricle. Doppler studies allow an assessment of the severity of regurgitation.

CARDIAC CATHETERIZATION is usually necessary if surgery is considered, to give further information about ventricular function and to examine the coronary anatomy.

Management
Mild symptoms may respond to diuretics and vasodilators. The timing of surgery and valve replacement is critical and must not be delayed until there is irreversible left ventricular dysfunction.

Tricuspid and pulmonary valve disease

Tricuspid and pulmonary valve disease are both uncommon. Tricuspid stenosis is almost always the result of rheumatic fever and is frequently associated with mitral and aortic valve disease which tend to dominate the clinical picture.

Tricuspid regurgitation is usually functional and secondary to dilatation of the right ventricle (and hence tricuspid valve ring) in severe right ventricular failure. Much less commonly it is caused by rheumatic heart disease, infective endocarditis or carcinoid syndrome (page 46). On examination there is a pansystolic murmur heard at the lower left sternal edge, the jugular venous pressure is elevated with giant 'v' waves (produced by the regurgitant jet through the tricuspid valve in systole), and the liver is enlarged and pulsates in systole. There may be severe peripheral oedema and ascites. In functional tricuspid regurgitation these signs improve with diuretic therapy.

Pulmonary regurgitation results from pulmonary hypertension and dilatation of the valve ring. Occasionally it is the result of endocarditis (usually in intravenous drug abusers). Auscultation reveals an early diastolic murmur heard at the upper left sternal edge (Graham Steell murmur) and similar to that of aortic regurgitation. Usually there are no symptoms and treatment is rarely required. Pulmonary stenosis is usually a congenital lesion but may present in adult life with fatigue, syncope and right ventricular failure.

INFECTIVE ENDOCARDITIS

Infective endocarditis is an infection of the endocardium or vascular endothelium of the heart. It may occur as a fulminating or acute infection but more commonly runs an insidious course and is known as subacute (bacterial) endocarditis (SBE).

Infection occurs in the following:

- On valves which have a congenital or acquired defect (usually on the left side of the heart). Right-sided endocarditis is more common in intravenous drug addicts

- On normal valves

- On prosthetic valves when infection may be 'early' (acquired at surgery) or 'late' (following bacteraemia). Infected prosthetic valves often need to be replaced

- In association with a ventricular septal defect or persistent ductus arteriosus

Aetiology
The most common organisms causing endocarditis are the following:

- *Streptococcus viridans* (in 50% of cases): this organism is a normal commensal of the upper respiratory tract; bacteraemia occurs following dental extractions, tonsillectomy and bronchoscopy. However, most patients have no history of recent surgery

- *Enterococcus faecalis*: implicated in endocarditis affecting older men with prostatic disease or following pelvic surgery

- *Staphylococcus aureus*: this often produces an acute fulminating illness seen particularly in intravenous drug addicts (using dirty needles) and in patients with central venous lines

Uncommon organisms: other bacteria, fungi, *Coxiella burnetii* (causative organism of Q fever, page 341) and *Chlamydia psittaci*.

Pathology

A mass of fibrin, platelets and infectious organisms form vegetations along the edges of the valve. Virulent organisms destroy the valve producing regurgitation and worsening heart failure.

Clinical features

Symptoms and signs result from:

- Infection producing an insidious onset of malaise, fever, night sweats, weight loss and anaemia. Splenomegaly is seen in 40% of cases and clubbing in 10%

- Valve destruction leading to heart failure and new or changing heart murmurs (in 90% of cases)

- Embolization of vegetations and metastatic abscess formation in the brain, spleen and kidney. Embolization from right-sided endocarditis causes pulmonary infarction and pneumonia

- Immune complex deposition in blood vessels producing a vasculitis and petechial haemorrhages in the skin, under the nails (splinter haemorrhages) and on the retinae (Roth's spots). Osler's nodes (tender subcutaneous nodules in the fingers) and Janeway lesions (painless erythematous macules on the palms) are uncommon. Immune complex deposition in the joints causes arthralgia and, in the kidney, acute glomerulonephritis. Microscopic haematuria occurs in 70% of cases but renal failure is uncommon

Endocarditis should always be considered in any patient with a heart murmur and fever.

Investigation

BLOOD COUNT shows a normochromic/normocytic anaemia with a raised ESR and often a leukocytosis.

BLOOD CULTURES (multiple sets) must be taken before antibiotics are started. Six sets taken over 24 hours will identify the organism in 75% of cases. Special culture techniques and serological tests are occasionally necessary if blood cultures are negative and unusual organisms suspected.

SERUM IMMUNOGLOBULINS are increased and complement levels decreased as a result of immune complex formation.

URINE STIX TESTING shows haematuria in most cases.

ECHOCARDIOGRAPHY identifies vegetations and underlying valvular dysfunction. Small vegetations may be missed and a normal echocardiogram does not exclude endocarditis.

Management
DRUG THERAPY
The first 2 weeks of antibiotic treatment is given intravenously and oral treatment continued for a further 2–4 weeks. While awaiting results of blood cultures, a combination of intravenous benzylpenicillin and gentamicin will cover most organisms. In acute fulminating cases, initial treatment should include flucloxacillin and fusidic acid to cover *Staph. aureus*. Subsequent treatment depends on the results of blood cultures and antibiotic sensitivity of the organism. Antibiotic doses are adjusted to ensure adequate bactericidal activity (microbiological assays of minimum bactericidal concentrations) and plasma concentrations of gentamicin are measured twice weekly to ensure that levels are within the therapeutic range.

SURGERY, to replace the valve, should be considered when there is severe heart failure, early infection of prosthetic material and worsening renal failure.

Prophylaxis
Patients at risk of endocarditis should receive antibiotic therapy before undergoing a procedure likely to result in bacteraemia. The choice of antibiotic depends on the procedure and the likelihood of endocarditis [CM p. 10].

PULMONARY HEART DISEASE

Pulmonary hypertension

Elevation of the pulmonary artery pressure (pulmonary hypertension) occurs with chronic lung disease, increased pulmonary blood flow (which occurs with atrial septal defect, ventricular septal defect and patent ductus arteriosus), left ventricular failure, mitral stenosis, recurrent pulmonary emboli and primary pulmonary hypertension (rare condition of unknown aetiology predominantly affecting young women).

Clinical features
Chest pain, fatigue, dyspnoea and syncope are common symptoms. The physical signs include a right ventricular parasternal heave and a loud pulmonary second sound. In advanced disease there is right heart failure. There are also features of the underlying disease.

Investigations
CHEST RADIOGRAPH shows enlarged proximal pulmonary arteries which taper distally. It may also reveal the underlying cause (e.g. emphysema, calcified mitral valve).

ECG shows right ventricular hypertrophy and P pulmonale.

Management

The treatment is that of the cause. In primary pulmonary hypertension there is a progressive downhill course and heart–lung transplantation is indicated for young patients with end-stage disease.

Pulmonary embolism

Pulmonary embolism is usually a consequence of thrombosis in the ileofemoral veins (deep venous thrombosis, page 316). More rarely it results from clot formation in the right atrium in patients with right-sided cardiac failure, particularly if there is atrial fibrillation.

Pathology

After pulmonary embolism, lung tissue is ventilated but not perfused, resulting in impaired gas exchange. A massive embolism suddenly increases pulmonary vascular resistance, causing acute right heart failure. A small embolus may be clinically silent unless it causes pulmonary infarction. This affects only a minority of cases because oxygen continues to be supplied by the bronchial arterial supply and the airways.

Clinical features

Massive pulmonary embolism presents as a medical emergency; the patient has severe central chest pain and suddenly becomes shocked, pale and sweaty, with marked tachypnoea and tachycardia. Syncope may result if the cardiac output is transiently but dramatically reduced. Death may follow rapidly. On examination the patient is shocked with central cyanosis. There is elevation of the jugular venous pressure, a right ventricular heave, accentuation of the second heart sound and a gallop rhythm. Smaller emboli present with dyspnoea and, if there is pulmonary infarction, haemoptysis, pleuritic chest pain and a pleural rub.

Investigations

RADIOLOGY. The chest radiograph is often normal but may show decreased vascular markings and a raised hemidiaphragm (caused by loss of lung volume). With pulmonary infarction, a late feature is development of a wedge-shaped opacity adjacent to the pleural edge sometimes with a pleural effusion.

ECG is usually normal except for sinus tachycardia. In massive embolism the features of acute right strain may be seen: tall peaked P waves in lead II, right axis deviation and right bundle-branch block.

BLOOD GASES show hypoxaemia and hypocapnia in massive embolism.

RADIONUCLIDE LUNG SCAN ($\dot{V}/\dot{Q}$ SCAN) demonstrates areas of ventilated lung with perfusion defects (ventilation–perfusion mismatch).

PULMONARY ANGIOGRAPHY is the definitive method of diagnosis but is usually only undertaken if surgery is considered in acute massive embolism. It shows obstructed vessels or obvious filling defects in the artery.

Treatment

Treatment (Table 8.11) is often started on the basis of clinical suspicion pending investigation. Immediate surgical embolectomy is considered in severe cases of massive embolism.

Table 8.11 Management of acute pulmonary embolism

60% oxygen if hypoxaemic

Analgesia
   Morphine (5–10mg i.v.) to relieve pain and anxiety

Prevention of further emboli
   Intravenous heparin and oral warfarin (page 142)

Thrombolytic therapy (page 142)
   Consider intravenous streptokinase in massive embolism

Chronic cor pulmonale

Cor pulmonale is right heart failure resulting from chronic pulmonary hypertension.

Aetiology

Chronic obstructive pulmonary disease caused by bronchitis and emphysema is responsible for most cases (Table 8.12). Pulmonary vascular resistance is increased because of destruction of the pulmonary vascular bed and pulmonary vasoconstriction caused by acidosis and hypoxia. Eventually, increased resistance leads to right heart strain and right ventricular failure.

Table 8.12 Causes of cor pulmonale

Intrinsic lung disease, e.g. chronic bronchitis and emphysema, pulmonary fibrosis

Recurrent pulmonary emboli

Skeletal abnormalities, e.g. kyphoscoliosis

Hypoventilation, e.g. morbid obesity

Neuromuscular disease, e.g. poliomyelitis, myasthenia gravis

Obstruction, e.g. sleep apnoea syndrome

Treatment
Treatment is directed towards the underlying pulmonary disease as well as right ventricular failure. Acute chest infections must be treated promptly. Oxygen therapy over a long period may reduce established pulmonary hypertension with improvement in overall prognosis (page 305).

MYOCARDIAL DISEASE

Myocarditis

Myocarditis is an inflammation of the myocardium. The most common cause in the UK is viral, particularly Coxsackie virus infection, but it may also occur with diphtheria, rheumatic fever, radiation injury and some drugs.

Clinical features
Patients present with an acute illness characterized by fever and varying degrees of biventricular failure. Cardiac arrhythmias and pericarditis may also occur.

Investigations
CHEST RADIOGRAPH may show cardiac enlargement.

ECG shows non-specific T-wave and ST changes.

The diagnosis is supported by demonstration of an increase in serum viral titres and inflammation on cardiac biopsy. The findings rarely influence management and biopsy is not usually performed.

Management
Treatment is with bed rest and treatment of cardiac failure. The prognosis is generally good.

Cardiomyopathy

The cardiomyopathies are a group of chronic heart muscle disorders of unknown cause. They are classified according to their clinical presentation as:

- Dilated cardiomyopathy – ventricular dilatation
- Hypertrophic cardiomyopathy – myocardial hypertrophy
- Restrictive cardiomyopathy – impaired ventricular filling

Dilated cardiomyopathy

Dilated cardiomyopathy (DCM) is characterized by dilated ventricles which contract poorly.

Clinical features
Patients present with the symptoms and signs of biventricular failure. Atrial and ventricular arrhythmias are common. Mural thrombi may form within the dilated ventricular chambers and give rise to systemic and pulmonary emboli.

Investigations
CHEST RADIOGRAPH demonstrates cardiac enlargement.

ECG is often abnormal. The changes are non-specific and include arrhythmias and T-wave flattening.

ECHOCARDIOGRAPHY shows dilated ventricles with global hypokinesis (compare ischaemia with regional contractile impairment).

CARDIAC BIOPSY is occasionally performed to exclude myocardial storage diseases and infiltrations, which may present with the clinical features of DCM (Table 8.13).

Management
Heart failure and arrhythmias are treated in conventional manner. A history of embolization is an indication for anticoagulant treatment. Severe congestive cardiomyopathy in young adults is treated with cardiac transplantation.

Table 8.13 Systemic heart muscle disease presenting with features of DCM

Cardiovascular disease
   Ischaemia
   Systemic hypertension
   Congenital heart disease
   Rheumatic heart disease
Drugs and toxins
   Alcohol
   Doxorubicin
Connective tissue disorders
   Systemic sclerosis
   Systemic lupus erythematosus
Neuromuscular diseases
   Muscular dystrophy
   Friedrich's ataxia
Infiltrations
   Glycogen storage disease
   Amyloidosis
   Haemochromatosis

Hypertrophic cardiomyopathy

Hypertrophic cardiomyopathy is characterized by marked ventricular hypertrophy of unknown cause, usually with disproportionate involvement of the interventricular septum. The hypertrophic non-compliant ventricles impair diastolic filling. It is sometimes a familial condition and there may be a history of heart disease or sudden death in relatives.

Clinical features
Symptoms include dyspnoea, angina and syncope. Arrhythmias are common and there is a high risk of sudden death. The carotid pulse is jerky because of rapid ejection and sudden obstruction to the ventricular outflow during

systole. An ejection systolic murmur occurs because of left ventricular outflow obstruction and the pansystolic murmur of functional mitral regurgitation may also be heard.

Investigations
The diagnosis is made on echocardiography which shows the ventricular hypertrophy with disproportionate involvement of the septum.

Management
The risk of death is reduced by antiarrhythmic drug therapy; amiodarone is the treatment of choice. Syncope or chest pain may be treated with β-blockers. Occasionally resection of septal myocardium may be indicated.

Restrictive cardiomyopathy

This is rare in the UK; the rigid myocardium restricts diastolic ventricular filling and the clinical features resemble those of constrictive pericarditis (see later). In the UK, the most common cause is amyloidosis. The ECG, chest radiograph and echocardiogram are often abnormal but the findings are non-specific. Diagnosis is by cardiac catheterization which shows characteristic pressure changes. An endomyocardial biopsy may be taken during the catheter procedure, thus providing histological diagnosis. There is no specific treatment. Cardiac transplantation is performed in severe cases.

PERICARDIAL DISEASE

Acute pericarditis

Aetiology
Acute inflammation of the pericardium is usually from Coxsackie viral infection or acute myocardial infarction. Other causes include uraemia, connective tissue diseases, trauma, tuberculosis and malignancy (breast, lung, leukaemia and lymphoma).

Clinical features
There is sharp retrosternal chest pain characteristically relieved by leaning forwards. Pain may be worse on inspiration and radiate to the neck and shoulders. The cardinal clinical sign is a pericardial friction rub which may be transient.

Diagnosis
ECG shows ST segment elevation in all the leads except AVR and V1. The elevated ST segments are characteristically concave upwards (convex upwards in infarction) and return towards baseline as inflammation subsides.

Management
Treatment is of the underlying disorder plus NSAIDs. Systemic corticosteroids are used in resistant cases.

Pericardial effusion and tamponade

Pericardial effusion is an accumulation of fluid in the pericardial sac which may result from any of the causes of pericarditis. Pericardial tamponade is a medical emergency and occurs when a large amount of pericardial fluid (which has often accumulated rapidly) restricts diastolic ventricular filling and causes a marked reduction in cardiac output.

Clinical features
The signs of pericardial tamponade are hypotension, tachycardia and an elevated jugular venous pressure which paradoxically rises with inspiration (Kussmaul's sign). There is invariably pulsus paradoxus (fall in blood pressure of more than 10 mmHg on inspiration). This is the result of increased venous return to the right side of the heart during inspiration. The increased right ventricular volume thus occupies more space within the rigid pericardium and impairs left ventricular filling.

Investigations
A CHEST RADIOGRAPH shows a large globular heart.

ECG shows low voltage complexes.

ECHOCARDIOGRAM is diagnostic showing an echo-free space around the heart.

Management
The treatment of tamponade is emergency pericardiocentesis. Pericardial fluid is drained percutaneously by introducing a needle into the pericardial sac. If the effusion recurs, in spite of treatment of the underlying cause, excision of a pericardial segment may be necessary. Fluid is then absorbed through the pleural and mediastinal lymphatics.

Constrictive pericarditis

In the UK, most cases of constrictive pericarditis are idiopathic in origin or result from intrapericardial haemorrhage during heart surgery. Tuberculous infection is no longer the most common cause.

Clinical features
The heart becomes encased within a rigid fibrotic pericardial sac, which prevents adequate diastolic filling of the ventricles. The clinical features resemble those of right-sided cardiac failure with jugular venous distension, dependent oedema, hepatomegaly and ascites. Kussmaul's sign is usually present and there may be pulsus paradoxus, atrial fibrillation and, on auscultation, a pericardial knock caused by rapid ventricular filling.

Investigations
RADIOLOGY. A chest radiograph shows a normal heart size and pericardial calcification (best seen on the lateral film).

Diagnosis is made by CT which shows pericardial thickening and calcification.

Management
Treatment is by surgical excision of the pericardium.

SYSTEMIC HYPERTENSION

The level of blood pressure can be said to be abnormal when it is associated with a clear increase in morbidity and mortality from heart disease, stroke and renal failure. This level varies with age, sex, race and country. The World Health Organization has used a definition of hypertension as blood pressure of more than 160/95 mmHg. The validity of a single blood pressure measurement is unclear (blood pressure rises acutely in certain situations, e.g. visiting the doctor) and usually several readings are required to confirm a diagnosis of hypertension. Occasionally, ambulatory blood pressure monitoring (blood pressure is measured throughout the day using a non-invasive technique) is used if doubt exists as to the level of blood pressure.

Aetiology

ESSENTIAL HYPERTENSION
More than 90% of cases of hypertension have no known underlying cause and the terms 'primary' or 'essential' hypertension are used. Several factors may play an aetiological role:

- Familial tendency
- Obesity
- High alcohol intake
- High salt intake?

SECONDARY HYPERTENSION
This should always be considered particularly in those presenting under the age of 35. Causes of secondary hypertension are the following:

- Renal disease accounts for over 80% of cases of secondary hypertension. Chronic glomerulonephritis, chronic pyelonephritis, congenital polycystic kidneys and renal artery stenosis are the diseases usually involved
- Endocrine disease (page 418): Conn's syndrome, Cushing's syndrome, phaeochromocytoma, and acromegaly
- Coarctation of the aorta which should be suspected in young people presenting with hypertension
- Pre-eclampsia occurring in the third trimester of pregnancy [CM p. 620]
- Drugs including oestrogen-containing oral contraceptives, other steroids and vasopressin

Clinical features

Hypertension is generally asymptomatic, although malignant or accelerated hypertension (usually BP > 200/130 mmHg) may present with characteristic symptoms. These include visual impairment, nausea, vomiting, fits, headaches or symptoms of acute cardiac failure. Secondary causes of hypertension may be suggested by specific features such as attacks of sweating and tachycardia in phaeochromocytoma.

EXAMINATION

In most patients the only finding is high blood pressure, but in others signs relating to the cause (e.g. abdominal bruit in renal artery stenosis, delayed femoral pulses in coarctation of the aorta) or the end-organ effects of hypertension may be present, e.g. loud second heart sound, left ventricular heave, fourth heart sound in hypertensive heart disease and retinal abnormalities. The latter are graded according to severity:

Grade 1 – increased tortuosity and reflectiveness of the retinal arteries (silver wiring)

Grade 2 – grade 1 plus arteriovenous nipping

Grade 3 – grade 2 plus flame-shaped haemorrhages and soft 'cotton-wool' exudates

Grade 4 – grade 3 plus papilloedema

Investigations

Investigations are carried out to identify end-organ damage and those patients with secondary causes of hypertension.

A CHEST RADIOGRAPH may show heart failure. Rib notching indicates coarctation of the aorta.

SERUM UREA AND ELECTROLYTES may show evidence of renal impairment. Hypokalaemia occurs in Conn's syndrome.

ECG may show evidence of left ventricular hypertrophy or myocardial ischaemia.

URINE STIX TESTING is performed to look for haematuria and proteinuria which may indicate renal disease (either the cause or the effect of hypertension).

Young patients with hypertension (< 35 years) or those where a secondary cause is suspected (e.g. from clinical examination or abnormal baseline investigations) should undergo further investigation, e.g. urinary catecholamines for phaeochromocytoma, full renal investigation for renovascular hypertension.

Management

Treatment of moderate-to-severe hypertension reduces the incidence of stroke, heart failure and renal damage but has less effect on coronary artery disease. The value of treating mild hypertension is less clear-cut. Recent studies have shown the benefits of treating elderly patients with hypertension (up to 80 years). Patients with severe hypertension or moderate hypertension with evidence of end-organ damage should be treated early. Treatment should also be given to other patients where the blood pressure is persistently high on prolonged follow-up.

GENERAL MEASURES include:

- Weight reduction
- Reduction of heavy alcohol consumption
- No added salt diet
- Regular exercise

DRUG THERAPY: a large number of drugs may be used in treatment and these are usually selected on the basis of efficacy, tolerance and compliance. Commonly used first-line agents are thiazide diuretics, β-blockers, calcium channel blockers and ACE inhibitors. Combination treatment may be needed in patients not controlled with one drug.

Diuretics increase renal sodium and water excretion and directly dilate arterioles. Loop diuretics, e.g. frusemide, and thiazide diuretics, e.g. bendrofluazide, are equally effective in lowering blood pressure although thiazides are usually preferred as the duration of action is longer, the diuresis is not so severe and they are cheaper. Side effects of thiazide diuretics include hypokalaemia, hyperuricaemia and impairment of glucose tolerance.

β-Adrenergic blocking agents: the mechanism of action of these agents is unclear. Although they reduce the force of cardiac contraction and renin production, they probably act predominantly via the central nervous system. There are a wide range of β-blocking agents with different properties such as cardioselectivity, intrinsic sympathomimetic activity and lipid solubility. Complications include aggravation of left ventricular failure, bradycardia, cold extremities, fatigue and weakness.

Calcium antagonists, e.g. nifedipine, diltiazem and verapamil, are increasingly used and act predominantly by dilatation of peripheral arterioles. Side effects are few and include bradycardia and cardiac conduction defects (verapamil and diltiazem), headaches, flushing and fluid retention.

ACE INHIBITORS, e.g. captopril, enalapril and lisinopril, block the conversion of angiotensin I to angiotensin II which is a more powerful vasoconstrictor, and block degradation of bradykinin which is a vasodilator. Side effects include first-dose hypotension and cough, proteinuria, rashes and leukopenia in high doses. ACE inhibitors are contraindicated in renal artery stenosis because inhibition of the renin–angiotensin system in this instance may lead to loss of renal blood flow and infarction of the kidney.

OTHER AGENTS: α-blocking agents (e.g. prazosin, doxazosin), hydralazine, and centrally acting agents (e.g. methyldopa and clonidine) may be indicated in specific circumstances.

Management of severe hypertension

Patients with severe hypertension (diastolic BP > 130 mmHg), hypertensive encephalopathy or severe complications such as left ventricular failure or aortic dissection should be admitted to hospital for urgent treatment. The aim should be to reduce the diastolic blood pressure slowly (over 24 hours) to about 100–110 mmHg. Oral nifedipine and β-blockers are usually successful. If more urgent reduction in blood pressure is necessary, as in aortic dissection, treatment is with intravenous nitroprusside, diazoxide or labetalol.

ARTERIAL AND VENOUS DISEASE

Aortic aneurysms

Aortic aneurysms are usually abdominal and result from atheroma.

Abdominal aortic aneurysm

Abdominal aortic aneurysms may be asymptomatic and found as a pulsating mass on abdominal examination or as calcification on a plain radiograph. An expanding aneurysm may cause epigastric or back pain. A ruptured aortic aneurysm is a surgical emergency presenting with epigastric pain radiating to the back and hypovolaemic shock. Diagnosis is by ultrasonography or CT scan. Surgery is indicated for a symptomatic aneurysm or large asymptomatic aneurysms (> 5 cm).

Thoracic aortic aneurysms

Cystic medial necrosis and atherosclerosis are the usual causes of thoracic aneurysms. Cardiovascular syphilis is no longer a common cause.

Clinical features

Thoracic aneurysms may be asymptomatic, cause pressure on local structures (causing back pain, dysphagia and cough) or result in aortic regurgitation if the aortic root is involved. Aortic dissection results from a tear in the intima, blood under high pressure creates a false lumen in the diseased media. Typically there is an abrupt onset of severe, tearing, central chest pain, radiating through to the back. Involvement of branch arteries may produce neurological signs, absent pulses and unequal blood pressure in the arms.

Management

The chest radiograph shows a widened mediastinum in dissection. The diagnosis is made by CT scanning or transoesophageal echocardiography (page 317). Management involves urgent control of blood pressure and surgical repair for proximal aortic dissection.

Raynaud's disease and phenomenon

Intermittent spasm occurs in the arteries supplying the fingers and toes. There is initial pallor (resulting from vasoconstriction) followed by cyanosis and, finally, redness from hyperaemia. Raynaud's disease (no underlying disorder) occurs most commonly in young women and must be differentiated from secondary causes of Raynaud's phenomenon, e.g. connective tissue diseases and β-blockers. Treatment is by keeping the hands and feet warm, stopping smoking and nifedipine in some cases.

Venous disease

Superficial thrombophlebitis

Superficial thrombophlebitis usually occurs in the leg. The vein is painful, tender and hard with overlying redness. Treatment is with simple analgesia, e.g. NSAIDs. Anticoagulation is not necessary as embolism does not occur.

Deep venous thrombosis

Thrombosis can occur in any vein but the veins of the pelvis and leg are the most common sites. Deep vein thrombosis (DVT) is often a result of prolonged immobility in bed, particularly following abdominal or pelvic surgery. Other risk factors are cardiac failure, pregnancy and childbirth, oral contraceptive drugs, malignant disease, chronic pulmonary disease and hypercoagulable states.

Clinical features

DVT is often asymptomatic but the leg may be warm and swollen with calf tenderness and superficial venous distension.

Investigations

Diagnosis of iliofemoral thrombosis is made by Doppler ultrasonography. This method is not reliable for calf vein thrombosis which is diagnosed by venography (not always performed as management is not affected, see below).

Management

For discussion of management see page 142.

The main aim of therapy is to prevent pulmonary embolism and all patients with thrombi above the knee must be anticoagulated. Anticoagulation for below-knee thrombi is controversial.

Anticoagulation is initially with heparin and subsequently with warfarin, usually continued for 3 months. Thrombolytic therapy is occasionally used for patients with a large iliofemoral thrombosis.

DICTIONARY OF TERMS: CARDIOVASCULAR DISEASE

CHRONOTROPIC: positively chronotropic means to increase the *rate* of contraction of the heart, negatively chronotropic is the opposite.

INOTROPIC: positively inotropic means increasing the *force* of cardiac muscle contraction.

PRELOAD is the extent to which the heart muscle is stretched before contraction; this is in effect the end-diastolic volume.

AFTERLOAD is the load against which the muscle exerts its contractile force, i.e. peripheral vascular tree.

EJECTION FRACTION is the fraction of the ventricular end-diastolic volume that is ejected during systole. It is usually equal to about 60%.

END-DIASTOLIC VOLUME is the volume of blood in the ventricle at the end of diastole.

ECHOCARDIOGRAPHY is a non-invasive method of recording the position and motion of the structures of the heart by echo obtained from beams of ultrasonic waves directed through the chest wall.

Transoesophageal echocardiography uses miniaturized transducers incorporated into special endoscopes. It allows better visualization of some structures and pathology, e.g. aortic dissection, prosthetic valve endocarditis.

Doppler echocardiography uses the Doppler principle (in this case, the frequency of ultrasonic waves reflected from blood cells is related to their velocity and direction of flow) to identify and assess the severity of valve lesions.

NUCLEAR IMAGING uses radiotracers (injected intravenously) which diffuse freely into myocardial tissue or attach to red blood cells.

Thallium-201 is taken up by cardiac myocytes. Ischaemic areas (produced by exercising the patient) with reduced tracer uptake are seen as 'cold spots' when imaged with a gamma camera.

Technetium-99m is used to label red blood cells and produce images of the left ventricle during systole and diastole.

CARDIAC CATHERIZATION is the passage of a small catheter through a peripheral vein (for study of right heart structures) or artery (for study of left heart structures) into the heart, permitting the securing of blood samples, measurement of intracardiac pressures and determination of cardiac anomalies.

FINAL MEDICINE EXAMINATION: CARDIOLOGY

The most common cardiology questions asked are about the investigation and management of hypertension (often in relatively young patients), the differential diagnosis of chest pain and the management of cardiac arrhythmias particularly atrial fibrillation. Other common questions are the presenting features and diagnosis of infective endocarditis and the management of heart failure.

1. What simple screening tests are justified in a 45-year-old man presenting with hypertension? What are the causes of secondary hypertension and how could your investigations demonstrate them?

2. Discuss the causes of acute chest pain in a 40-year-old man. What additional clinical features may help to establish a diagnosis?

3. A 28-year-old married man with a family history of ischaemic heart disease presents with exertional chest pain. Discuss investigation and management.

4. How would you try to differentiate acute pericarditis from acute myocardial infarction clinically?

5. A 60-year-old woman presents with breathlessness and clinical features of mild heart failure. She is found to have atrial fibrillation with an uncontrolled ventricular response (130 beats/min).

   (a) Give four possible causes for the atrial fibrillation.
   (b) Name three drugs that may be used to control the ventricular response.
   (c) What investigations would you order?

6. A 44-year-old woman is admitted to hospital with malaise and fever. She has felt unwell for 6 months. Examination shows pallor, an apical pansystolic murmur and splenomegaly. A blood count sent by the general practitioner shows a haemoglobin of 8.4 g/dl, WBC 7.2×10^9/l and platelets 394×10^9/l.
   What investigations are required?
   How might treatment be monitored?

7. Discuss the clinical features of an acute attack of left ventricular failure. Name three physical findings that would be of most value in distinguishing it from other causes of severe shortness of breath.

8. What are the key points to the management of acute pulmonary oedema?

9. A 50-year-old man complains of a painful red swollen calf. What factors may be responsible? How would you discriminate between the causes?

10. A 61-year-old man is admitted following a year's history of dizziness on exertion culminating in a black-out while cutting the lawn. On admission he has a slow rising pulse and a systolic ejection murmur. There was no history of angina.
What is the likely diagnosis?
How would you estimate its clinical severity?
What is the most probable pathology?
What is the treatment?

ANSWERS

1. If the history or physical examination does not suggest a secondary cause for hypertension the screening tests in a middle-aged man are a chest radiograph, serum urea, creatinine and electrolytes, and stix testing of the urine to look for protein and blood. The secondary causes of hypertension are listed on page 312 and relevance of these investigations discussed on page 313. An ECG is also performed to look for end-organ damage (left ventricular hypertrophy) which is an indication for early treatment rather than observation in a patient with mild hypertension.

2. The causes of chest pain are listed on page 262. The question does not give any clues as to the site of the chest pain which would narrow the differential diagnosis. Myocardial ischaemia must always be considered, particularly if there are risk factors. Additional symptoms are breathlessness (often occurs with pneumonia, pneumothorax and sometimes with myocardial infarction), nausea and vomiting (with infarction), cough (with pneumonia) and fever (with pericarditis).

3. The nature of the chest pain and the positive family history suggest a diagnosis of angina resulting from ischaemic heart disease. He is very young and every effort should be made to confirm the diagnosis, identify risk factors and determine the extent and site of coronary artery stenosis. A resting ECG and usually an exercise ECG is performed (page 287). Risk factors (page 286) are identified from the history, physical examination and measurement of serum cholesterol and blood glucose; every effort must be made to correct abnormalities. In younger

people (< 50 years) coronary angiography is often performed to document the site and extent of coronary artery stenosis which will guide future management. In patients with left main stem or multivessel disease, coronary artery bypass grafting is of clear prognostic benefit compared to medical therapy. Treatment is medical (page 288) in the first instance in the absence of these lesions. His siblings and children should also be screened for risk factors, e.g. familial hypercholesterolaemia.

4. Acute pericarditis and myocardial infarction are discussed on pages 310 and 289. They can usually be differentiated on the basis of the nature, the site and radiation of the pain, and the presence of associated symptoms and signs (e.g. nausea, vomiting, breathlessness, pericardial rub on auscultation).

5. The causes of atrial fibrillation are listed on page 270. In an elderly woman, probable causes are ischaemic heart disease, mitral valve disease, thyrotoxicosis and cardiomyopathy. The drugs usually used to control the ventricular rate are those that slow conduction through the AV node: digoxin, β-blockers and verapamil. Digoxin is the only one not to have a negative inotropic action and thus can be used in heart failure. Investigations are an ECG (which will show fibrillation and may show evidence of ischaemia or mitral valve disease, Figure 8.7), a chest radiograph (which will confirm the clinical diagnosis of heart failure and may show evidence of mitral valve disease, Figure 8.14), an echocardiogram and thyroid function tests.

6. This combination of clinical signs suggests infective endocarditis affecting the mitral valve. Investigations are discussed on page 304. Treatment is monitored clinically (patient well-being, temperature charts, evidence of heart failure) and by regular blood counts, ESR and echocardiography. Antibiotic doses are adjusted according to bacteriological studies (minimum bactericidal concentration) and gentamicin levels (to ensure therapeutic levels are obtained but without toxic levels likely to cause side effects).

7. Clinical features of acute left ventricular failure are listed on page 280. A gallop rhythm, widespread crackles and pulsus alternans differentiate pulmonary oedema from other causes of acute

shortness of breath (listed in Table 9.1). In pulsus alternans the arterial pressure alternates between high and low systolic peaks. Its presence indicates severe left ventricular failure.

8. The key points to the management of pulmonary oedema are listed in Table 8.6.

9. The differential diagnosis of a swollen calf includes deep venous thrombosis, cellulitis or a ruptured Baker's cyst. Oedema in heart failure or hypoalbuminaemia also causes a swollen calf but this is usually bilateral. A Baker's cyst is a synovial cyst in the popliteal fossa which sometimes occurs in rheumatoid arthritis. Rupture of the cyst produces calf swelling but not usually redness. It can sometimes be difficult to distinguish clinically between cellulitis and a DVT, and a venogram may be needed.

10. The history and examination are typical of aortic stenosis (page 300). As in this case, presentation is usually in the sixth decade. The most likely pathology is a calcified bicuspid aortic valve. The presence of symptoms indicates at least moderately severe aortic stenosis. A longer ejection systolic murmur, clinical and ECG evidence of left ventricular hypertrophy all indicate more severe stenosis. The severity may be more accurately assessed by Doppler echocardiography. Treatment in a symptomatic patient is valve replacement.

CHAPTER 9

Respiratory Disease

Symptoms of respiratory disease

The common symptoms of respiratory disease are cough, sputum production, breathlessness, haemoptysis and wheeze.

COUGH is a non-specific symptom and the most common manifestation of lower respiratory tract disease. It may be the only symptom of asthma when it is typically worse at night, on waking and after exercise. A chronic cough is common in smokers; however, a worsening cough may be the presenting symptom of bronchial carcinoma and needs investigation.

DYSPNOEA. This is the subjective sensation of shortness of breath. *Orthopnoea* is breathlessness that occurs when lying flat and is the result of both abdominal contents pushing the diaphragm into the thorax and redistribution of blood from the lower extremities to the lungs. *Paroxysmal nocturnal dyspnoea* is a manifestation of left heart failure: the patient wakes up gasping for breath and finds some relief by sitting upright. The mechanism is similar to orthopnoea but, because sensory awareness is depressed during sleep, severe interstitial pulmonary oedema can accumulate.

The speed of onset of breathlessness is useful when formulating a differential diagnosis (Table 9.1).

Table 9.1 Differential diagnosis of dyspnoea

Sudden	Over hours	Over days	Over months/years
Inhaled foreign body	Asthma	Pleural effusion	Chronic airflow limitation
Pneumothorax	Pneumonia	Lung cancer	Pulmonary fibrosis
Pulmonary embolism	Pulmonary oedema		Anaemia
	Extrinsic allergic alveolitis		

WHEEZE. Wheezing is the result of airflow limitation of any cause. It should be distinguished from *stridor* caused by obstruction of the trachea or major bronchi, e.g. by tumour.

HAEMOPTYSIS (coughing blood) requires thorough investigation. The common causes are bronchial carcinoma, pulmonary infarction, tuberculosis and pulmonary oedema (pink frothy sputum). Rust-coloured sputum may occur with pneumococcal pneumonia, but haemoptysis should not be attributed to infection without investigation. Less common causes include bronchiectasis, benign tumour, bleeding disorder and, rarely, Wegener's granulomatosis and

Goodpasture's syndrome. A chest radiograph should be performed in all patients and subsequent investigations (e.g. bronchoscopy, CT, isotope lung scan) decided from the history and examination.

Respiratory function tests

Respiratory function tests are simple outpatient investigations carried out to assess airflow limitation and lung volumes. The normal values vary for age, sex and height, and between individuals.

PEAK EXPIRATORY FLOW RATE (PEFR) is measured with a peak flowmeter. It records the maximum expiratory flow rate during a forced expiration after full inspiration. It is useful in detecting airflow limitation and in monitoring response to treatment.

FORCED EXPIRATORY VOLUME (FEV) and FORCED VITAL CAPACITY (FVC) are measured with a spirometer. The patient exhales as fast and as long as possible from a full inspiration, the volume expired in the first second is the FEV_1 and the total volume expired is the FVC. The ratio FEV_1:FVC is a measure of airflow limitation and is normally about 75%.

- Airflow limitation: FEV1:FVC < 75%
- Restrictive lung disease: FEV_1:FVC > 75%

More sophisticated techniques allow measurement of *total lung capacity* (TLC) and *residual volume* (RV). These are increased in obstructive lung disease because of air trapping and reduced in lung fibrosis.

TRANSFER FACTOR (T_{CO}) measures transfer of a low concentration of carbon monoxide in the inspired air to haemoglobin. The transfer coefficient (K_{CO}) is the value corrected for differences in lung volume. Gas transfer is reduced early on in emphysema and lung fibrosis.

Assessment of lung function is also made by measurement of arterial blood gases and with exercise tests to assess walking distance in a 6-minute time period.

DISEASES OF THE UPPER RESPIRATORY TRACT

The common cold (acute coryza)

The common cold is caused by infection with one of the many strains of rhinovirus. Spread is by droplets and close personal contact. After an incubation period of 12 hours to 5 days the major symptoms are malaise, slight pyrexia, sore throat and a watery nasal discharge which becomes mucopurulent after a few days. Treatment is symptomatic. The differential diagnosis is mainly from rhinitis.

Sinusitis

Sinusitis is an infection of one of the paranasal sinuses (maxillary, frontal or ethmoid) and may complicate allergic rhinitis or an upper respiratory tract infection (caused by mucosal oedema and blockage of the ostium). Acute infections are usually caused by *Streptococcus pneumoniae* or *Haemophilus influenzae*. Symptoms are frontal headache, facial pain and tenderness, and nasal discharge. The diagnosis is usually clinical and treatment is with antibiotics, e.g. cefaclor and nasal decongestants. Rare complications include local and cerebral abscesses.

Rhinitis

The symptoms of rhinitis are sneezing, watery nasal discharge and nasal blockage. *Perennial rhinitis* occurs throughout the year and may be allergic (the allergens are similar to those for asthma) or non-allergic. *Seasonal allergic rhinitis* (hay fever) occurs during the summer months and is caused by allergy to grass and tree pollen and a variety of mould spores (e.g. *Aspergillus fumigatus*) which grow on cultivated plants. The diagnosis of rhinitis is clinical. Skin-prick testing and measurement of specific serum IgE antibody in conjunction with a detailed clinical history will identify causal antigens. The management involves avoidance of allergens if practical and topical antihistamines, decongestants and steroids. A low dose of oral prednisolone may be necessary when other treatments fail.

Acute pharyngitis

Viruses, particularly one from the adenovirus group, are the most common cause of acute pharyngitis. Symptoms are sore throat and fever which are self-limiting and only require symptomatic treatment. More persistent and severe pharyngitis may imply bacterial infection, often secondary invaders, of which the most common organisms are *Streptococcus pneumoniae, Haemophilus influenzae* and *Staphylococcus aureus*. This requires appropriate antibiotic therapy, e.g. oral cefaclor.

Acute laryngotracheobronchitis

This is usually the result of infection with one of the parainfluenza viruses or measles virus. Symptoms are most severe in children under 3 years of age. Inflammatory oedema involving the larynx causes a hoarse voice, barking cough (croup) and stridor. Tracheitis produces a burning retrosternal pain. Treatment is with oxygen and inhaled steam; tracheotomy is needed in severe cases.

Influenza

The influenza virus belongs to the orthomyxovirus group and exists in two main forms – A and B. The surface of the virion is coated with haemagglutinin (H) and an enzyme, neuraminidase (N), which are important for attachment to the host respiratory epithelium. Human immunity develops against the H and N antigens. Influenza A has the capacity to undergo antigenic 'shift' and major changes in the H and N antigens are associated with pandemic infections which may cause millions of deaths worldwide. Minor antigenic 'drifts' are associated with less severe epidemics.

Clinical features

After an incubation period of 1–3 days there is an abrupt onset of fever, myalgia, headache, sore throat and dry cough, which may last several weeks.

Diagnosis

Laboratory diagnosis is not always necessary but serology shows a fourfold rise in antibody titre over a 2-week period.

Management

Treatment is usually symptomatic (aspirin, bed rest, maintenance of fluid intake). Amantadine hydrochloride may be useful in patients who have not been immunized.

Complications

Pneumonia is the most common complication. This is either viral or the result of secondary infection with bacteria, of which *Staphylococcus aureus* is the most serious with a mortality rate of up to 20%.

Prophylaxis

Influenza vaccine is prepared from current strains. It is effective in 70% of people and lasts for only about a year. It is reserved for chronically sick people, elderly people and medical staff during a pandemic.

Inhalation of foreign bodies

Children inhale foreign bodies, frequently peanuts, more often than adults. In adults it is usually associated with a depressed conscious level such as after an alcoholic binge. A large object will totally occlude the airways and rapidly result in death. Smaller objects impact more peripherally (usually the right main bronchus because it is more vertical than the left) and cause choking, or patients may present at a later stage with persistent suppurative pneumonia or lung abscess. In an emergency the foreign body is dislodged from the airway using the Heimlich manoeuvre: the subject is gripped from behind with the arms around the upper abdomen, a sharp forceful squeeze pushes the diaphragm into the thorax and the rapid airflow generated may be sufficient to force the foreign body out of the trachea or bronchus. In the non-emergency situation bronchoscopy is used to remove the foreign body.

DISEASES OF THE LOWER RESPIRATORY TRACT

Asthma

Asthma is a common chronic inflammatory condition of the lung airways the cause of which is incompletely understood. It has three characteristics: reversible airflow limitation, airway hyperresponsiveness to a range of stimuli and airway inflammation.

Epidemiology

At one time it was thought that about 5% of the population had asthma at some time in their lives. This figure is probably higher with increased recognition of the disease. There is a geographical variation; asthma is more common in New Zealand and much rarer in Far Eastern countries.

Aetiology

There are two major factors involved in the development of asthma:

- ATOPY. This is the term used to describe those individuals who readily develop antibodies of immunoglobulin E (IgE) class against common environmental antigens such as the house dust mite, grass pollen and fungal spores from *Aspergillus fumigatus*

- INCREASED RESPONSIVENESS OF THE AIRWAYS of the lung (as measured by a fall in FEV_1) to stimuli such as inhaled histamine and methacholine (bronchial provocation tests)

Asthma has traditionally been divided into extrinsic (atopic) and intrinsic (non-atopic) on the basis that in extrinsic asthma allergens can be identified by positive skin-prick reactions to common inhaled allergens. It is now recognized that almost all asthmatic patients show some degree of atopy and this classification is used less often.

Precipitating factors

The major allergen (Der p1) is contained in the faecal particles of the house dust mite – *Dermatophagoides pteronnysinus* – which is found in dust throughout the house. Non-specific factors which may cause wheezing are viral infections, cold air, exercise, irritant dusts, vapours and fumes (cigarette smoke, perfume, exhaust fumes), emotion and drugs (non-steroidal anti-inflammatory drugs, β-blockers).

Over 200 materials encountered at the workplace may give rise to wheezing which typically improves at weekends and during holidays (occupational asthma). Common occupations associated with asthma are vets and animal handlers (allergens are mouse, rat and rabbit urine and fur), bakers (wheat, rye) and laundry workers (biological enzymes).

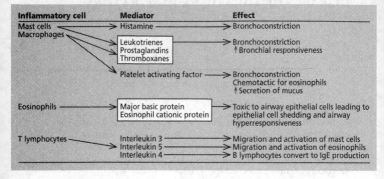

Inflammatory cell	Mediator	Effect
Mast cells Macrophages	Histamine	Bronchoconstriction
	Leukotrienes Prostaglandins Thromboxanes	Bronchoconstriction ↑ Bronchial responsiveness
	Platelet activating factor	Bronchoconstriction Chemotactic for eosinophils ↑ Secretion of mucus
Eosinophils	Major basic protein Eosinophil cationic protein	Toxic to airway epithelial cells leading to epithelial cell shedding and airway hyperresponsiveness
T lymphocytes	Interleukin 3 Interleukin 5 Interleukin 4	Migration and activation of mast cells Migration and activation of eosinophils B lymphocytes convert to IgE production

Figure 9.1 The pathogenesis of asthma.

A rare cause of asthma is the air-borne spores of *Aspergillus fumigatus* (a soil mould). There are fleeting shadows on the chest radiograph and peripheral blood eosinophilia (*allergic bronchopulmonary aspergillosis* – not to be confused with the severe aspergillus pneumonia occurring in the immuno-compromised).

Pathogenesis
The pathogenesis of asthma is complex and not fully understood. It involves a number of cells, mediators, nerves and vascular leakage (Figure 9.1) which can be activated by several mechanisms of which exposure to allergens is the most important.

The *cellular* component of the inflammatory response includes eosinophils, T lymphocytes, macrophages and mast cells which release a number of inflammatory mediators. Mast cell degranulation is produced by the union of antigen with IgE antibody which is bound to the mast cell surface.

Clinical features
Symptoms are episodic wheezing, cough and shortness of breath which are typically worse at night and in the early morning. A cough may be the only presenting symptom. Some patients have just one or two attacks a year whereas others have chronic symptoms. On examination, during an attack, there is reduced chest expansion, prolonged expiratory time and expiratory polyphonic wheezes.

Investigations
The diagnosis of asthma is often made on the history and response to bronchodilators. There is no single satisfactory diagnostic test for all asthmatic patients.

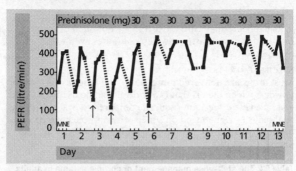

Figure 9.2 Classical diurnal variation of asthma, showing the effect of steroids. The arrows indicate the morning 'dips'. M, morning; N, noon; E, evening.

LUNG FUNCTION TESTS. Demonstration of a greater than 15% improvement in FEV_1 or PEFR following inhalation of a bronchodilator.

PEAK FLOW CHARTS. Measurement of PEFR by the patient on waking, during the day and before bed shows the characteristic variability in airflow limitation. Most asthmatic individuals will show obvious diurnal variation with lowest values occurring in the early morning (the 'morning dip', Figure 9.2).

HISTAMINE OR METHACHOLINE BRONCHIAL PROVOCATION TESTS. Bronchial hyperreactivity is demonstrated by asking the patients to inhale gradually increasing doses of histamine or methacholine and demonstrating a fall in FEV_1 Patients with clinical symptoms of asthma respond to very low doses.

CHEST RADIOGRAPH is performed at diagnosis and usually only repeated in an acute severe asthma attack.

SKIN-PRICK TESTS are used to identify allergens to which the patient is sensitive. A weal develops 15 minutes after allergen injection in the epidermis of the forearm.

Management
The effective treatment of asthma centres on patient education, avoidance of precipitating factors and specific drug treatment.

AVOIDANCE OF PRECIPITATING FACTORS
Patients should be discouraged from smoking and avoid allergens, e.g. household pets, which have been shown to provoke attacks. Avoidance of the house dust mite may be possible with frequent house cleaning and the use of effective covers for bedding. It is important to identify occupational

asthma because early diagnosis and removal of the patient from exposure may cure the asthma. Continued exposure may lead to severe asthma which continues even when exposure ceases.

SPECIFIC DRUG TREATMENT

Most drugs are delivered directly into the lungs as aerosols or powders which means that lower doses can be used and systemic side effects are reduced compared to oral treatment. Asthma is now managed on a step-wise approach which depends partly on repeated measurements of PEFR by the patient (Table 9.2).

Table 9.2 The step-wise management of chronic asthma in adults

Step	Treatment
1. Occasional symptoms	Inhaled short acting β-agonist as required
2. Daily symptoms	Low dose (up to 400 µg twice daily) inhaled corticosteroids
3. Severe symptoms	High dose (up to 1000 µg twice daily) inhaled corticosteroids
4. Severe symptoms not controlled	Add in long-acting inhaled β-agonist, or slow release theophylline
5. Severe symptoms not controlled	Add in oral steroids once daily

- Patient measures PEFR at home to guide treatment
- Short acting inhaled bronchodilators taken at any step as required
- A rescue course of oral prednisolone may be given at any time for acute exacerbation
- Acute severe asthma (PEFR < 30% of predicted) required hospital attendance

- β_2-Adrenoreceptor agonists, e.g. salbutamol, terbutaline and the longer-acting salmeterol, relax bronchial smooth muscle and cause bronchial dilatation
- Anticholinergic bronchodilators, e.g. ipratropium bromide or oxitropium bromide cause bronchodilatation and may be additive to adrenoreceptor stimulants
- Corticosteroids are powerful anti-inflammatory agents. They are used as maintenance treatment in all but very mild asthmatic individuals
- Anti-inflammatory agents, e.g. sodium cromoglycate, prevent activation of inflammatory cells and may be useful in mild asthma
- Sustained relief theophylline may be useful in some patients (Table 9.2). The side effects (tachycardia,

Table 9.3 Treatment of acute severe asthma
Monitor: pulse, respiratory rate, blood pressure, PEFR, oximetry, arterial blood gases

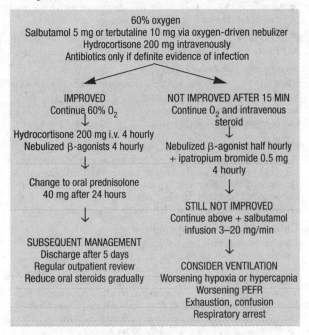

60% oxygen
Salbutamol 5 mg or terbutaline 10 mg via oxygen-driven nebulizer
Hydrocortisone 200 mg intravenously
Antibiotics only if definite evidence of infection

IMPROVED
Continue 60% O_2

Hydrocortisone 200 mg i.v. 4 hourly
Nebulized β-agonists 4 hourly

Change to oral prednisolone
40 mg after 24 hours

SUBSEQUENT MANAGEMENT
Discharge after 5 days
Regular outpatient review
Reduce oral steroids gradually

NOT IMPROVED AFTER 15 MIN
Continue O_2 and intravenous steroid

Nebulized β-agonist half hourly
+ ipatropium bromide 0.5 mg
4 hourly

STILL NOT IMPROVED
Continue above + salbutamol
infusion 3–20 mg/min

CONSIDER VENTILATION
Worsening hypoxia or hypercapnia
Worsening PEFR
Exhaustion, confusion
Respiratory arrest

arrhythmias and nausea) are seen less than with rapid-release preparations. Intravenous aminophylline (a water-soluble preparation of theophylline and ethylenediamine) is sometimes used in acute severe asthma

● The immunosuppressive drug methotrexate in low doses has been used in severely asthmatic individuals as a steroid-sparing agent

Acute severe asthma

Acute severe asthma is diagnosed when a patient has severe progressive asthmatic symptoms over a number of hours or days. It is a medical emergency that must be recognized and treated immediately at home with subsequent transfer to hospital (Table 9.3). In the UK, 1500 patients still die annually from this condition.

Clinical features
Features of acute severe asthma are the following:

- Inability to complete a sentence in one breath
- Tachycardia ≥ 110 beats/min
- Pulsus paradoxus, i.e. systolic blood pressure falls by more than 10 mmHg on inspiration
- Wheezing; the chest may be silent in very severe asthma
- PEFR < 50% of predicted value or < 50% of patient's best

Investigations and monitoring

CHEST RADIOGRAPH to exclude a pneumothorax.

BLOOD GASES: a rising P_aCO_2 and falling P_aO_2 indicate that ventilation may be necessary.

SERIAL PEFR as a guide to treatment.

Acute bronchitis

Acute bronchitis is usually viral but may be complicated by bacterial infection, particularly in smokers and patients with chronic airflow limitation. Symptoms are cough, retrosternal discomfort, chest tightness and wheezing, which usually resolve spontaneously over 4–8 days.

Chronic bronchitis and emphysema

Chronic bronchitis is defined symptomatically as cough productive of sputum on most days for at least 3 months of the year for more than 1 year. *Emphysema* is a pathological diagnosis and is defined as dilatation and destruction of the lung tissue distal to the terminal bronchioles. Although it has been suggested that these definitions separate patients into two different clinical groups (the 'pink puffers' with predominant emphysema and the 'blue bloaters' with predominant chronic bronchitis), most patients have both emphysema and chronic bronchitis, irrespective of the clinical signs. Chronic airflow limitation (CAL) is the collective term used for this group of patients.

Epidemiology

Chronic bronchitis and emphysema develop over many years and patients are rarely symptomatic before middle age. It is common (17% of men and 8% of women in the 40–60 year age group) in the UK, where it is one of the leading causes of lost working days.

Pathology

In *chronic bronchitis* there is airway narrowing, and hence airflow limitation, as a result of hypertrophy and hyperplasia of mucous glands, bronchial wall inflammation and mucosal oedema. The epithelial cell layer may ulcerate and, when the ulcers heal, squamous epithelium may replace columnar epithelium (squamous metaplasia).

Emphysematous changes lead to 'loss of elastic recoil' which normally keeps airways open during expiration; this is associated with expiratory airflow limitation and air trapping.

Aetiology and pathogenesis
- *Smoking* is the dominant causal agent. Persistent irritation by cigarette smoke causes hypertrophy of mucous glands. In addition, the lungs of smokers are infiltrated by granulocytes which may damage lung tissue by releasing proteases.
- *Atmospheric pollution* plays a minor role compared to smoking.
- α_1-*Antitrypsin deficiency* (page 89) is a rare cause of early onset emphysema. α_1-Antitrypsin is normally present in lung secretions and inhibits proteases. Deficiency, in theory, allows lung breakdown to proceed unchecked.

Clinical features
The main symptoms are cough, sputum, wheeze and breathlessness. Frequent infective exacerbations (from *Streptococcus pneumoniae* or *Haemophilus influenzae*) occur. On examination the patient with severe disease is breathless at rest with prolonged expiration and using the accessory muscles of respiration; chest expansion is poor and the lungs are hyperinflated. There may be a wheeze or quiet breath sounds. In 'pink puffers' breathlessness is the predominant problem; they are not cyanosed. 'Blue bloaters' hypoventilate; they are cyanosed, may be oedematous and have features of CO_2 retention (warm peripheries with a bounding pulse, flapping tremor of the outstretched hands and confusion in severe cases).

Investigations
The diagnosis is usually made clinically in a life-time smoker.
LUNG FUNCTION TESTS: the ratio of FEV_1 to FVC is reduced (< 70%) and the PEFR is low. Lung volumes are normal or increased.
CHEST RADIOGRAPH: typical features are hyperinflation, flat diaphragms, reduced peripheral lung markings and bullae, although the chest radiograph may be normal.
HAEMOGLOBIN AND PCV may be high as a result of secondary polycythaemia (page 127).
ARTERIAL BLOOD GASES may be normal or show hypoxia and hypercapnia.

Complications
- Respiratory failure (page 370)
- Cor pulmonale, i.e. right heart failure secondary to lung disease (page 307)

Management
The most important aspect of management is to persuade the

patient to stop smoking which will slow down the rate of deterioration. Drug therapy is similar to that of asthma.

ASSESSMENT OF REVERSIBILITY is made with a 2-week course of oral prednisolone (30 mg daily) with measurement of lung function before and after the treatment period. If there is objective evidence of benefit (> 15% improvement in FEV_1), oral steroids are gradually reduced and replaced with inhaled steroids.

BRONCHODILATORS. Inhaled β_2-agonists and the anticholinergic agent, ipratropium bromide, may produce symptomatic improvement even with little change in lung function tests.

LONG-TERM DOMICILLARY OXYGEN THERAPY will reduce mortality if given for 19 hours per day (every day) at a flow rate of 1–3 l/min to increase arterial oxygen saturation to > 90%. It is prescribed to patients who no longer smoke with an FEV_1 < 1.5 l/min and a P_aO_2 < 7.3 kPa.

ADDITIONAL TREATMENTS include venesection for polycythaemia (page 127) and diuretics for oedema. Exacerbations of CAL are usually the result of a superimposed respiratory infection (often *Haemophilus influenzae*) and are treated in a similar manner to asthma. However, these patients often depend on a degree of hypoxaemia to maintain respiratory drive and therefore, if oxygen is necessary, low concentrations (24%) are given so as not to reduce respiratory drive. The oxygen concentration may be increased in increments (28% and then 35%) if clinical examination and repeated arterial blood gases do not show hypoventilation and carbon dioxide retention. Exacerbations are occasionally the result of pneumothorax, heart failure or pulmonary embolism, and these must be considered and excluded.

Prognosis
Fifty per cent of patients with severe breathlessness die within 5 years.

Obstructive sleep apnoea

Obstructive sleep apnoea (OSA) is characterized by repetitive apnoeas (cessation of breathing for 10 seconds or more) as a result of obstruction of the upper airway during sleep.

Epidemiology
OSA affects about 1% of the population and is most common in overweight middle-aged men. It can occur in children, particularly those with large tonsils.

Aetiology
Apnoeas occur if the upper airway at the back of the throat is sucked closed when the patient breathes in. This occurs

during sleep because the muscles that hold the airway open are hypotonic. Airway closure continues until the patient is woken up by the struggle to breathe against a blocked throat. Contributing factors include alcohol ingestion before sleep, obesity and CAL. It is more common in hypothyroidism and acromegaly.

Clinical features

The major symptoms are snoring, apnoeas witnessed by bed partners and excessive daytime sleepiness which may lead to impairment of work performance and driving. Other symptoms are morning headaches, impotence and nocturnal choking.

Diagnosis

OVERNIGHT OXIMETRY shows frequent falls in arteriolar oxygen saturation in some but not all patients.

POLYSOMNOGRAPHY is a detailed sleep study performed in a sleep laboratory and provides a definitive diagnosis. It includes measurement of sleep quality, nasal and oral airflow, thoracoabdominal movements and arterial oxygen saturation.

Management

- Predisposing factors, e.g. obesity, tonsillar hypertrophy and facial deformities, should be treated

- CPAP (continuous positive airway pressure) to the airway via a tight-fitting nasal mask – nasal CPAP – during sleep keeps the pharyngeal walls open and is a very effective treatment

Bronchiectasis

Bronchiectasis is defined as dilatation of the bronchi. It may be localized to a lobe or generalized throughout the bronchial tree. There is impaired clearance of bronchial secretions with secondary bacterial infection.

Aetiology

- INFLAMMATORY: infective processes, e.g. measles, whooping cough, klebsiella pneumonia, may damage and weaken the bronchial wall leading to dilatation and ciliary damage

- OBSTRUCTION: proximal obstruction of an airway, e.g. inhaled foreign body, enlarged tuberculous lymph nodes, leads to distal accumulation of secretions which then become infected, resulting in localized bronchiectasis

- CONGENITAL FACTORS: these include cystic fibrosis (page 337), Kartagener's syndrome (bronchiectasis associated with immotile cilia, transposition of viscera and sinusitis) and immunoglobulin deficiencies which lead to recurrent infections

- IDIOPATHIC in which there is progressive bronchiectasis with no underlying cause

Epidemiology
Most cases arise in childhood but the incidence has decreased in all age groups with effective antibiotic treatment of pneumonia.

Clinical features
Cough and sputum production are the most common symptoms. In severe bronchiectasis there is production of copious amounts of thick, foul-smelling green sputum. Other symptoms are haemoptysis, breathlessness and wheeze. On examination there is clubbing and coarse crackles over the affected area, usually the lung bases.

Investigations
RADIOLOGY: the chest radiograph may be normal or show dilated bronchi with thickened bronchial walls and sometimes multiple cysts containing fluid. High-resolution CT (slices are between 1 and 2 mm thick compared to conventional CT slice of 10 mm) is the investigation of choice and may show bronchial wall thickening that is not shown on a standard chest radiograph. Bronchography is only used to assess extent of disease before surgery (see treatment).

SPUTUM CULTURE is essential during an infective exacerbation. The common organisms are *Staphylococcus aureus, Pseudomonas aeruginosa* and *Haemophilus influenzae.*

FURTHER INVESTIGATIONS, e.g. serum immunoglobulins, sweat test, in patients where an underlying cause is suspected.

Management
PHYSIOTHERAPY AND DAILY POSTURAL DRAINAGE are of vital importance. The patient is taught to carry them out at home.

ANTIBIOTICS, e.g. cefaclor, for infective exacerbations. If there is no improvement it is probable that there is infection with *Pseudomonas aeruginosa* which requires specific antibiotics, e.g. ceftazidime, administered by aerosol or parenterally. Oral ciprofloxacin is an alternative.

BRONCHODILATORS are used for those with demonstrable airflow limitation.

SURGERY is reserved for the very small minority with localized disease.

Complications
The main complications are pneumonia, cerebral abscess and life-threatening haemoptysis.

Cystic fibrosis

Cystic fibrosis is an autosomal recessive condition occurring in 1:2000 live births. It is characterized by a generalized abnormality of all exocrine glands, resulting in the production of unusually viscous secretions which block and damage the glands.

Table 9.4 Pathogenesis and approaches to treatment of respiratory disease in cystic fibrosis

Amiloride, DNAase, antiprotease and ATP are given by aerosol.

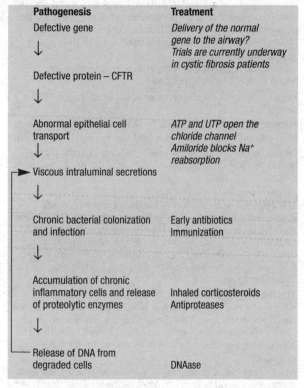

Pathogenesis	Treatment
Defective gene ↓	*Delivery of the normal gene to the airway? Trials are currently underway in cystic fibrosis patients*
Defective protein – CFTR ↓	
Abnormal epithelial cell transport ↓	*ATP and UTP open the chloride channel Amiloride blocks Na⁺ reabsorption*
Viscous intraluminal secretions ↓	
Chronic bacterial colonization and infection ↓	Early antibiotics Immunization
Accumulation of chronic inflammatory cells and release of proteolytic enzymes ↓	Inhaled corticosteroids Antiproteases
Release of DNA from degraded cells	DNAase

Aetiology

There is defective opening of chloride channels at the luminal surface of epithelial cells, resulting in decreased excretion of chloride into the airway lumen. Associated with this is increased sodium and hence water absorption from the lumen which results in thick tenacious secretions. The genetic defect in cystic fibrosis has been localized to the long arm of chromosome 7. A large gene is responsible for production of a 1480 amino acid protein – the cystic fibrosis transmembrane conduction regulator (CFTR) – which probably represents the chloride channel. The most common mutation is ΔF_{508} (deletion, phenylalanine at position 508).

Clinical features

Neonates may present with meconium ileus. In children and young adults the most common presenting symptoms are those of bronchiectasis and recurrent chest infections. There may be steatorrhoea and diabetes mellitus as a result of pancreatic insufficiency. Males are infertile because of failure of development of the vas deferens. Chronic ill health in children leads to impaired growth and delayed puberty.

Investigations

GENETIC SCREENING and counselling are offered to couples with a family history of the disease.

PRENATAL DIAGNOSIS by amniocentesis or chorionic villous sampling.

NEONATAL DIAGNOSIS is made by demonstration of low levels of immunoreactive trypsin in a heel-prick specimen of blood.

IN CHILDREN the diagnosis is made by demonstration of a high sweat sodium > 60 mmol/l. In adults the results are more difficult to interpret.

Management

Management of bronchiectasis and exocrine pancreatic insufficiency has been described previously (page 336). More recently, an understanding of the basic defect and pathogenesis of cystic fibrosis has led to newer treatments which are described in Table 9.4. Some patients with severe respiratory disease have received lung or heart/lung transplantations.

The recent emergence of *Pseudomonas cepacia* is a problem for patients and doctors alike. It is associated with accelerated lung disease and resistance to antibiotics with some strains. Close contact promotes cross-infection, so siblings with cystic fibrosis may pass the organism from one to another.

Prognosis

Ninety per cent of children now survive into their teens and the mean survival is 29 years. Most mortality is the result of pulmonary disease.

DISEASES OF THE LUNG PARENCHYMA

Pneumonias

Pneumonia may be defined as an inflammation of the substance of the lung and is usually caused by bacteria.

Pneumonia can be classified both anatomically, e.g. lobar (*affecting the whole of one lobe*) and bronchopneumonia (*affecting the lobules and bronchi*), or on the basis of aetiology (Table 9.5). *Mycobacterium tuberculosis* is an important cause of pneumonia; it is considered separately as both mode of presentation and treatment are different from the infective agents shown in the table.

Table 9.5 Aetiology of pneumonia in UK

Type of pneumonia	Clinical circumstance
Community acquired	Usually occurs in otherwise fit patients.
Streptococcus pneumoniae	*Streptoccocus* sp. is the most common
Mycoplasma pneumoniae	cause of pneumonia (50% of cases),
Influenza A virus (usually with	*Mycoplasma* sp. is the next most
a bacterial component)	common (6%)
Haemophilus influenzae	Pre-existing chronic lung disease
Chlamydia sp.	*Chlamydia psittaci* contacted from
	infected birds
Staphylococcus aureus	Occurs in children, intravenous drug
	abusers and after influenza
Legionella pneumophila	Acquired from contaminated water,
	e.g. showers in hotels and hospitals
Coxiella burnetii	Transmitted from animals; occurs in
	abattoir and animal hide workers
Hospital acquired	
Gram-negative bacteria	Causative organisms differ from
Staphylococcus aureus	community-acquired, predominantly
Anaerobes	Gram-negative organisms (e.g.
	Pseudomonas, *Klebsiella* spp.)
In the immunosuppressed	
Pneumocystis carinii	Occur in patients with AIDS,
Aspergillus fumigatus	leukaemia, congenital
Cytomegalovirus	immunodeficiency

Clinical features
Precipitating factors for pneumonia are underlying lung disease, smoking, alcohol abuse, immunosuppression and other chronic illnesses. Symptoms and signs vary according to the infecting agent and to the immune state of the patients. Most commonly there is pyrexia, pleuritic chest pain and a dry cough which may later become productive. Signs of consolidation and a pleural rub may be present.

Investigations
SPUTUM should be sent for culture and Gram stain.

BLOOD COUNT. The white cell count is raised in 50% of those with pneumococcal pneumonia but in only 10% of those with legionella or mycoplasma pneumonia.

BLOOD CULTURE is positive in 15–25% even if the sputum is negative and indicates a poorer prognosis.

CHEST RADIOGRAPHY confirms consolidation but these changes may lag behind the clinical course. A chest radiograph which remains persistently abnormal (> 6 weeks) suggests an underlying abnormality, usually a carcinoma.

Management

In mild cases treatment can be started immediately with oral cefaclor and erythromycin. More severe cases should be admitted to hospital and treated with intravenous cefuroxime and erythromycin. Penicillin and ampicillin/amoxycillin is no longer used because many of the common organisms are resistant. Pleuritic pain requires analgesia, and oxygen therapy should be given if there is severe hypoxia. Treatment should be modified in the light of subsequent investigations.

Specific forms of pneumonia

MYCOPLASMA PNEUMONIAE

Mycoplasma pneumonia commonly presents in young adults with generalized features such as headaches and malaise which may precede chest symptoms by 4 or 5 days. Physical signs in the chest may be scanty, and chest radiographic appearances frequently do not correlate with the clinical state of the patient. The white cell count is not raised and cold agglutinins are raised in 50%. Diagnosis is usually based on clinical suspicion and subsequently confirmed by a rising antibody titre (paired sera taken at presentation and 10 days later). Treatment is with erythromycin or tetracycline. Extrapulmonary complications (myocarditis, erythema multiforme, haemolytic anaemia and meningoencephalitis) will occasionally dominate the clinical picture.

HAEMOPHILUS INFLUENZAE

This is commonly the cause of pneumonia in patients with chronic bronchitis and emphysema. There are no other features to differentiate it from other causes of bacterial pneumonia.

CHLAMYDIA SPECIES

Chlamydia pneumoniae is a recently recognized organism and a more common cause of pneumonia than previously thought.

Patients with *C. psittaci* pneumonia may give a history of contact with infected birds, particularly parrots. Symptoms include malaise, fever, cough and muscular pains which may be low grade and protracted over many months. Occasionally the presentation mimics meningitis with high fever, prostration, photophobia and neck stiffness. Diagnosis is confirmed by demonstrating a rising serum titre of complement-fixing antibody and treatment is with erythromycin or tetracycline.

STAPHYLOCOCCI

Staphylococcus aureus usually causes pneumonia only after a preceding influenza viral illness or in intravenous drug users. It results in patchy areas of consolidation which may break down to form abscesses that appear as cysts on the radiograph. Pneumothorax, effusions and empyemas are frequent, and septicaemia may develop with metastatic abscesses in other organs. All patients with this form of pneumonia are extremely ill and the mortality rate is in excess of 25%. Treatment is with intravenous flucloxacillin.

LEGIONELLA PNEUMOPHILA
Infection with this organism may be sporadic, occur in institutions such as hotels or hospitals *(contamination of water and cooling systems)* or occur as outbreaks in immunocompromised patients. Infection is spread by the aerosol route and affects men twice as commonly as women. Clinical features include malaise, myalgia, headache and fever with rigors. Nausea, vomiting and diarrhoea are common, and patients may be acutely ill with mental confusion and other neurological signs. Respiratory symptoms include tachypnoea and a dry cough which later becomes purulent. Diagnosis is by direct immunofluorescent staining of the organism in the pleural fluid, sputum or bronchial washings, and confirmed by a rise in serum antibody titre. The treatment of choice is tetracycline although rifampicin is also used. Mortality rate may be up to 30% in elderly patients although most recover spontaneously.

COXIELLA BURNETII (Q FEVER)
There are systemic symptoms of fever, malaise and headache, often associated with multiple lesions on the chest radiograph. The illness may run a chronic course and may be associated with endocarditis. Diagnosis is made with a rising serum titre of complement-fixing antibody and treatment is with erythromycin or tetracycline.

PSEUDOMONAS AERUGINOSA
Pseudomonas aeruginosa is seen in the immunocompromised and in patients with cystic fibrosis, in whom its presence is associated with a worsening of the clinical condition and increasing mortality. Treatment is with ceftazidime or ciprofloxacin (page 336). These antibiotics can be inhaled via nebulizers in patients with cystic fibrosis.

PNEUMOCYSTIS CARINII
Pneumocystis carinii is the most common opportunistic infection in patients with the acquired immune deficiency syndrome (AIDS). The clinical features and treatment are described on page 22.

Aspiration pneumonia
Aspiration of gastric contents into the lungs can produce a severe destructive pneumonia as a result of the corrosive effect of gastric acid – the Mendelson's syndrome. Aspiration

usually occurs into the posterior segment of the right lower lobe because of the bronchial anatomy. It is associated with periods of impaired consciousness, structural abnormalities, such as tracheo-oesophageal fistulae or oesophageal strictures, or bulbar palsy.

Lung abscess and empyema

A lung abscess results from localized suppuration of the lung associated with cavity formation, often with a fluid level on the chest radiograph. Empyema means the presence of pus in the pleural cavity, usually from rupture of a lung abscess into the pleural cavity or from bacterial spread from a severe pneumonia.

Aetiology
A lung abscess develops in the following circumstances:

- As a complication of pneumonia
- Secondary to bronchial obstruction by tumour or foreign body
- From septic emboli from a focus elsewhere (usually staphylococcus)
- Secondary to infarction

Clinical features
There is a persisting or worsening pneumonia, often with the production of copious amounts of foul-smelling sputum. With empyema the patient is usually very ill with a high fever and neutrophil leukocytosis. There may be malaise, weight loss and clubbing of the digits.

Investigations
Bacteriological investigation is best conducted on specimens obtained by transtracheal aspiration, bronchoscopy or percutaneous transthoracic aspiration.

Management
Antibiotics are given to cover both aerobic and anaerobic organisms. Intravenous cefuroxime, erythromycin and metronidazole are given for 5 days followed by oral cefaclor and metronidazole for several weeks. Empyemas should be treated by prompt tube drainage or rib resection and drainage of the empyema cavity. Abscesses occasionally require surgery.

Tuberculosis ND

Epidemiology
Tuberculosis is now the most common cause of death worldwide from a single infectious disease, and the disease is on the increase in most parts of the world. This primarily results from inadequate programmes for disease control, multiple drug resistance, co-infection with HIV and a rapid

rise in the world's population of young adults – the group with the highest mortality from tuberculosis. In the UK, the incidence of tuberculosis is 40 times greater in immigrants from the Asian population than in the native white population.

Pathology
The initial infection with *Mycobacterium tuberculosis* is known as *primary tuberculosis*. It usually occurs in the lung but may occur in the gastrointestinal tract, particularly the ileocaecal region. The primary focus in the lung is subpleural in the mid to upper zones (Figure 9.3) and is characterized by exudation and infiltration with neutrophil granulocytes. These are replaced by macrophages which engulf the bacilli and result in the typical granulomatous lesions which consist of central areas of caseation surrounded by epithelioid cells and Langhans' giant cells (both derived from the macrophage). The primary focus is almost always accompanied by caseous lesions in the regional lymph nodes (mediastinal and cervical). In most people the primary infection and the lymph nodes heal completely and become calcified. Some of these calcified primary lesions harbour tubercle bacilli which may become reactivated if there is depression of the host defence system. Occasionally there is dissemination of the primary infection producing *miliary tuberculosis*.

Reactivation results in typical *postprimary tuberculosis*. Postprimary tuberculosis refers to all forms of tuberculosis that develop after the first few weeks of the primary infection when immunity to the mycobacteria has developed.

Clinical features
Primary TB is usually symptomless; occasionally there may be erythema nodosum (page 516), a small pleural effusion or pulmonary collapse from compression of a lobar bronchus by enlarged nodes (Figure 9.3). Most commonly clinical tuberculosis represents delayed reactivation. Symptoms begin insidiously with malaise, anorexia, weight loss, fever and cough. Sputum is mucoid purulent or blood-stained, but night sweats are uncommon. There are often no physical signs although occasionally signs of a pneumonia or pleural effusion may be present.

Investigations
CHEST RADIOGRAPHY typically shows patchy or nodular shadows in the upper zones with loss of volume and fibrosis with or without cavitation.

SPUTUM is stained with Ziehl–Neelsen stain for acid- and alcohol-fast bacilli and cultured on Dover's or Lowenstein–Jensen medium. This takes 4–8 weeks.

BRONCHOSCOPY with washings of the affected lobes is useful if no sputum is available.

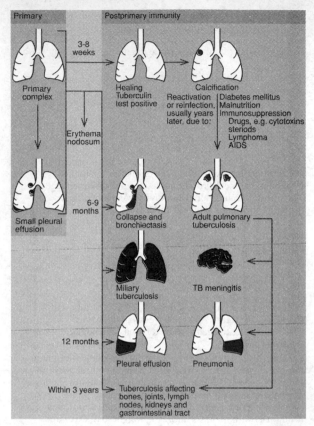

Figure 9.3 The manifestations of primary and postprimary tuberculosis.

BIOPSY with histological examination and culture of pleura, lymph nodes and solid lesions within the lung (tuberculomas) may be required for diagnosis.

Management

Pulmonary tuberculosis assumed to be caused by sensitive organisms is treated with rifampicin and isoniazid for 6 months along with pyrazinamide for the first 2 months until drug sensitivities are available. Treatment duration should be extended to 9 months for bone tuberculosis and to 12 months for tuberculous meningitis. Ethambutol is included in a treatment regimen if resistance is suspected. Streptomycin is now rarely used in the UK, but it may be added if the organism is resistant to isoniazid. Significant side effects are uncommon and are listed in Table 9.6. A transient asymptomatic rise in the serum transferase level may occur with rifampicin but treatment is only stopped if hepatitis develops.

Table 9.6 Side effects of drug treatment

Rifampicin	Stains body secretions and urine pink
	Induces liver enzymes and accelerates metabolism of some drugs including phenytoin, warfarin and oestrogens. Oestrogen-containing contraceptive pills are thus unreliable
	Hepatitis
	Rarely thrombocytopenia
Isoniazid	Polyneuropathy; prophylactic pyridoxine is recommended
	Allergic reactions
	Hepatitis
Pyrazinamide	Hepatitis
	Hyperuricaemia and gout
	Rash and arthralgia
Ethambutol	Dose-related retrobulbar neuritis. Patients are asked to report visual problems and to undergo regular specialist ophthalmic examination

The major causes of treatment failure are incorrect prescribing by the doctor and inadequate compliance by the patient. Treatment should be supervised by a specialist physician. All cases of TB must be notified to the local Public Health Authority so that contact tracing and screening can be arranged. Close contacts of a case are screened for evidence of diseases with a chest radiograph and a Mantoux test (intradermal injection of purified protein derivative of *M. tuberculosis* produces induration and inflammation in individuals with active infection or who have previously been immunized with BCG).

Prevention

Immunization with BCG (Bacille Calmette–Guèrin) decreases the risk of developing tuberculosis by about 15–70%. It is a bovine strain of *Mycobacterium tuberculosis* which has lost its virulence after growth in the laboratory for many years. Routine immunization is becoming less common in the UK as the incidence of tuberculosis is decreasing in the indigenous population. Immunization produces cellular immunity and a positive tuberculin test, and is the main reason why the Mantoux test is now of little value for diagnosis of active disease in the UK. BCG immunization of the newborn is still given in developing countries where TB is more prevalent.

Chemoprophylaxis

Patients with chest radiographic changes compatible with previous tuberculosis and who are about to undergo treatment with an immunosuppressive agent should receive chemoprophylaxis with isoniazid.

Granulomatous lung disease

A granuloma is a mass or nodule of chronic inflammatory tissue and is characterized by the presence of epithelioid multinucleate giant cells. Sarcoidosis is the most common cause of lung granulomas.

Sarcoidosis

Sarcoidosis is a multisystem granulomatous disorder, commonly affecting young adults and usually presenting with bilateral hilar lymphadenopathy (BHL), pulmonary infiltrations and skin or eye lesions.

Epidemiology

The disease has been identified in all ethnic groups but is much more common in patients of Afro-Caribbean origin than in Caucasians. The disease may also be clinically more severe in this group. It is most common in young adults and is more prevalent in females than males.

Aetiology

This is unknown although genetic, environmental and infective factors have all been implicated.

Immunopathology

- The typical non-caseating (compare TB) sarcoid granuloma consists of a focal accumulation of epithelioid cells, macrophages and lymphocytes, mainly T cells

- There is a depressed cell-mediated immunity to antigens, such as tuberculin and *Candida albicans*, and an overall lymphopenia with low circulating T cells and slightly increased B cells (as a result of sequestration of lymphocytes within the lung)

- There is an increased number of cells in the bronchoalveolar lavage: particularly CD4 helper cells

- Transbronchial biopsies show infiltration of alveolar walls and interstitial spaces with mononuclear cells before granuloma formation

Clinical features

The most common presentation is with bilateral hilar lymphadenopathy which may be found incidentally on a routine chest radiograph or be associated with mild fever, malaise, arthralgia and erythema nodosum (page 516).

Pulmonary infiltration may predominate and, in a minority of patients, there is progressive fibrosis resulting in increasing effort dyspnoea, cor pulmonale and death. The chest radiograph is negative at presentation in up to 20% of non-respiratory cases. Skin and ocular sarcoidosis are the most common extrapulmonary problems (Table 9.7). Asymptomatic hypercalcaemia is found on routine blood tests in 10% of established cases, but is less commonly a clinical problem. Hepatitis and hepatosplenomegaly are uncommon but granulomata may often be found if a liver biopsy is performed. Cardiac involvement is rare.

Table 9.7 Extrapulmonary features of sarcoidosis

Skin	Erythema nodosum, skin papules, lupus pernio (red/blue infiltration of the nose)
Eye	Anterior uveitis, conjunctivitis, keratoconjunctivitis sicca, uveoparotid fever (bilateral uveitis, parotid gland enlargement and facial nerve palsy)
Bone	Arthralgias, bone cysts
Metabolic	Hypercalcaemia as a result of high circulating levels of $1,25(OH_2)D_3$ from activated sarcoid macrophages
Liver	Granulomatous hepatitis, hepatosplenomegaly
CNS	Seventh cranial nerve palsy, hypothalamic involvement, hypopituitarism
Heart	Ventricular arrhythmias, conduction defects, cardiomyopathy with cardiac failure

Investigations

Diagnosis depends on a compatible clinical picture, exclusion of other causes of granulomatous diseases, such as tuberculosis and beryllium poisoning, and histological evidence of non-caseating granulomata.

TRANSBRONCHIAL BIOPSY is the most useful investigation and gives positive histological evidence in 90% of cases of pulmonary sarcoidosis.

LUNG FUNCTION TESTS in pulmonary infiltration show a restrictive lung defect with a decreased total lung capacity, FEV_1, FVC and gas transfer.

SERUM ANGIOTENSIN-CONVERTING ENZYME (ACE) is raised in 75% of patients. It is useful in assessing activity of disease, but is not of diagnostic value because it is also elevated in patients with lymphoma, tuberculosis, asbestosis, silicosis and Gaucher's disease.

TUBERCULIN TEST is negative in 80% of patients. It is of no diagnostic value.

BIOPSY and histological examination of involved lymph nodes, liver or skin lesions are sometimes necessary for diagnosis.

THE KVEIM TEST involves an intradermal injection of sarcoid spleen and subsequent (4–6 weeks later) histological examination for non-caseating granulomata. It is rarely used because of the risk of transmission of infection and reduced sensitivity and specificity compared to other tests.

Differential diagnosis

The differential diagnosis of BHL includes lymphoma, pulmonary tuberculosis and bronchial carcinoma with secondary spread. The combination of symmetrical BHL and erythema nodosum only occurs in sarcoidosis.

Management

The requirement for treatment and the role of steroids are presently contested in many aspects of this disease. Hilar lymphadenopathy without any other evidence of lung involvement does not require treatment. Infiltration or abnormal lung functions test which persists for 6 months after diagnosis should be treated with 30 mg prednisolone for 6 weeks, reducing to 15 mg prednisolone on alternate days for 6–12 months. Most patients with hypercalcaemia or other evidence of extrapulmonary sarcoidosis probably require treatment with prednisolone. Topical steroids are used for eye involvement.

Prognosis

In patients of Afro-Caribbean origin, mortality rate may be up to 10%, but is less than 5% in Caucasians. Death is mainly as a result of respiratory failure or renal damage from hypercalciuria. The prognosis is best in those with BHL and no infiltration on the chest radiograph: more than 90% recover spontaneously.

Wegener's granulomatosis

Wegener's granulomatosis is a vasculitis of unknown aetiology characterized by lesions involving the upper respiratory tract, the lungs and the kidneys. The disease often starts with rhinorrhoea with subsequent nasal mucosal ulceration, cough, haemoptysis and pleuritic pain. Chest radiography shows nodular masses or pneumonic infiltrates with cavitation which often show a migratory pattern. Antineutrophil cytoplasmic antibodies (page 196) are found in the serum in over 90% of cases with active disease, and measurement is useful both diagnostically and as a guide to disease activity in the treated patient. Typical histological changes are best shown in the kidney where there is a necrotizing glomerulonephritis. Treatment is with cyclophosphamide.

Pulmonary fibrosis and honeycomb lung

Pulmonary fibrosis is the end result of many diseases of the respiratory tract. It may be one of the following types:

- Localized, e.g. following unresolved pneumonia
- Bilateral, e.g. in TB
- Widespread, e.g. in cryptogenic fibrosing alveolitis

Honeycomb lung is the radiological appearance seen with widespread fibrosis. Dilated and thickened terminal and respiratory bronchioles produce cystic airspaces giving a honeycomb appearance on chest radiography.

Cryptogenic fibrosing alveolitis

Cryptogenic fibrosing alveolitis is a rare disorder of unknown aetiology which causes gradual diffuse fibrosis throughout the lung fields usually in late middle age.

Clinical features

There is progressive breathlessness and cyanosis leading eventually to respiratory failure. Finger clubbing occurs in two-thirds of cases, and fine bilateral basal crackles are heard on auscultation. Rarely, an acute form known as the Hamman–Rich syndrome occurs.

Investigation

CHEST RADIOGRAPHIC appearances are initially of a ground-glass appearance progressing to fibrosis and honeycomb lung.

LUNG FUNCTION TESTS show a restrictive defect. The lung volumes are reduced, FEV_1:FVC ratio is normal to high (with both values being reduced) and gas transfer is reduced.

BRONCHOALVEOLAR LAVAGE shows increased numbers of cells, particularly neutrophils.

BLOOD GASES show hypoxaemia with a normal P_aCO_2.

HISTOLOGICAL CONFIRMATION with transbronchial or open lung biopsies may be required in younger people.

AUTOANTIBODIES such as antinuclear factor and rheumatoid factor may be positive.

Differential diagnosis

This is from other causes of lung fibrosis: rheumatoid lung, sarcoidosis, radiation, pneumoconiosis, chronic extrinsic allergic alveolitis and drugs (amiodarone, busulphan, methysergide).

Treatment

Large doses of prednisolone are used (prednisolone 30 mg daily), and azathioprine and cyclophosphamide may also be tried. Single lung transplantation is now an established treatment for some individuals and current survival rate figures are 60% at one year after transplantation.

Prognosis

The median survival is approximately 5 years.

Extrinsic allergic alveolitis

Extrinsic allergic alveolitis is characterized by a widespread diffuse inflammatory reaction in the alveoli and small airways of the lung as a response to inhalation of a range of different antigens. By far the most common is farmers' lung which affects up to one in 10 of the farming community in poor wet areas around the world (Table 9.8).

Table 9.8 Extrinsic allergic bronchiolar alveolitis

Disease	Situation	Antigens
Farmers' lung	Forking mouldy hay or other vegetable material	*Faenia rectivirgula* (*Micropolyspora faeni*)
Bird fanciers' lung	Handling pigeons, cleaning lofts or budgerigar cages	Proteins present in feathers and excreta
Malt workers' lung	Turning germinating barley	*Aspergillus clavatus*
Humidifier fever	Contaminated humidifying systems in air conditioners or humidifiers	A variety of bacteria or amoebae

Clinical features
There is fever, malaise, cough and shortness of breath several hours after exposure to the causative antigen. Physical examination reveals tachypnoea, and coarse end-inspiratory crackles and wheezes. Continuing exposure leads to a chronic illness with weight loss, effort dyspnoea, cough and the features of fibrosing alveolitis.

Investigations
FULL BLOOD COUNT shows a raised white cell count in acute cases.

CHEST RADIOGRAPH shows fluffy nodular shadowing with subsequent development of streaky shadows, particularly in the upper zones.

LUNG FUNCTION TESTS show a restrictive defect with a decrease in gas transfer.

PRECIPITATING ANTIBODIES are present in the serum. (These are evidence of exposure and not disease.)

BRONCHOALVEOLAR LAVAGE shows increased lymphocytes and granulocytes.

Management
Prevention is the aim with avoidance if possible of exposure to the antigen. Prednisolone in large doses (30–60 mg daily) may be required to cause regression of the disease in the early stages.

Pneumoconiosis

Most inhaled particles cause no damage to the lung because they are trapped in the nose, removed by the mucociliary clearance system or destroyed by alveolar macrophages. Small inorganic dust particles that reach the acinus and damage macrophages initiate an inflammatory reaction and subsequent fibrosis. Pneumoconiosis (Table 9.9) is the term used for the lung disease that develops. The incidence of pneumoconiosis has decreased since the introduction of improved working conditions.

Table 9.9 The common pneumoconioses

Disease	Cause	Occupation
Coal workers' pneumoconiosis	Coal dust	Coal mining
Asbestosis	Asbestos	Building trade, pipe fitters
Silicosis	Silica	Mining, sand blasting, stone masons
Berylliosis	Beryllium	Atomic reactors, electronics

Coal workers' peumoconiosis

The disease is subdivided into *simple pneumoconiosis* and *progressive massive fibrosis* (PMF). Simple pneumoconiosis produces small (< 1.5 mm) pulmonary nodules on the chest radiograph. It is unclear whether symptoms and a decline in respiratory function are the result of the disease *per se* or of associated smoking and chronic airflow limitation. The importance of simple pneumoconiosis is that it may lead to the development of PMF with continued exposure. PMF is characterized by large (1–10 cm), often confluent fibrotic masses predominantly in the upper lobes. Unlike simple pneumoconiosis the disease may progress after exposure to coal dust has ceased. Symptoms are dyspnoea and cough productive of black sputum. Eventually respiratory failure may supervene. There is no specific treatment and further exposure must be prevented. Patients with PMF and some with simple pneumoconiosis (depending on severity of chest radiographic changes) are eligible for disability benefit.

Asbestosis

Asbestos is a mixture of fibrous silicates which have the common properties of resistance to heat, acid and alkali, hence their widespread use at one time. Chrysotile or white asbestos comprises 90% of the world production and is less fibrogenic than the other forms – crocidolite (blue asbestos) and amosite (brown asbestos). The diseases caused by asbestos (Table 9.10) are all characterized by a long latency period (20–40 years) between exposure and disease.

Table 9.10 The effects of asbestos on the lung

Disease	Pathology and clinical features
Asbestos bodies in the lung	They produce no symptoms or change in lung function and serve only as a marker of exposure
Pleural plaques	Fibrotic plaques on the parietal pleura which usually produce no symptoms
*Bilateral diffuse pleural thickening	Thickening of the parietal and visceral pleura which produces effort dyspnoea and a restrictive ventilatory defect
*Mesothelioma	Tumour arising from mesothelial cells of the pleura, peritoneum and pericardium. Often presents with a pleural effusion. There is no treatment and median survival is 2 years
*Asbestosis	Characterized by progressive dyspnoea associated with finger clubbing and bilateral basal end-inspiratory crackles. There is a restrictive ventilatory defect on lung function testing
*Lung cancer, often adenocarcinoma	Presentation and treatment is that of lung cancer (see below)

* The diseases indicated are all eligible for compensation under the Social Security Act of 1975.

CARCINOMA OF THE LUNG

Epidemiology
Bronchial carcinoma is the most common malignant tumour in the Western World and is the third most common cause of death after heart disease and pneumonia in the UK. There is a 3.5:1 male to female ratio, but although the rising mortality of this disease has levelled off in men, it continues to rise in women.

Aetiology
Smoking is by far the most important aetiological factor, although there is a higher incidence in urban areas compared to rural areas even when allowances are made for smoking. Other aetiological factors are passive smoking, exposure to asbestos and possibly also contact with arsenic, chromium, iron oxides and products of coal combustion.

Pathology

These are broadly divided into small cell and non-small cell cancer. Non-small cell tumours are further subdivided as shown in Table 9.11.

Table 9.11 Types of bronchial carcinoma

Cell type	Percentage lung tumours	Characteristics
Non-small cell		
Squamous	40	The most common cancer, occasionally cavitates, widespread metastases occur late
Large cell	25	Less well-differentiated tumour that metastasizes early
Adenocarcinoma	10	More common in non-smokers and as a result of asbestos exposure. Usually occurs peripherally
Alveolar cell	1–2	Presents as a peripheral nodule or as diffuse nodular lesions of multicentric origin
Small cell	20–30	Arises from endocrine cells (Kulchitsky cells) which often secrete polypeptide hormones. Rapidly growing and highly malignant but the only bronchial cancer that responds to chemotherapy

Clinical features

LOCAL EFFECTS OF TUMOUR WITHIN A BRONCHUS
Cough, chest pain, haemoptysis and breathlessness are typical symptoms.

SPREAD WITHIN THE CHEST
Tumour may directly involve the pleura and ribs, causing pain and bone fractures. Spread to involve the brachial plexus causes pain in the shoulder and inner arm (Pancoast's tumour), spread to the sympathetic ganglion causes Horner's syndrome (page 451), and spread to the left recurrent laryngeal nerve causes hoarseness and a bovine cough. In addition the tumour may directly involve the oesophagus, heart or superior vena cava (causing upper limb oedema, facial congestion and distended neck veins).

METASTATIC DISEASE
Metastases present as bone pain, epilepsy or with focal neurological signs.

These are rare apart from finger clubbing (Table 9.12).

There may, in addition, be non-specific features such as malaise, lethargy and weight loss. On examination of the chest there are often no physical signs, although lymphadenopathy, signs of a pleural effusion, lobar collapse or unresolved pneumonia may be present.

Table 9.12 Non-metastatic extrapulmonary manifestations of bronchial carcinoma

Endocrine	Ectopic ACTH secretion (Cushing's syndrome) Ectopic antidiuretic hormone secretion (dilutional hyponatraemia) Secretion of PTH-like substance (hypercalcaemia)
Neurological	Cerebellar degeneration Myopathy, polyneuropathies Myasthenic syndrome (Eaton–Lambert syndrome)
Vascular/haematological	Thrombophlebitis migrans Non-bacterial thrombotic endocarditis Anaemia Disseminated intravascular coagulation
Skeletal	Clubbing (30%) Hypertrophic osteoarthropathy (clubbing with painful wrists and ankles)
Cutaneous	Dermatomyositis Acanthosis nigricans (pigmented overgrowth of skin in axillae or groin) Herpes zoster

Investigations

The aim of investigation is to confirm the diagnosis, determine the histology and assess tumour spread as a guide to treatment.

CONFIRM THE DIAGNOSIS

Chest radiograph is the most valuable initial test although tumours need to be between 1 and 2 cm to be recognized reliably. They usually appear as a round shadow, the edge of which often has a fluffy or spiked appearance. There may be evidence of cavitation, lobar collapse, a pleural effusion or secondary pneumonia. Spread through the lymphatic channels gives rise to *lymphangitis carcinomatosis*, appearing as streaky shadowing throughout the lung.

DETERMINE THE HISTOLOGY

Sputum is examined for malignant cells. Bronchoscopy is

used to obtain samples for histological investigation and for obtaining washings for cytology. Transthoracic fine needle aspiration biopsy under radiographic or CT screening is useful for obtaining tissue diagnosis from peripheral lesions.

ASSESS SPREAD OF THE TUMOUR
At bronchoscopy involvement of the first 2 cm of either main bronchus or of the recurrent laryngeal nerve (vocal cord paresis) indicates inoperability. CT is useful for assessing the mediastinum and extent of tumour spread. Mediastinoscopy and lymph node biopsy may be necessary before surgery if the scan shows lymphadenopathy which can be reactive or involved by tumour. The presence of bony and liver metastases is determined by serum alkaline phosphatase and other liver biochemistry. Liver ultrasonography and isotope bone scan are only necessary if these screening tests are abnormal.

DETERMINE PATIENT SUITABILITY FOR MAJOR OPERATION
Physical examination and respiratory function tests.

Treatment
SURGERY is the only treatment of any value for non-small cell cancer. In the 20% of cases that are suitable for resection the 5-year survival rate is 25–30%.

RADIOTHERAPY in high doses can produce results that are equal to surgery in patients with localized tumours but who are otherwise unfit for surgery, e.g. poor lung function testing. Palliative radiotherapy is useful for bone pain, haemoptysis and superior vena caval obstruction.

CHEMOTHERAPY is only of value in small cell cancer and has resulted in a fivefold increase in median survival from 3 to 15 months. A small number of patients achieve several years of remission.

LOCAL TREATMENTS. Endoscopic laser therapy, endobronchial irradiation and transbronchial stenting are being increasingly employed to deal with distressing symptoms in inoperable cases. Malignant pleural effusions should be aspirated to dryness and a sclerosing agent (e.g. tetracycline, bleomycin) instilled into the pleural space. In the terminal stages the quality of life must be maintained as far as possible. In addition to general nursing and medical care, patients may need oral or intravenous opiates for pain (given with laxatives to prevent constipation) and prednisolone may improve the appetite.

Differential diagnosis
In most cases the diagnosis is straightforward. A solitary round shadow on the radiograph may also be the result of a benign growth, a secondary deposit, tuberculoma or hydatid cyst.

Metastatic tumours in the lung

Metastases in the lung are common, usually presenting as round shadows 1.5–3 cm in diameter. The most common primary sites are kidney, prostate, breast, bone, gastrointestinal tract, cervix or ovary.

DISEASES OF THE PLEURA

Dry pleurisy

Dry pleurisy is the term used to describe inflammation of the pleura when there is no effusion. This results in localized sharp pain made worse on deep inspiration, coughing and bending or twisting movements. Common causes are pneumonia, pulmonary infarct and carcinoma.

Epidemic myalgia (Bornholm's disease) is the result of infection with Coxsackie B virus. It is characterized by an upper respiratory tract infection followed by pleuritic pain and abdominal pain with tender muscles. The chest radiograph remains normal and the illness clears in one week.

Pleural effusion

A pleural effusion is an excessive accumulation of fluid in the pleural space. It can be detected clinically when there is more than 500 ml present and by radiography when there is more than 300 ml. The physical signs and chest radiographic appearances are shown in Figure 9.4.

Aetiology

Serous effusions may be *transudates* (protein content < 30 g/l) or *exudates* (> 30 g/l). The causes of a serous effusion are shown in Table 9.13. More rarely effusions consist of blood (*haemothorax*), pus (*empyema*) or lymph (*chylothorax*). Chylous effusions are caused by leakage of lymph from the thoracic duct as a result of trauma or infiltration by carcinoma.

Table 9.13 Causes of a pleural effusion

Transudates	Exudates
Heart failure	Bacterial pneumonia
Hypoproteinaemia	Carcinoma of the bronchus
Constrictive pericarditis	Pulmonary infarction
Hypothyroidism	Tuberculosis
Meigs' syndrome (ovarian fibroma with right-sided pleural effusion and ascites)	Connective tissue disease
	Postmyocardial infarction syndrome
	Acute pancreatitis
	Mesothelioma
	Sarcoidosis (rarely)

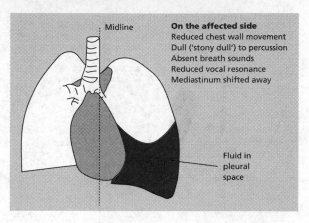

Midline

On the affected side
Reduced chest wall movement
Dull ('stony dull') to percussion
Absent breath sounds
Reduced vocal resonance
Mediastinum shifted away

Fluid in pleural space

Figure 9.4 The physical signs and chest radiographic appearances of a pleural effusion.

Investigations
Diagnosis is by pleural aspiration and pleural biopsy. Fluid is sent for the following:

● Protein estimation

● Bacteriological examination: Gram stain and culture, Ziehl–Neelson stain and culture

● Cytology for malignant cells

● Occasionally: amylase, rheumatoid factor, glucose

Management
This depends on the underlying cause.

Pneumothorax

Pneumothorax means the presence of air in the pleural space and this may occur spontaneously or secondary to trauma. A 'tension pneumothorax' is rare unless the patient is on positive pressure ventilation. In this situation the pleural tear acts as a one-way valve through which air passes only during inspiration. Positive pressure builds up causing increasing cardiorespiratory embarrassment and eventually cardiac arrest. Treatment is immediate intercostal tube drainage.

Aetiology
Spontaneous pneumothorax usually occurs in young men as a result of rupture of a pleural bleb, usually in the apex of the lung. A bleb is thought to be a congenital defect in the connective tissue of the alveolar wall which may occur in both lungs with equal frequency. Often these patients are tall

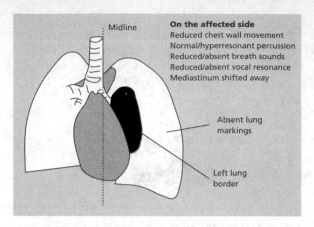

Figure 9.5 The physical signs and chest radiographic appearances of pneumothorax.

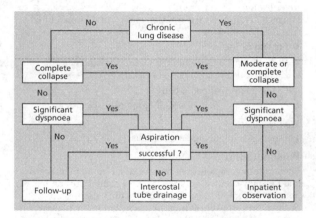

- Moderate pneumothorax = lung collapsed half-way towards heart border.
- Complete = airless lung, separate from diaphragm.
- Simple aspiration performed with local anaesthetic and larger-bore intravenous cannula. Insert cannula in second intercostal space in midclavicular line.
- Intercostal tube inserted in fifth intercostal space in midaxillary line.

Figure 9.6 Management of a pneumothorax.

and thin. In patients over 40 years of age the usual cause is underlying chronic bronchitis and emphysema.

Clinical features

There is a sudden onset of pleuritic pain with increasing breathlessness.

The physical signs, chest radiographic appearances and management are shown in Figures 9.5 and 9.6.

Disorders of the diaphragm

The most common cause of *unilateral diaphragmatic paralysis* is the result of involvement of the phrenic nerve (C2–C4) in the thorax by a bronchial carcinoma. Other common causes of phrenic paralysis are trauma, surgery and motor neuron disease. Unilateral paralysis produces no symptoms.

The characteristic features of *bilateral diaphragmatic weakness* are orthopnoea, paradoxical (inward) movement of the abdominal wall on inspiration and a large fall in FVC on lying down. It may be the result of trauma or occur as part of a generalized muscular or neurological condition such as motor neuron disease, muscular dystrophy or Guillain–Barré syndrome. Treatment is either diaphragmatic pacing or night-time assisted ventilation.

FINAL MEDICINE EXAMINATIONS: RESPIRATORY MEDICINE

Questions related to the respiratory system are common and appear frequently as long answers or as part of a short answer section. The most common questions related to the diagnosis and management of asthma are:

1. How would you assess the severity of an acute attack of bronchial asthma, and how would your findings influence the treatment?

2. A 45-year-old woman develops breathlessness and wheezing following a cold. What features would you seek to support a diagnosis of asthma?

3. An 18-year-old girl, known to have asthma, is brought to the accident and emergency department by a friend. She became breathless the previous night but was told that this was the result of 'hyperventilation'. She improved that morning but is again breathless. On arrival she is panicky, distressed and breathless with a rapid respiratory rate:

   (a) How would you assess the presence and severity of asthma?

   (b) If this is asthma, what treatment would you give?

(c) How would you assess the effectiveness of this treatment?

(d) How would you decide whether or not admission to the ward is required?

Pneumonia appears frequently:

4. List the causes of pneumonia in a previously healthy young adult. Describe the clinical features and laboratory tests that would help to establish the aetiology.

5. Describe your approach to the investigation and management of pneumonia in a 50-year-old ventilation engineer.

Other common questions relate to the differential diagnosis and appropriate investigations which should be performed in patients presenting with common respiratory symptoms and signs.

6. What are the main causes of haemoptysis? How would you investigate a patient with this complaint?

7. List the four conditions which you consider most likely to account for acute shortness of breath in a 50-year-old man. What are the most important physical signs for each condition? Indicate briefly how else the differential diagnosis may be made.

8. What are the features and common causes of erythema nodosum? How would you investigate a patient with this condition?

Finally single respiratory diseases (other than asthma and pneumonia) are favourite examination questions, particularly the management of a pneumothorax.

9. Discuss in reasonable detail your management of a 25-year-old man presenting with acute right pleural pain, in whom the radiograph shows air in the pleural cavity and a completely collapsed right lung.

10. Describe the clinical presentations of sarcoidosis, indicating their relative frequency.

11. What is cystic fibrosis? How may it be diagnosed and managed?

ANSWERS

1. The severity is assessed clinically: tachycardia, pulsus paradoxus and cyanosis indicate a severe attack. Measurement of PEFR (page 324) and blood gases should be undertaken. These decide initially whether the patient needs hospital assessment and what treatment is given in hospital (page 330).

2. A positive family history, previous wheezing on exposure to allergens and other clinical features discussed on page 328 support a diagnosis of asthma.

3. This is discussed on page 331 under the heading of acute severe asthma.

4,5. The causes of pneumonia in a healthy adult are listed on page 339. Pneumonia in a ventilation engineer may be the result of any of the causes of community-acquired pneumonia, but he is particularly at risk of infection with *Legionella* sp. The initial treatment must cover this organism and investigations performed particularly must look for evidence of infection (page 341). Additional treatment includes oxygen therapy to correct hypoxaemia and treatment of complications, e.g. acute renal failure, hyponatraemia.

6. The causes of haemoptysis and investigation are listed on page 323.

7. Acute means onset over hours or days. The most probable causes are pulmonary oedema, pneumothorax and pneumonia (although cough is often the predominant symptom). Pulmonary embolism may occur, particularly in a patient with risk factors (page 306).

8. Clinical features and causes are listed on page 517. The initial investigation is a chest radiograph. Subsequent tests depend very much on the history, physical examination and radiographic appearances. For example, in a patient with diarrhoea and a normal radiograph, a small bowel follow-through is appropriate to look for Crohn's disease. In a patient with one episode who is otherwise well no further investigation is necessary.

9–11. These are discussed on pages 357, 346, and 337, respectively.

CHAPTER 10

Intensive Care Medicine

Intensive care medicine (or 'critical care medicine') is concerned predominantly with the management of patients with acute life-threatening conditions ('the critically ill') in a specialized unit. It also encompasses the resuscitation and transport of those who become acutely ill, or are injured, either elsewhere in the hospital or in the community. An intensive care unit (ICU) has the necessary facilities and expertise required to provide cardiorespiratory support to these sick patients. Some of these patients, in addition, have kidney or liver failure and management of this is described in the relevant chapters.

All patients admitted to the ICU require skilled nursing care (patient to nurse ratio of 1:1) and physiotherapy. Many require nutritional support. General medical management includes the prevention of venous thrombosis (page 142), pressure sores and constipation. A number of scoring systems are in use to evaluate the severity of the patient's illness. [CM p. 735]

ACUTE DISTURBANCES OF HAEMODYNAMIC FUNCTION (SHOCK)

The term 'shock' is used to describe acute circulatory failure with inadequate or inappropriately distributed tissue perfusion resulting in generalized cellular hypoxia. The causes of shock are listed in Table 10.1.

Table 10.1 Causes of shock

Cardiogenic	Myocardial infarction, myocarditis, arrhythmias
Mechanical	Obstruction to outflow, e.g. pulmonary embolus Restricted cardiac filling, e.g. cardiac tamponade

Peripheral circulation	Hypovolaemic
	    Exogenous losses, e.g. haemorrhage, burns
	    Endogenous losses, e.g. sepsis, anaphylaxis
	Normovolaemic, e.g. sepsis, anaphylaxis

Pathophysiology

SYMPATHOADRENAL

In response to hypotension there is a reflex increase in sympathetic nervous activity and catecholamine release from the adrenal medulla. The resulting vasoconstriction, increased myocardial contractility and heart rate help restore blood pressure and cardiac output. Activation of the renin–angiotensin system leads to vasoconstriction and salt and water retention, which help to restore circulating volume.

NEUROENDOCRINE RESPONSE

There is release of anterior pituitary hormones and glucagon which are insulin antagonists. They raise blood sugar and may be responsible for some of the cardiovascular changes.

RELEASE OF MEDIATORS

In septic shock components of microorganisms (e.g. endotoxin of Gram-negative bacteria) release cytokines (tumour necrosis factor, interleukin-1 and interferon-γ) from macrophages and white cells, activate the complement system and cause release of the vasodilator, nitric oxide, from vascular endothelium. The end result of these processes is vasodilatation, increased vascular permeability, endothelial cell damage and platelet aggregation.

Vasodilatation and increased vascular permeability are also seen in shock secondary to anaphylaxis.

MICROCIRCULATORY CHANGES

If shock (from whatever cause) persists, there is eventually relaxation of the precapillary sphincters leading to capillary sequestration of blood. Fluid is forced into the extravascular space causing interstitial oedema, haemoconcentration and an increase in plasma viscosity.

In all forms of shock there may be activation of the coagulation pathway with development of disseminated intravascular coagulation (DIC, see page 139).

Clinical features

The history will often indicate the cause of shock, e.g. a patient involved in a motorway pile-up is likely to have serious injuries (often internal and thus concealed) and be developing hypovolaemic shock. A patient with a history of peptic ulceration may now be bleeding into the gastrointestinal tract and rectal examination will show melaena. Anaphylactic shock may develop in susceptible individuals after insect stings and eating certain foods, e.g. peanuts.

HYPOVOLAEMIC SHOCK

Inadequate tissue perfusion causes blue cold skin with slow capillary refill. The blood pressure may be maintained initially but later hypotension supervenes (systolic BP < 100mmHg) with oliguria (< 30 ml of urine/h), confusion and restlessness. Increased sympathetic tone causes tachycardia (pulse > 100/min) and sweating.

CARDIOGENIC SHOCK
Additional clinical features are those of myocardial failure,
e.g. raised jugular venous pressure (JVP), pulsus alternans,
'gallop' rhythm (see page 281).

MECHANICAL SHOCK
Muffled heart sounds, pulsus paradoxus, elevated JVP and
Kussmaul's sign occur in cardiac tamponade. In pulmonary
embolism there are signs of right heart strain with a raised
JVP with prominent 'a' waves, right ventricular heave and
loud pulmonary second sound.

ANAPHYLACTIC SHOCK
Profound vasodilatation leads to *warm* peripheries and low
blood pressure. Erythema, urticaria, angio-oedema,
bronchospasm, and oedema of the face and larynx may all be
present.

SEPTIC SHOCK
In the early stages there is vasodilatation, pyrexia and rigors.
At a later stage there are features of hypovolaemic shock.
Sepsis in elderly people is common without the classic clinical
features.

Monitoring
This is both by clinical and invasive means.

CLINICAL
An assessment of skin perfusion, measurement of pulse, BP,
JVP and urinary flow rate will guide treatment in a
straightforward case. Additional invasive monitoring will be
required in seriously ill patients who do not respond to initial
treatment.

INVASIVE
● Blood pressure: a continuous recording may be made with
  an intra-arterial cannula, usually in the radial artery.

● Central venous pressure (CVP) is related to right
  ventricular end-diastolic pressure which depends on
  circulating blood volume, venous tone, intrathoracic
  pressure and right ventricular function. CVP is measured
  by inserting a catheter percutaneously into the superior
  vena cava and connecting the catheter to a manometer
  system. The normal range is 0–4 cm H_2O above the
  manubriosternal angle in a supine patient. In shock, CVP
  may be normal, because in spite of hypovolaemia there is
  increased venous tone. A better guide to circulating
  volume is the response to a fluid challenge (Figure 10.1).

● Left atrial pressure: in uncomplicated cases, the CVP is an
  adequate guide to the filling pressures of both sides of the
  heart. However, if there is disparity in function between
  the two ventricles (e.g. infarction of the left ventricle) left
  atrial pressure must be measured. A Swan–Ganz catheter

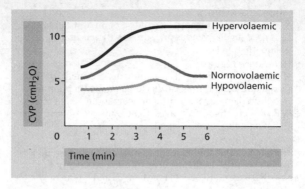

Figure 10.1 The effect of rapid administration (200 ml of 0.9% saline over 1–3 minutes) of a fluid challenge to patients with a CVP within the normal range.

is introduced percutaneously into a central vein and then guided through the chambers of the heart into the pulmonary artery. By inflating a balloon at the tip of the catheter, pulmonary artery wedge pressure (PAWP) is measured which is a reflection of left atrial pressure (Table 10.2).

● Cardiac output is measured, using a modified Swan–Ganz catheter, by recording temperature changes in the pulmonary artery after injecting a bolus of cold dextrose into the right atrium.

Table 10.2 Cardiac catheterization reference values

	Pressure (mmHg)
Pulmonary artery	
Systolic	15–30
End-diastolic	3–12
Mean	9–16
Wedge pressure	1–10
Cardiac output	5 l/min

Management

This is summarized in Table 10.3. The underlying cause must be identified and treated appropriately. Whatever the aetiology of shock, tissue blood flow and blood pressure must be restored.

EXPANSION OF THE CIRCULATING VOLUME
Volume replacement is obviously important in hypovolaemic

Table 10.3 Management of shock

RESTORE DELIVERY OF OXYGEN TO THE TISSUES

Ensure adequate oxygenation and ventilation	Restore cardiac output and BP
Maintain patent airway	Expand circulating volume
Administer oxygen	Support cardiovascular function
Support respiratory function	

MONITOR	MONITOR
• Respiratory rate	• Skin colour
• Blood gases	• Capillary refill time
• Chest radiograph	• Peripheral temperature
	• Urine flow
	• Blood pressure
	• ECG
	• CVP in most cases
	• Swan–Ganz catheter, in selected cases

Investigations	Treat underlying cause	Treat complications
All cases		
FBC and coagulation screen	Control haemorrhage	e.g. Coagulopathy, renal failure
Urea and electrolytes		
Blood glucose	Sepsis ⎱ see	
Liver biochemistry	Anaphylaxis ⎰ above	
Blood gases		
Selected cases		
Infection screen		
Blood lactate		
Fibrinogen degradation products		
Cross-match blood		

shock but also in anaphylactic and septic shock where there is vasodilatation, sequestration of blood and loss of circulating volume secondary to capillary leakage. High filling pressures may also be needed in mechanical shock. Care must be taken to prevent volume overload which leads to a reduction in stroke volume and a rise in left atrial pressure with a risk of pulmonary oedema. The choice of fluid depends on the clinical situation:

- Whole blood is the fluid of choice for haemorrhage. Cross-matched blood must be used if possible but, in extreme emergencies, the 'universal donor' group O rhesus negative blood is used. Complications of massive blood transfusion are hypothermia, thrombocytopenia, hypocalcaemia and depletion of clotting factors.

- *Colloids* are osmotically active and stay longer in the circulation than *crystalloid*. Polygelatin solutions (e.g. gelatin and Haemaccel) are the most widely used. Human albumin solution and dextrans are used less commonly because of the expense (albumin) and higher complication rate (dextrans).

Table 10.4 Inotropic agents used in the management of shock: the effect of each inotrope on the adrenergic receptors is shown

	α	β₁	β₂	Dopamine	Main use
Dopamine					
1–3 µg/kg per min				++	Often used as the first choice for treating shock as it increases inotropy while restoring perfusion pressure to vital organs (kidney, brain, heart and gut). It is also useful at low dose for augmenting renal blood flow in combination with other agents. However, at high doses (> 10 µg/kg per min) there is vasoconstriction which may result in ischaemia
3–10 µg/kg per min		++		++	
> 10 µg/kg per min	++	++		++	
Dobutamine	+	+++	++	0	Dobutamine is used in cardiogenic shock because it combines an inotropic action with decreased peripheral resistance
Adrenaline	+++	+++	++	0	A potent inotrope used in patients not responding to dobutamine or dopamine. At high doses vasoconstriction may increase renal perfusion pressure and urine output but as dose is further increased marked vasoconstriction leads to decreased cardiac output, oliguria and peripheral gangrene
Noradrenaline	++	+++	0	0	Particularly useful in septic shock as administration leads to increased inotropy and an increase in peripheral vascular resistance
Isoprenaline	0	+++	+++	0	Rarely used
Dopexamine	0	0	+++	++	Useful where a low cardiac output is associated with vasoconstriction
Enoximone	Phosphodiesterase inhibitor; does not act at adrenergic receptors				Inotropic and vasodilatory action is occasionally useful in acute heart failure

0 = no agonism, + = mild agonism, ++ = moderate agonism, +++ = pronounced agonism.

- Crystalloids, e.g. 5% dextrose, 0.9% saline, are readily available and cheap. Once in the circulation they quickly redistribute into the interstitial fluid. Therefore large volumes are needed to restore circulating volume and the excess fluid in the interstitial space may contribute to pulmonary oedema. Large volumes of crystalloid (> 1 l) are best avoided.

MYOCARDIAL CONTRACTILITY AND INOTROPIC AGENTS
Myocardial contractility is impaired in cardiogenic shock and at a later stage in other forms of shock as a result of hypoxaemia, acidosis and release of mediators. When a patient remains hypotensive despite adequate volume replacement inotropic agents are administered. These must be administered via a large central vein and the effects carefully monitored. The inotropic agents used and their clinical effects are shown in Table 10.4.

ADDITIONAL TREATMENT
Vasodilators, e.g. sodium nitroprusside and isosorbide dinitrate may be useful in selected patients who remain vasoconstricted and oliguric despite adequate volume replacement and a satisfactory blood pressure. Finally, in patients with a potentially reversible depression of left ventricular function (e.g. cardiogenic shock secondary to a ruptured interventricular septum), intra-aortic balloon counterpulsation (IABCP) may be used as a temporary measure to maintain life until definitive surgical treatment. [CM p. 553–554]

SPECIFIC TREATMENT OF THE CAUSE
In all cases the cause of shock must be identified if possible and specific treatment given when indicated.

- Septic shock: antibiotic therapy should be directed towards the probable cause. In the absence of helpful clinical guidelines, 'blind' antibiotic therapy (e.g. cefuroxime and gentamicin) should be started after performing an infectious screen: chest radiograph and culture of blood, urine and sputum. Lumbar puncture, ultrasonography and CT of the chest and abdomen are useful in selected cases. Abscesses require drainage. Steroids are now felt to have no role in the treatment of septic shock.

   Anti-tumour necrosis factor antibodies, anti-endotoxin antibodies and nitric oxide synthetase inhibitors are under evaluation for use in septic shock

- Anaphylactic shock must be identified and treated immediately with:

   Adrenaline: 0.3–0.5 mg i.v. given over 5 minutes with full ECG monitoring

Hydrocortisone: 100–200 mg i.v.

Chlorpheniramine: 10 mg i.v.

If the patient is seen before shock or severe dyspnoea has developed, adrenaline is administered by *subcutaneous* or *intramuscular injection*. Patients who have had an attack of anaphylaxis and are at risk of developing another, should carry a preloaded syringe of adrenaline for subcutaneous administration.

RESPIRATORY FAILURE

Respiratory failure occurs when pulmonary gas exchange is sufficiently impaired to cause hypoxaemia with or without hypercapnia.

It can be divided into two types (Table 10.5):

- Type 1 respiratory failure in which the P_aO_2 is low (<8kPa) and the P_aCO_2 is normal or low
- Type 2 respiratory failure caused by poor ventilation of the lung. The P_aO_2 is low and the P_aCO_2 is high (>7kPa)

Table 10.5 Causes of respiratory failure

Type 1 respiratory failure	Type 2 respiratory failure
Pulmonary oedema	Chronic bronchitis and emphysema
Pneumonia	Severe asthma
Asthma	Muscle weakness, e.g.
Pulmonary embolism	Guillain–Barré syndrome
Adult respiratory distress syndrome	Respiratory centre depression
Fibrosing alveolitis	Chest wall deformities

Monitoring

CLINICAL

Assessment should be made on the following criteria: tachypnoea, tachycardia, sweating, pulsus paradoxus, use of accessory muscles of respiration and inability to speak. Signs of carbon dioxide retention may be present such as asterixis *(coarse tremor)*, bounding pulse, warm peripheries and papilloedema.

PULSE OXIMETRY

Light weight oximeters placed on an ear lobe or finger can give a continuous reading of oxygen saturation by measuring the changing amount of light transmitted through arterial blood. Although simple and reliable, these instruments are not very sensitive to changes in oxygenation.

ARTERIAL BLOOD GAS ANALYSIS

Analysis of arterial blood gives definitive measurements of P_aO_2, P_aCO_2, oxygen saturation, pH and bicarbonate. In type

2 respiratory failure, retention of carbon dioxide causes $P_a CO_2$ and $[H^+]$ to rise resulting in *respiratory acidosis*. The kidney compensates by retaining bicarbonate reducing the $[H^+]$ towards normal. In type 1 respiratory failure or in hyperventilation, there may be a fall in $P_a CO_2$ and $[H^+]$ resulting in *respiratory alkalosis*. Other abnormalities of acid–base balance are discussed in Chapter 6.

Table 10.6 Normal arterial blood gas analysis

$P_a O_2$ (pressure of oxygen in arterial blood gas)	10.0–13.3 kPa
$P_a CO_2$ (pressure of carbon dioxide in arterial blood gas)	4.8–6.1 kPa
Oxygen saturation	> 92%
pH	7.35–7.45
Bicarbonate	22–30 mmol/l

Management

This includes administration of supplemental oxygen, control of secretions, treatment of pulmonary infection, control of airway obstruction and limiting pulmonary oedema. In most patients oxygen is given by a face mask or nasal cannulae. With these devices, inspired oxygen concentration varies from 35% to 55% with flow rates between 6 and 10/l. However, in patients with chronically elevated carbon dioxide, hypoxia rather than hypercapnia maintains the respiratory drive and thus *fixed performance masks* (e.g. *Venturi masks*) should be used in which the concentration of oxygen can be accurately controlled. Respiratory stimulants such as doxapram have a very limited role in treatment.

RESPIRATORY SUPPORT

Respiratory support should be considered when the above measures are not sufficient. The type of respiratory support depends on the underlying disorder and clinical severity. Careful consideration should be given to ventilating patients with severe chronic lung disease as those who are severely incapacitated may be difficult to wean from the ventilator.

INTERMITTENT POSITIVE PRESSURE VENTILATION (IPPV)

IPPV requires tracheal intubation and therefore anaesthesia if the patient is conscious. The beneficial effects of IPPV include improved carbon dioxide elimination, improved oxygenation and relief from exhaustion as the work of ventilation is removed. High concentrations of oxygen (up to 100%) may be administered accurately. If adequate oxygenation cannot be achieved, a positive airway pressure can be maintained at a chosen level throughout expiration by attaching a threshold resistor valve to the expiratory limb of the circuit. This is known as positive end-expiratory pressure (PEEP) and its primary effect is to re-expand under-ventilated lung areas thereby reducing shunts and increasing $P_a O_2$.

Table 10.7 Indications for IPPV

Indication	Comment
Acute respiratory failure	Particularly when exhaustion, confusion, agitation or decreased consciousness are present
Acute ventilatory failure	e.g. Myasthenia gravis, Guillain–Barré syndrome
Prophylactic postoperative ventilation	In poor risk patients
Head injury	With acute brain oedema. Intracranial pressure is decreased by elective hyperventilation as this reduces cerebral blood flow
Trauma	e.g. Chest injury and lung contusion
Severe left ventricular failure	
Coma with breathing difficulties	e.g. Following drug overdose

CONTINUOUS POSITIVE AIRWAY PRESSURE (CPAP)
Oxygen is delivered to the spontaneously breathing patient under pressure via a tightly fitting face mask or endotracheal tube. Oxygenation and vital capacity improves and the lungs become less stiff.

INTERMITTENT MANDATORY VENTILATION (IMV)
This technique allows the ventilated patient to breathe spontaneously between mandatory tidal volumes delivered by the ventilator. These coincide with the patient's own respiratory effort. It is used as a method of weaning patients from artificial ventilation or as an alternative to IPPV.

The major complications of intubation and assisted ventilation are:

● Trauma to the upper respiratory tract from the endotracheal tube

● Secondary pulmonary infection

● Barotrauma: overdistension of the lungs and alveolar rupture may present with pneumothorax (page 357) and surgical emphysema

● Reduction in cardiac output: the increase in intrathoracic pressures during controlled ventilation impedes cardiac filling and lowers cardiac output

Adult respiratory distress syndrome (ARDS)

ARDS is defined as diffuse bilateral pulmonary infiltrates, refractory hypoxaemia, stiff lungs and respiratory distress in the *absence of cardiogenic pulmonary oedema* (i.e. the pulmonary capillary wedge pressure is less than 18 mmHg).

Aetiology

It is usually a non-specific reaction to a variety of insults including sepsis, trauma, burns, pancreatitis, fat or amniotic fluid embolism, aspiration pneumonia or cardiopulmonary bypass.

Pathophysiology

The cardinal feature is pulmonary oedema as a result of increased vascular permeability caused by release of inflammatory mediators. Oedema may induce vascular compression resulting in pulmonary hypertension which is later exacerbated by vasoconstriction in response to increased autonomic nervous activity. A haemorrhagic intra-alveolar exudate forms which is rich in platelets, fibrin and clotting factors. This inactivates surfactant, stimulates inflammation and promotes hyaline membrane formation. These changes may result in progressive pulmonary fibrosis.

Clinical features

Tachypnoea, increasing hypoxia and laboured breathing are the initial features. The chest radiograph shows diffuse bilateral shadowing, which may progress to a complete 'white-out'.

Management

This is based on the treatment of the underlying condition. Pulmonary oedema should be limited with fluid restriction, and the use of diuretics.

Steroids currently have no role in the treatment or prophylaxis of this condition. The role of the vasodilator nitric oxide which can improve V/Q matching by increasing perfusion of ventilated lung units has yet to be determined.

Prognosis

Overall there is a 50% mortality rate, most patients dying from sepsis. The prognosis is very dependent on the underlying cause and rises steeply with age and with the development of multiorgan failure.

FINAL MEDICINE EXAMINATIONS: INTENSIVE CARE

Frequently there are questions related to the management of certain conditions, e.g. severe asthma not responding to initial therapy, where part of the management involves admission to an ICU and possibly ventilatory support. Less frequently there were questions entirely concerned with the diagnosis and management of shock or rarely respiratory failure and ventilatory support.

1. A man aged 55 years who underwent right hemicolectomy for carcinoma of the caecum 4 days ago has developed acute circulatory failure ('shock') with an arterial pressure of 65/40 mmHg and heart rate of 120/min. List the probable causes of this occurrence. Indicate the clinical features that would aid you in distinguishing between them and outline your initial management of the situation.

2. Write short notes on the management of cardiogenic shock.

3. Compare the clinical manifestations of acute haemorrhagic, acute cardiogenic and acute bacterial (septicaemic) shock.

ANSWERS

1. The two most likely causes are sepsis or a massive pulmonary embolism. Less likely are gastrointestinal haemorrhage and a perioperative myocardial infarction complicated by cardiogenic shock. The clinical features of each of these conditions are discussed on pages 365. 306. 39 and 289. respectively. Management involves:

   Emergency resuscitation with 60% oxygen, large bore intravenous cannulae and administration of colloid.

   Make a diagnosis. Temperature charts and physical examination will often reveal the cause. Consider: ECG, blood gases, chest radiograph.

   Further treatment. Depends on the response to fluids and the likely cause.

2. Cardiogenic shock is an extreme form of cardiac failure ('pump failure') often secondary to a myocardial infarction in which there has been extensive damage to the left ventricular muscle. The mortality rate is 90%. Management therefore involves admission to ICU, oxygen therapy, relief of pain and intensive monitoring (Table 10.3) including a Swan–Ganz catheter (page 366). Dobutamine and dopamine are given for their inotropic action and to promote renal perfusion (Table 10.4). If PCWP is below 18 mmHg, fluid is cautiously infused so as to optimize the filling pressures of the heart. Vasodilators are sometimes given (page 369).

3. This is discussed on pages 364–365.

CHAPTER 11

Poisoning, Drug and Alcohol Abuse

POISONING

In most hospitals in the Western World the most common reason for acute admission of young people to a medical ward is acute poisoning. The types of poisoning are shown in Table 11.1. In adults with self-poisoning the most common drugs taken are benzodiazepines and antidepressants, followed by paracetamol and then aspirin. Patients often take more than one drug including alcohol.

Self-poisoning is the most common way by which people commit or attempt suicide (these categories are encompassed by the term 'deliberate self-harm'), other means are usually by violent methods, e.g. hanging, shooting or drowning. Attempted suicide by a violent method is associated with future suicide and these patients must be assessed by a psychiatrist (page 379).

Table 11.1 Types of poisoning

Self-poisoning refers to the deliberate ingestion of an overdose of a drug or some other substance not meant for consumption

Suicide is the term applied to all self-poisoned patients who die whether it was their intention to kill themselves or not

Accidental poisoning occurs mostly in children below 5 years of age, but can occur in adults, e.g. from the accidental inhalation of a gas, ingestion of fluid from a wrongly labelled bottle, stings and bites, or eating poisonous foods (such as mushrooms)

Non-accidental poisoning is the deliberate administration of a poison, often to a child

Homicidal poisoning

Clinical features
Eighty per cent of adults are conscious on arrival at hospital and the diagnosis of self-poisoning can usually be made early from the history. In the unconscious patient a history from friends or relatives is helpful, and the diagnosis can often be inferred from tablet bottles or a suicide note brought by the ambulance attendants. In any patient with altered consciousness, drug overdose must always be considered in the differential diagnosis. A full physical examination must include an assessment of cardiorespiratory status and conscious level (page 463). The physical signs that may aid

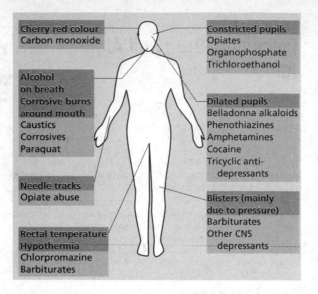

Figure 11.1 Physical signs in poisoning.

identification of the agent responsible for poisoning are
shown in Figure 11.1.

Investigations

Blood and urine samples should always be taken on
admission. They are useful in medicolegal cases and are vital
for the correct management of poisoning with paracetamol or
salicylates. As a guide to treatment, levels must be repeated if
the patient presents early as drug absorption is still taking
place. Further investigations depend on the drugs ingested.

Management

Most patients with self-poisoning require only general care
and specific treatment is not necessary. In the UK the
Regional Poisons Centre provide a round the clock service
for advice about the management of overdose; the telephone
number is found in the *British National Formulary*. The
management of a patient with overdose is summarized in
Table 11.2.

EMERGENCY RESUSCITATION

● Turn the patient semiprone to reduce the risk of aspiration

● Administer 60% oxygen by face mask

● Clear the airway and intubate if the gag reflex is absent

Table 11.2 Principles of management of patients with self-poisoning

1	Emergency resuscitation
2	Prevent further drug absorption
3	Increase drug elimination
4	Administration of specific drug antidotes
5	Psychiatric assessment

- Artificial ventilation is sometimes necessary if ventilation is inadequate
- Treat hypotension (page 366), arrhythmias (page 293) and convulsions (usually with diazepam)
- Hypothermia ($< 35°C$) should be sought with a low-reading rectal thermometer and treated with 'space blankets' and warm intravenous fluids

PREVENTION OF FURTHER DRUG ABSORPTION

- *Gastric lavage* is used to remove the drug from the stomach. It is of little value after 4 hours except in the case of salicylates, tricyclic antidepressants and paracetamol, which may remain within the stomach for many hours. The main danger of gastric lavage is aspiration and the unconscious patient must be intubated, with a cuffed endotracheal tube, if the gag reflex is absent
- *Induction of vomiting* with ipecacuanha syrup is an alternative to lavage, particularly in small children where lavage is difficult. It is contraindicated in the unconscious patient. Both lavage and induced vomiting are contraindicated for corrosives, petrol and paraffin because of the risk of further damage to the oesophageal mucosa (corrosives) and lung aspiration and chemical pneumonitis (petrol and paraffin)
- *Activated charcoal* reduces the gastrointestinal absorption of many drugs and is useful, in addition to emesis or lavage, or when these are contraindicated. It can be administered by mouth or nasogastric tube

INCREASING DRUG ELIMINATION

Forced alkaline diuresis depends on the principle that ionization of acid drugs (e.g. salicylates) is increased in alkaline urine and thus renal tubular reabsorption is reduced (as only lipophillic non-ionized drugs cross the lipid membrane readily). It is a potentially dangerous procedure which is usually only undertaken in cases of severe salicylate poisoning (Table 11.3). Careful clinical and laboratory monitoring is necessary.

Dialysis (peritoneal or haemodialysis, page 249) is used with some drugs in cases of severe poisoning, e.g. salicylates, barbiturates and lithium.

Haemoperfusion involves the passage of heparinized blood through devices containing absorbent particles such as activated charcoal or resins, to which drugs are absorbed. Its use should be considered in patients severely poisoned with certain drugs (e.g. theophylline, short- and medium-acting barbiturates and glutethimide) who fail to improve despite the use of adequate supportive measures.

Table 11.3 Forced alkaline diuresis

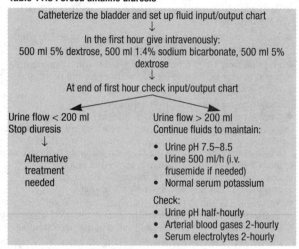

Catheterize the bladder and set up fluid input/output chart
↓
In the first hour give intravenously:
500 ml 5% dextrose, 500 ml 1.4% sodium bicarbonate, 500 ml 5% dextrose
↓
At end of first hour check input/output chart

Urine flow < 200 ml
Stop diuresis
↓
Alternative treatment needed

Urine flow > 200 ml
Continue fluids to maintain:

- Urine pH 7.5–8.5
- Urine 500 ml/h (i.v. frusemide if needed)
- Normal serum potassium

Check:
- Urine pH half-hourly
- Arterial blood gases 2-hourly
- Serum electrolytes 2-hourly

ANTAGONIZING THE EFFECTS OF POISONS
Specific antidotes are available for a small number of drugs; these will be considered under the individual drugs.

PSYCHIATRIC ASSESSMENT
All suicide attempts must be taken seriously and an assessment made of suicidal intent. In some patients, often young females, the act was not premeditated, they have no wish to die and the tablets were taken in response to an acute situation, e.g. an argument with the boyfriend. The risk of suicide is low and formal psychiatric assessment is not always necessary. In the absence of potential medical problems, these patients may not necessarily need to be admitted to hospital providing there is the necessary social and emotional back-up at home.

In other patients there is clear suicide intent; the act was planned, a suicide note was written and efforts were made not to be discovered (Table 11.4). These patients must be assessed by a psychiatrist before leaving hospital. Other factors which are associated with a risk of suicide are listed in Table 11.4 and these patients must also be considered for psychiatric referral.

Table 11.4 Guidelines for psychiatric referral in deliberate self-harm

Absolute indications for referral to a psychiatrist
Clinical depression
Psychotic illness of any kind
Clearly suicidal attempt: premeditated act, suicide note, attempts made not to be discovered during act
Persistent suicidal intent

Factors that increase the risk of suicide
Addiction to alcohol or drugs
Patients over 45, especially if male
Those with a family history of suicide
Those with serious physical disease
Those living alone or otherwise unsupported
Those in whom there is a major unresolved crisis
Persistent suicide attempts

Specific drug problems

Salicylates

Salicylates uncouple oxidative phosphorylation leading to increased oxygen consumption and carbon dioxide production. Hypercapnia and salicylates directly stimulate the respiratory centre causing hyperventilation and a respiratory alkalosis. Compensatory mechanisms, which include renal excretion of bicarbonate accompanied by sodium, potassium and water, exacerbate the subsequent metabolic acidosis. Interference with carbohydrate, fat and protein metabolism gives rise to increased lactate, pyruvate and ketone bodies. This, combined with the fact that aspirin itself is an organic acid, produces a metabolic acidosis.

Clinical features
The symptoms and signs of salicylate poisoning include tinnitus, nausea and vomiting, overbreathing, hyperpyrexia and sweating with a tachycardia. Alternatively the patient may appear completely well even with high blood levels of salicylate. The ingestion of 10–20 g of aspirin in an adult is likely to cause moderate to severe toxicity. Impaired clotting factors and platelet function are sometimes seen but bleeding is rare. In severe poisoning there may be cerebral and pulmonary oedema resulting from increased capillary permeability. Coma and respiratory depression are late signs.

Management
- Gastric lavage up to 24 hours after ingestion in severe cases
- Activated charcoal 50 g and repeated 4-hourly in severe cases
- Correct dehydration and hypokalaemia with intravenous fluids
- In severe cases (blood salicylate level > 500 mg/l [3.6 mmol/l]) consider forced alkaline diuresis (Figure 11.2)
- Intramuscular vitamin K to correct hypoprothrombin-aemia.

Paracetamol

Paracetamol in overdose may cause fatal hepatic necrosis and is responsible for over 200 deaths per year in the UK. Paracetamol is converted to a toxic metabolite, *N*-acetyl-*p*-benzoquinoimine, which is normally inactivated by conjugation with reduced glutathione. After a large overdose, glutathione is depleted and the toxic metabolite binds covalently with sulfhydryl groups on liver cell membranes causing necrosis. Marked liver cell necrosis can occur with as little as 10 g (20 tablets) and death with 15 g. The prothrombin time or international normalized ratio (INR) is the best guide to the severity of the liver damage.

Clinical features
The main danger is liver failure which usually becomes apparent in 72–96 hours after drug ingestion. Acute renal failure may occur in the absence of severe liver failure.

Management
Treatment depends on the interval between overdose and presentation and on the plasma concentrations of paracetamol (Figure 11.2). The investigation and management of paracetamol poisoning are summarized in Figure 11.2. The two antidotes in use for paracetamol poisoning increase the availability of glutathione. Intravenous acetylcysteine is the treatment of choice; there are few side effects other than occasional hypersensitivity reactions. Oral methionine is an alternative but absorption and efficacy are erratic if the patient is vomiting. Patients who develop liver damage with a raised INR should remain in hospital until the values are returning to normal. A poor prognosis is indicated by an INR value above 3, raised serum creatinine concentration or a blood pH below 7.3 recorded more than 24 hours after overdose. If any of these abnormalities are present, advice should be sought from a specialist liver unit. Patients with severe hepatic damage may require liver transplantation.

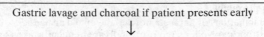

Gastric lavage and charcoal if patient presents early

↓

Start intravenous acetylcysteine infusion if potentially
serious overdose (> 7.5 g)

↓

Measure plasma paracetamol levels in all patients

↓

Decision to continue treatment based on the nomogram
below

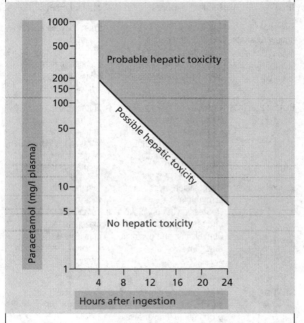

All patients at risk measure: liver biochemistry,
prothrombin time, blood sugar, urea and electrolytes.

Figure 11.2 The investigation and treatment of paracetamol poisoning.
Plasma paracetamol levels are unreliable within 4 hours after ingestion;
absorption is still taking place and peak levels are not yet attained.
Levels are unreliable more than 16 hours after ingestion, and
acetylcysteine is still given if a potentially toxic overdose has been taken
and the patient presents within 24 hours.

Co-proxamol

Combinations of paracetamol and the opioid analgesic, dextropropoxyphene (co-proxamol) are frequently taken in overdose. The initial features are those of opioid overdose (see later); patients may die from respiratory depression and acute heart failure unless they are given naloxone as an antidote to the dextropropoxyphene. Paracetamol hepatotoxicity may develop later and should be anticipated and treated as indicated above.

Table 11.5 Clinical features and management of overdose

Drug	Clinical features	Management
Tricyclic antidepressants	Tachycardia, hypotension, fixed dilated pupils, convulsions, urinary retention, arrhythmias, decreased conscious level	Treat convulsions with diazepam. Arrhythmias may respond to correction of acidosis and hypoxia
Benzodiazepines	Drowsiness, ataxia, dysarthria and coma. Potentiate the effect of other CNS depressants taken concomitantly	Flumazenil, a benzodiazepine antagonist given intravenously is used in cases of severe respiratory depression
Phenothiazines	Hypotension, hypothermia, arrhythmias. Depression of consciousness and respiration. Convulsions and dystonic reactions	Symptomatic treatment of complications, e.g. diazepam for convulsions. Dystonic reactions treated with intravenous benztropine
NSAIDs	Mefenamic acid is the most significant member of this group taken in overdose. Convulsions are the most important feature	Convulsions treated with diazepam
β-Blockers	Bradycardia and hypotension. Coma, convulsions and hypoglycaemia with severe overdose	Atropine for hypotension and arrhythmias. In resistant cases intravenous glucagon which has a positive inotropic effect

Other drugs

Table 11.5 outlines the clinical features and management of the other drugs which are commonly taken in cases of overdose. For all of those drugs that are taken by mouth the initial management should include gastric lavage or induced vomiting and charcoal if the patient presents in time.

Carbon monoxide

Carbon monoxide (CO) poisoning is usually the result of inhalation of smoke, car exhaust or fumes caused by combustion of any fuel in the absence of adequate oxygen and ventilation. CO combines readily with haemoglobin to form carboxyhaemoglobin, thus preventing the formation of oxyhaemoglobin. The clinical features include headache, mental impairment and coma in severe cases. In spite of hypoxaemia the skin is pink. Treatment consists of removing the patient from the CO source, and giving as high a concentration of oxygen as possible. Referral for hyperbaric oxygen treatment should be considered if the victim is or has been unconscious or has a blood carboxyhaemoglobin concentration of more than 40%.

Alcohol

Acute intoxication with alcohol produces severe depression of consciousness and hypoglycaemia, particularly in children. Treatment usually only consists of gastric lavage with an endotracheal tube in position. Blood glucose is measured and glucose given if indicated.

DRUG ABUSE

Under the Misuse of Drugs Regulations of 1985, drugs with a high abuse potential, drugs of addiction and other drugs with non-therapeutic psychotropic activity are categorized as *controlled drugs*. These include opiates, cocaine, barbiturates, lysergide, amphetamines and related drugs. Any patient who is believed to be dependent or addicted to controlled drugs must, by law, be notified to the Home Office.

Opioids

Opioid drugs produce physical dependency, such that an acute withdrawal syndrome develops ('cold turkey') if the drugs are stopped. These severe symptoms – profuse sweating, tachycardia, dilated pupils, leg cramps, and diarrhoea and vomiting – may be reduced by giving methadone.

Drug addicts frequently overdose themselves causing varying degrees of coma, respiratory depression and pinpoint pupils. Treatment is with intravenous naloxone, an opiate antagonist. The drug is short acting and repeated doses or an infusion may be necessary, with the rate titrated according to the clinical response.

Cannabis

Cannabis is usually smoked and often taken casually. It is a mild hallucinogen seldom accompanied by a desire to increase the dose; withdrawal symptoms are uncommon.

Lysergide

Lysergic acid diethylamine (LSD) is a much more potent hallucinogen; its use can lead to severe psychotic states in which life may be at risk. Even in overdose severe physiological reactions do not seem to occur. Adverse reactions are treated with repeated reassurance, a sedative, e.g. diazepam, is sometimes necessary. Phenothiazines may be necessary in severe cases.

Cocaine

Cocaine can be taken by injection, inhalation ('crack') or ingestion. It stimulates the central nervous system producing euphoria, agitation and tachycardia. Convulsions, pyrexia and cardiorespiratory depression may occur in severe cases of overdose and management is supportive.

Amphetamines

Amphetamines are taken for their stimulatory effect. In overdose there is confusion, delirium, hallucinations and violent behaviour. Cardiac arrhythmias can be a major problem. Treatment is with sedatives, such as diazepam. Forced acid diuresis may be used but is rarely required.

Ecstasy (MDMA, 3,4-methylenedioxymethamphetamine) is a synthetic amphetamine derivative taken orally as tablets or capsules. In Britain it is used almost exclusively as a 'dance drug' and the adverse effects are the result of the drug's pharmacological properties compounded by physical exertion. Serious acute complications are convulsions, hyperpyrexia, coagulopathy, rhabdomyolysis, renal failure and death. Treatment is supportive.

Solvents

The inhalation of organic solvents has become a common problem, particularly in teenagers. The patient presents either in the acute intoxicated state (with euphoria and excitement) or as a chronic abuser with excoriation and rashes over the face and a peripheral neuropathy. Sudden death can occur and is probably the result of cardiac arrhythmias.

ALCOHOL ABUSE

Drinking-related problems have increased in recent years. Approximately one in five male admissions to acute medical wards is directly or indirectly the result of alcohol. Over the past 20 years admissions to psychiatric hospitals for treatment of alcohol-related problems has increased 25-fold.

A number of medical, social and psychiatric problems are related to alcohol abuse (see below) and may be seen in the absence of actual physiological dependence. Alcohol dependence has seven essential elements:

- A compulsive need to drink
- A regular (daily) drinking routine to avoid or relieve withdrawal symptoms
- Drinking takes priority over other activities
- Increased tolerance to alcohol
- Repeated withdrawal symptoms often worse on waking in the morning
- Early morning drinking to avoid withdrawal symptoms (nausea, sweating, agitation)
- Reinstatement after abstinence

Guidelines for safe limits of drinking are 21 units per week in men, 14 units in women (one unit = a measure of spirits, a glass of wine or half a pint of standard strength beer). Slightly higher intake is probably unlikely to lead to harm but intake above 36 units per week in men and 24 units in women increases the risk to health. An elevated serum γGT (γ-glutamyltranspeptidase) (page 66) and raised red cell mean corpuscular volume (MCV, page 105) are useful screening tests for alcohol abuse and are helpful in monitoring progress. Blood and urine alcohol levels are sometimes measured to demonstrate high intake.

Consequences of alcohol abuse and dependence

Physical complications

These usually occur after a long period of heavy drinking, e.g. 10 years. Problems are generally seen earlier in women than in men. Damage is the result of direct tissue toxicity and the effects of malnutrition and vitamin deficiency which often accompany alcohol abuse.

CARDIOVASCULAR
A direct toxic effect in the heart leads to a cardiomyopathy and arrhythmias.

NEUROLOGICAL
Acute intoxication leads to ataxia, falls and head injury with intracranial bleeds. Long-term complications include polyneuropathy (page 501), myopathy, cerebellar degeneration (page 459), dementia (page 506) and epilepsy.

Wernicke–Korsakoff syndrome is the result of vitamin B_1 deficiency (thiamine) and thus may also be seen in severe starvation and prolonged vomiting. The clinical features include an acute onset of confusion, ataxia, nystagmus and ophthalmoplegia usually with sixth nerve palsies or defects of conjugate gaze (page 453). Untreated the patient becomes increasingly drowsy, lapses into a coma and dies. In less acute cases the characteristic features of Korsakoff's syndrome appear. There is a gross defect of short-term memory associated with confabulation. The diagnosis in these conditions is essentially clinical. Treatment is with thiamine (100 mg twice daily) which may reverse some of the early changes but the memory impairment is often irreversible. Treatment must be given to all patients in which the diagnosis is even considered.

GASTROINTESTINAL EFFECTS

These include liver damage (page 90), pancreatitis (page 99), oesophagitis and an increased incidence of oesophageal carcinoma.

HAEMATOLOGY
These include thrombocytopenia (alcohol inhibits platelet maturation and release from bone marrow), a raised MCV and anaemia from dietary deficiency of folate.

Psychiatric complications

There is an increased incidence of depression and deliberate self-harm among alcoholics. In these patients attempted suicide must always be taken seriously and psychiatric referral considered (page 379).

Social complications

These include marital and sexual difficulties, employment problems, financial difficulties and homelessness.

Alcohol withdrawal

Most heavy drinkers will experience some form of withdrawal symptoms if they attempt to reduce or stop drinking.

- Early mild features occur within 6–12 hours and include tremor, nausea and sweating. Treatment is with a reducing dose of chlormethiazole (see below).

- Late major features usually occur within 2–3 days but may take up to 2 weeks:

  Generalized tonic–clonic seizures (pages 474–475)

  Delerium tremens with fever, tremor, tachycardia, agitation and visual hallucinations ('pink elephants'). Treatment must be given urgently (Table 11.6)

Table 11.6 Management of delirium tremens

ADMIT PATIENT TO HOSPITAL
Chlormethiazole 9–12 capsules (each capsule contains 192 mg) for 24 hours, then reduced over 5 days, or diazepam 4–100 mg for 2 days then reduced
Correct dehydration, electrolyte imbalance
Treat infection
B vitamins intravenously

Intravenous chlormethiazole should be avoided and oral treatment should not be carried on long term.

FINAL MEDICINE EXAMINATION: POISONING, DRUG AND ALCOHOL ABUSE

1. After a disagreement with her boyfriend, a 20-year-old woman was seen to ingest 50 tablets of aspirin (i.e. 15 g total) and was brought to hospital 4 hours later. You find her alert and complaining of mild tinnitus only. The salicylate concentration in a blood sample taken in the accident and emergency department is within the therapeutic range. She wishes to return home and regrets the whole incident; in particular, she assures you that she has no suicidal intent. Briefly outline the major points of management.

2. A 50-year-old man, recently divorced, is admitted from the accident and emergency department having taken 50 soluble aspirin tablets about 6 hours previously:
   (a) Describe the clinical features that would alert you to severe toxicity.
   (b) What would be your management if severe toxicity were confirmed?
   (c) When he has recovered physically, what features would alert you to the danger of a further life-threatening event?

3. Outline the effects and management of paracetamol poisoning.

4. Outline the various physical disorders that may occur as a result of excessive consumption of alcohol. What features in a routine haematological screen would lead you to suspect alcohol abuse?

ANSWERS

1. Ingestion of 10–20 g of aspirin may produce severe toxicity. This case represents a very serious overdose and serum levels are within the normal range because intestinal absorption is still taking place (see page 380). Initial management is with gastric lavage and then administration of repeated doses of activated charcoal. Intravenous fluids should be started immediately to initiate a diuresis; further management depends on the salicylate concentration in a repeat blood sample taken 6 hours after drug ingestion (page 380). More than one drug is often taken in overdose cases and this should be sought from the history and measurement of plasma paracetamol levels. Several points suggest that the overdose is not a serious suicide attempt (page 378) and psychiatric referral is probably not necessary.

2. (a) The symptoms and signs of salicylate poisoning are listed on page 379; a patient with severe poisoning may initially have few symptoms.

   (b) The management of severe toxicity is discussed on page 380. In very severe poisoning (blood salicylate level > 1000 mg/l) or if forced alkaline diuresis is contraindicated or a diuresis not obtained, haemodialysis or haemoperfusion (page 378) may be necessary. Complications of salicylate poisoning (hypoglycaemia, hypoprothrombinaemia and pulmonary oedema) must be treated.

   (c) Attempted suicide in a middle-aged man with a recent life event must be taken seriously. Other risk factors for suicide are listed in Table 11.4.

3. This is discussed on pages 380–381.

4. The physical complications of alcohol abuse are discussed on page 385. Macrocytosis and, less commonly, thrombocytopenia are seen with alcohol abuse.

CHAPTER 12

Endocrinology

[CM p. 769]

Hormones were traditionally thought of as chemical messengers, released from endocrine cells into the circulation and acting at a site distant from their site of secretion. The situation is more complex and hormones may act in a variety of ways, such as (a) neurotransmitters, (b) a local hormone effect with action on adjacent cells *(paracrine action)* or (c) acting on the cell of origin *(autocrine)*. Hormones act by binding to specific receptors either on the target cell or within the cell (e.g. thyroid hormones, cortisol). The result is a cascade of intracellular reactions within the target cell which frequently amplifies the original stimulus and leads ultimately to a response by the target cell. Some hormones, e.g. growth hormone and thyroxine, act on most tissues of the body. Others act on only one tissue, e.g. thyroid-stimulating hormone (TSH) and adrenocorticotrophin (ACTH) are secreted by the anterior pituitary and have specific target tissues, namely the thyroid gland and the adrenal cortex.

THE HYPOTHALAMUS AND PITUITARY

The hypothalamus contains many vital centres for functions such as appetite, thirst, thermal regulation and sleep/waking. It also plays a role in circadian rhythm, the menstrual cycle, stress and mood. Releasing factors produced in the hypothalamus reach the pituitary via the portal system which runs down the pituitary stalk. These releasing factors stimulate or inhibit the production of hormones by the anterior pituitary which, in turn, stimulate the peripheral glands and tissues. This pattern is illustrated in Figure 12.1. The posterior pituitary acts as a storage organ for antidiuretic hormone (ADH, vasopressin) and oxytocin, which are synthesized in the supraoptic and paraventricular nuclei in the anterior hypothalamus and pass to the posterior pituitary along a single axon in the pituitary stalk. ADH is discussed on page 416; oxytocin produces milk ejection and uterine myometrial contractions.

Control and feedback

Most hormone systems are controlled by some form of feedback; an example is the hypothalamic–pituitary–thyroid axis (Figure 12.2). Thyrotrophin-releasing hormone (TRH),

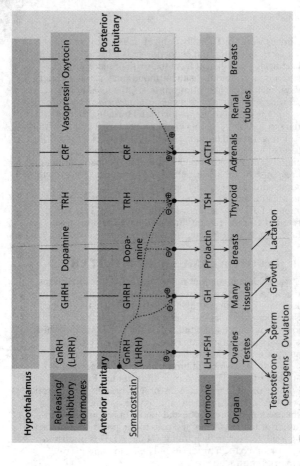

Figure 12.1 Hypothalamic-releasing hormones and the pituitary trophic hormones. +, stimulation; −, inhibition. See text for abbreviations.

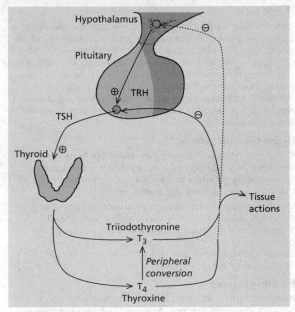

Figure 12.2 The hypothalamic–pituitary–thyroid feedback system. The dotted line indicates probable negative feedback at the hypothalamic level.

secreted in the hypothalamus, stimulates TSH secretion from the anterior pituitary which, in turn, stimulates synthesis and release of thyroid hormones from the thyroid gland. Circulating thyroid hormone feeds back on the pituitary and possibly the hypothalamus to suppress production of TRH and TSH, and hence a fall in thyroid hormone secretion. Conversely, a fall in thyroid hormone secretion (e.g. after thyroidectomy) leads to increased secretion of TRH and TSH.

A patient with a hormone-producing tumour fails to show negative feedback and this is useful in diagnosis, e.g. the dexamethasone suppression test in diagnosis of Cushing's syndrome.

Common presenting symptoms in endocrine disease

Hormonal abnormalities have a wide range of clinical effects and there are many presenting symptoms and signs of endocrine disease. Many of these symptoms are vague and non-specific, e.g. tiredness in hypothyroidism, weight loss, anorexia and malaise in Addison's disease, and the differential diagnosis is often wide.

Weight gain

Patients often ascribe weight gain to endocrine abnormalities. This is rarely the case and weight gain is usually the result of excessive food intake; occasionally, however, patients with Cushing's syndrome or hypothyroidism will present in this way. There are usually additional features in the history or on clinical examination which point to the correct diagnosis. Obesity is a feature of polycystic ovary syndrome and must always be considered in a female with irregular periods with or without hirsutism.

Delayed or early puberty

Precocious puberty (< 9 years) or delayed puberty (> 15 years) is often the result of a familial tendency although hypothalamic–pituitary disease may present in this way, and endocrine investigations are usually undertaken.

Other symptoms which often require specific endocrine investigations include hirsutism (page 400), menstrual irregularities with infrequent or absent periods (page 398), galactorrhoea and infertility. Carpal tunnel syndrome is usually idiopathic, but may be a presenting feature of acromegaly or hypothyroidism.

Pituitary tumours

Benign pituitary tumours are the most common form of pituitary disease. Symptoms may arise as a result of excess hormone secretion, inadequate hormone production or from pressure and local infiltration.

Overproduction

Overproduction of pituitary hormones may cause the following:

- Growth hormone (GH) excess resulting in acromegaly or gigantism (usually acidophil adenomas)
- Prolactin excess (chromaphobe adenomas)
- Cushing's disease resulting from excess ACTH production (basophil adenomas or hyperplasia)

Tumours producing luteinizing hormone (LH), follicle-stimulating hormone (FSH) or TSH are very rare.

Underproduction

This is the result of disease at either a hypothalamic or pituitary level, and it results in the clinical features of hypopituitarism (page 394).

Local effects

Local infiltration of or pressure on surrounding structures (Figure 12.3) may result in:

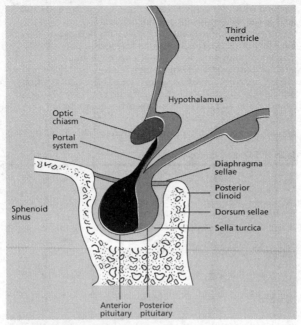

Figure 12.3 A sagittal section of the pituitary fossa, showing the important anatomical relationships.

- Visual loss with field defects. This is typically a bitemporal hemianopia caused by pressure on the optic chiasm (page 449)
- Headache produced by tumour involvement of the meninges and bony structures
- Obesity and altered appetite and thirst. This is from involvement of the hypothalamus. In children, hypothalamic involvement may lead to early puberty (precocious puberty)
- Hydrocephalus caused by interruption of CSF flow
- Cranial nerve lesions by infiltration of the cavernous sinus (see Table 14.1)

Hypopituitarism

Deficiency of hypothalamic-releasing hormones or pituitary hormones may be either selective or multiple. Multiple deficiencies usually result from tumour growth or other destructive lesions, and there is usually a progressive loss of function with LH and FSH being affected first and TSH and ACTH last. Rather than prolactin deficiency, hyperprolactinaemia occurs relatively early because of loss of tonic inhibitory control by dopamine (Figure 12.1). Panhypopituitarism refers to deficiency of all anterior pituitary hormones and is most commonly caused by tumours, surgery or radiotherapy. Vasopressin and oxytocin secretion will only be affected if the hypothalamus is involved by either hypothalamic tumour or extension of a pituitary lesion.

Aetiology

The causes of hypopituitarism are listed in Table 12.1.

Table 12.1 Causes of hypopituitarism

Neoplastic	Primary tumours
	Secondary deposits
	Craniopharyngioma
Infective	Meningitis
	Encephalitis
	Syphilis
Vascular	Pituitary apoplexy
	Sheehan's syndrome
Immunological	Pituitary antibodies
Traumatic	Skull fracture
	Surgery
Infiltrations	Sarcoidosis
	Haemochromatosis
Others	Radiation damage
	Chemotherapy
	'Empty sella' syndrome
'Functional'	Anorexia
	Starvation
	Emotional deprivation
Congenital	Kallman's syndrome

Clinical features

These depend on the extent of hypothalamic–pituitary deficiencies. Gonadotrophin deficiency results in loss of libido, amenorrhoea and impotence whereas hyperprolactinaemia results in galactorrhoea and hypogonadism. Growth hormone deficiency is usually silent except in children, although it may impair well-being in adults. Secondary hypothyroidism and adrenal failure lead to tiredness, slowness of thought and action, and mild hypotension. Long-standing hypopituitarism may give the classic picture of pallor with hairlessness *(alabaster skin)*.

Particular syndromes related to hypopituitarism are the following:

- KALLMAN'S SYNDROME: isolated gonadotrophin deficiency with anosmia, colour blindness, midline facial deformities and renal abnormalities

- SHEEHAN'S SYNDROME: this situation, now rare, is pituitary infarction following severe postpartum haemorrhage

- PITUITARY APOPLEXY: infarction or haemorrhage into a pituitary tumour which may result in life-threatening hypopituitarism

- 'EMPTY SELLA' SYNDROME: the sella turcica appears radiologically devoid of pituitary tissue; the pituitary is actually placed eccentrically and function is usually normal

Investigation

Each axis of the hypothalamic–pituitary system may require separate investigation. The presence of normal gonadal function (*ovulatory menstruation* or *normal libido/erections*) suggests that multiple defects of the anterior pituitary are unlikely. Tests range from measurement of basal hormone levels to stimulatory tests of the pituitary and tests of feedback for the hypothalamus. [CM pp. 781–782 and 1048–1050]

Management

Steroid and thyroid hormones are essential for life and are given as oral replacement drugs with the aim of restoring clinical and biochemical normality. Androgens and oestrogens are replaced for symptomatic control. If fertility is desired, LH and FSH analogues may be used. GH therapy is given to the growing child and it may also produce substantial benefits to the GH-deficient adult in terms of work capacity and psychological well-being.

MALE REPRODUCTION AND SEX

Luteinizing hormone-releasing hormone (LHRH, also called gonadotrophin-releasing hormone, GnRH) is synthesized in the hypothalamus. It is released episodically into the pituitary portal circulation (during and after puberty) and stimulates LH and FSH secretion from the anterior pituitary gland. LH and FSH stimulate production of testosterone and sperm respectively from the testes.

Normal puberty, delayed and precocious puberty [CM pp. 784–785]

Disorders of sexual differentiation [CM p. 787]

Male hypogonadism

Male hypogonadism is a descriptive term for the clinical features associated with androgen deficiency. The presentation depends on the age of onset of hypogonadism (Table 12.2). In prepubertal onset the patient presents with delayed puberty and eunuchoid body proportions resulting from the continued growth of long bones which occurs because of delayed fusion of the epiphyses.

Table 12.2 Consequences of androgen deficiency in the male

Prepubertal onset with eunuchoidism
Increased height and arm span
Lack of adult hair distribution
High-pitched voice
Small penis, testes and scrotum
Decreased muscle mass

Hypogonadism beginning after puberty
Decreased prostate size
Diminished rate of growth of beard and body hair
Fine feminine skin
Decreased potency and libido

A large number of diseases can lead to destruction or malfunction of the hypothalamic–pituitary–testicular axis (Table 12.3). Klinefelter's syndrome is the most common cause of male hypogonadism, with an incidence of 1 in 1000 live births. It is the result of the presence of an extra X chromosome (47, XXY). Accelerated atrophy of germ cells gives rise to sterility and small firm testes. The clinical picture varies; in the most severely affected there is complete failure of sexual maturation, eunuchoid body proportions, gynaecomastia and mental handicap.

Table 12.3 Causes of male hypogonadism

Hypothalamic	Isolated GnRH deficiency Kallman's syndrome
Pituitary	Hyperprolactinaemia Hypopituitarism
Testicular	*Congenital:* Klinefelter's syndrome, anorchia, Leydig cell agenesis, failure of testicular descent *Acquired:* trauma, torsion, chemotherapy, radiation
Target tissues	Androgen receptor deficiency
Systemic disease	Renal failure Liver cirrhosis

Investigations
Measurement of basal serum testosterone, LH and FSH will confirm the diagnosis and allow the distinction between primary gonadal (testicular) failure and hypothalamic–

pituitary disease. In testicular failure testosterone levels will be low, but LH/FSH levels high as a result of loss of the negative feedback of testosterone on the hypothalamus–pituitary. Further investigations, e.g. serum prolactin, chromosomal analysis, pituitary CT and pituitary function tests will depend on the site of the defect.

Management

The cause can rarely be reversed. The mainstay of treatment is androgen replacement. Although hypogonadotrophic patients have the potential for fertility, LH and FSH or pulsatile GnRH are only used (instead of testosterone) when fertility is desired as these regimens are expensive and complex.

Loss of libido and impotence

Impotence is defined as failure to initiate an erection or to maintain an erection until ejaculation. Erection is the result of increased vascularity of the penis controlled via the sacral parasympathetic outflow; it may be impaired by vascular disease, autonomic neuropathy and nerve damage after pelvic surgery. The nervous pathways for ejaculation are centred on the lumbar sympathetics, and abnormalities may occur with autonomic neuropathy and traumatic nerve damage. Psychological factors, endocrine factors (causes of hypogonadism described above), alcohol and drugs, e.g. cannabis, β-blockers and diuretics, may cause abnormalities at either stage. A careful history and examination will identify the cause in many patients. The presence of nocturnal emissions and morning erections excludes an endocrine cause. Many cases are the result of psychological factors and the patient may respond to psychosexual counselling.

Table 12.4 Causes of gynaecomastia

Physiological	Neonatal resulting from the influence of maternal hormones Pubertal Old age
Deficient testosterone secretion	Any cause of hypogonadism (see Table 12.3)
Oestrogen-producing tumours	Of the testis or adrenal gland
HCG-producing tumours	Of the testis or the lung
Drugs	Oestrogens, digitalis, cannabis, heroin, spironolactone, cyproterone, cimetidine
Other	Hyperthyroidism, liver disease

HCG = human chorionic gonadotrophin.

Gynaecomastia

The development of benign breast tissue in the male is the result of an increase in the oestrogen:androgen ratio (Table 12.4). Gynaecomastia is common in early puberty as a result of relative oestrogen excess, and usually resolves spontaneously. Unexplained gynaecomastia occurs, especially in elderly people, and is a diagnosis of exclusion after thorough examination and investigation. The treatment is either of the underlying cause or by removal of the drug if possible. Occasionally surgery is needed.

FEMALE REPRODUCTION AND SEX

In the adult female, higher brain centres impose a menstrual cycle of 28 days upon the activity of hypothalamic GnRH. Pulses of GnRH stimulate release of pituitary LH and FSH. LH stimulates ovarian androgen production and FSH stimulates follicular development and aromatase activity (an enzyme required to convert ovarian androgens to oestrogens). Oestrogens are necessary for normal pubertal development and maintenance of the menstrual cycle; they also have effects on a variety of tissues.

The menopause

The menopause, or cessation of periods, naturally occurs about the age of 45–55 years. During the·late forties, first FSH and then LH concentrations begin to rise, probably as follicle supply diminishes. Oestrogen levels fall and the cycle becomes disrupted. Menopause may also occur surgically, with radiotherapy to the ovaries and with ovarian disease (e.g. premature menopause in the twenties and thirties). Symptoms of the menopause are hot flushes, vaginal dryness and breast atrophy. There may also be vague symptoms of depression, loss of libido and weight gain. There is loss of bone density (osteoporosis, page 190) and the premenopausal protection against ischaemic heart disease disappears. Most of these effects may be reduced by hormone replacement therapy (HRT) which is now given long term to most women with menopausal symptoms; some authorities would recommend giving HRT to all women to protect against osteoporosis and ischaemic heart disease. HRT is always given to women with premature ovarian failure. Oestrogens, when given alone, increase the risk of endometrial cancer and so combination treatment with progestogens is given to women with an intact uterus.

Female hypogonadism and amenorrhoea

Amenorrhoea is the absence of menstruation. It is often physiological, e.g. during pregnancy and lactation, and after the menopause. *Primary amenorrhoea* is failure to start spontaneous menstruation by the age of 16 years. *Secondary amenorrhoea* is absence of menstruation for 3 months in a woman who has previously had menstrual cycles. In the female, hypogonadism almost always presents as amenorrhoea or oligomenorrhoea (irregular periods with long cycles). The other features of oestrogen deficiency include atrophy of the breasts and vagina, loss of pubic hair and osteoporosis.

Aetiology

The causes of amenorrhoea are listed in Table 12.5. Severe weight loss (e.g. anorexia nervosa) has long been associated with amenorrhoea but it is now recognized that less severe forms of weight loss, produced by dieting and exercise, are a common cause of amenorrhoea caused by abnormal secretion of GnRH.

Polycystic ovary syndrome is a common cause of oligomenorrhoea and amenorrhoea, hirsutes and acne in patients who have a history of irregular menses, often dating from the menarche. There are bilateral cystic ovaries associated with deficient production of oestrogens and excess androgen production. Ultrasonography examination shows multiple small cysts.

Table 12.5 Pathological causes of amenorrhoea

Hypothalamic	* GnRH deficiency (isolated or as part of Kallman's syndrome) Weight loss, physical exercise, stress Post-oral contraceptive therapy
Pituitary	Hyperprolactinaemia Hypopituitarism
Gonadal	Polycystic ovary syndrome Premature ovarian failure – autoimmune basis * Defective ovarian development (dysgenesis) Androgen-secreting ovarian tumours Radiotherapy
Other diseases	Thyroid dysfunction, Cushing's syndrome Adrenal tumours, severe illness
Uterine/vaginal abnormality	* Imperforate hymen or absent uterus

* Presents as primary amenorrhoea.

Investigations

The cause of amenorrhoea may be apparent after a full history and examination. Basal levels of serum FSH, LH, oestrogen and prolactin will allow a distinction between primary gonadal and hypothalamic–pituitary causes. Further investigations, e.g. ultrasonography of ovaries, laparoscopy and ovarian biopsy, pituitary C T or MRI and measurement of serum testosterone, will depend on the probable site of the defect and the findings on clinical examination.

Management

Treatment is of the cause where possible, e.g. increase weight, treat hypothyroidism and hyperprolactinaemia. In those patients where the underlying defect cannot be corrected, cyclical oestrogens are given to reverse the symptoms of oestrogen deficiency and prevent early osteoporosis. The treatment, however, is different in those patients who want to become pregnant. Patients with isolated GnRH deficiency or hypopituitarism are treated with human FSH/LH. Patients with polycystic ovaries are treated with clomiphene or, more rarely, wedge resection of the ovaries.

Hirsutism

This is an excess growth of hair in a male pattern – beard area, abdominal wall, thigh and around the nipples. In most patients no underlying disease can be found but in some cases hirsutism is the result of increased adrenal or ovarian androgen production (Table 12.6).

Table 12.6 Causes of hirsutism

Familial and racial	
Adrenal	Androgen-secreting tumours
	Congenital adrenal hyperplasia
Ovarian	Androgen-secreting tumours
	Polycystic ovarian syndrome
Androgenic drugs	Androgens, phenytoin, minoxidil, cyclosporin
Idiopathic	Target organ hypersensitivity

A short history, accompanying virilization (male secondary sexual characteristics), and severe menstrual disturbance are suggestive of significant androgen secretion with a more serious underlying cause, e.g. adrenal tumour. The management is to identify and treat the underlying cause. Excess hair can be removed or disguised by shaving, bleaching and waxing. Other treatments are the antiandrogen, cyproterone acetate, and oestrogens that reduce free androgens by increasing levels of the sex hormone-binding globulin.

Hyperprolactinaemia

Prolactin release, unlike other pituitary hormones, is tonically inhibited by dopamine from the hypothalamus via the pituitary stalk. There is a physiological increase in prolactin during pregnancy and postpartum breast feeding.

Aetiology

The most important pathological cause of high prolactin is a prolactin-secreting pituitary adenoma. Other pituitary or hypothalamic tumours may also cause hyperprolactinaemia by interfering with dopamine inhibition of prolactin release. Other causes include primary hypothyroidism (high TRH levels stimulate prolactin) and drugs: metoclopramide and phenothiazines caused by inhibition of dopamine, oestrogens and cimetidine.

Clinical features

There is galactorrhoea, oligo- or amenorrhoea, subfertility and impotence as a result of inhibition of GnRH by high levels of prolactin. If there is a pituitary tumour there may be headache and visual field defects.

Investigations

SERUM PROLACTIN LEVEL. Very high levels in the absence of pregnancy and drugs are suggestive of a prolactinoma.

THYROID FUNCTION TESTS.

CT OR MAGNETIC RESONANCE IMAGING OF THE PITUITARY.

VISUAL FIELDS AND PITUITARY FUNCTION should be checked if a pituitary tumour is the cause.

Management

Causative drugs should be withdrawn if possible and hypothyroidism treated. In the case of a prolactinoma, the dopamine agonist, bromocriptine, will reduce plasma prolactin concentrations and produce some shrinkage in tumour size. Definitive therapy is controversial and depends on the size of the tumour, the patient's wish for fertility and the facilities available. Trans-sphenoidal surgery, combined with postoperative radiotherapy for large tumours, often restores normoprolactinaemia but there is a high late recurrence rate (50% at 5 years). Small tumours (*microadenomas*) in asymptomatic patients may only need observation.

THE GROWTH AXIS

GH is secreted from the anterior pituitary and its tissue effects are mediated by insulin-like growth factor (IGF-1) synthesized in the liver and other tissues. Deficiency of GH produces short stature in children but, in adults, it is often clinically silent, although recent evidence suggests that it may result in significant impairment in well-being and work capacity. Excessive GH production leads to gigantism in children (if acquired before epiphyseal fusion) and acromegaly in adults.

Acromegaly

Acromegaly is rare and caused by a benign pituitary adenoma in almost all cases. Hyperplasia resulting from excess of

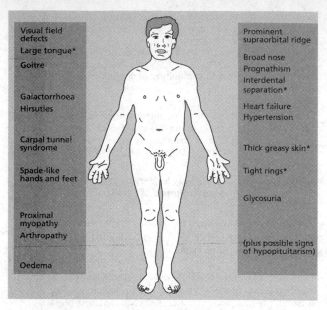

Figure 12.4 The symptoms and signs of acromegaly. *These indicate signs of greater discriminant value.

GH-releasing hormone (GHRH) is rare. Males and females are affected equally and the incidence is highest in middle age.

Clinical features

Symptoms and signs are shown in Figure 12.4. One-third of patients present with changes in appearance and one-quarter with visual field defects or headaches.

Investigations

GLUCOSE TOLERANCE TEST is diagnostic. In a positive test there is failure of the normal suppression of serum GH below 1 mU/l in response to a glucose load. Some show a paradoxical rise. Twenty-five per cent of individuals with acromegaly have a diabetic glucose tolerance test.

SERUM GH LEVELS are usually elevated but, if available, measurement of plasma IGF-1 may be more useful because plasma levels fluctuate less than those of GH.

LATERAL SKULL RADIOGRAPHS are abnormal in 90% with enlargement of the pituitary fossa, and are a good screening test.

VISUAL FIELD DEFECTS are common and should be plotted by perimetry.

CT AND MRI of the pituitary give good definition of tumour extent and anatomy.

PITUITARY FUNCTION TESTING usually shows evidence of hypopituitarism.

HYPERPROLACTINAEMIA occurs in 30%.

Management

Treatment is indicated in all except elderly people or those with minimal abnormalities because untreated acromegaly is associated with markedly reduced survival. Most deaths result from heart failure, coronary artery disease and hypertension related causes. The preferred treatment is controversial and complete cure if possible is often slow. The choice lies between:

- SURGERY: this is the treatment of choice in suitable cases and may be trans-sphenoidal, or transfrontal if the tumour is large. Surgery is usually combined with radiotherapy because excision is rarely complete

- RADIOTHERAPY when given alone takes 1–10 years to be effective

- DRUGS: octreotide, a long-acting somatostatin analogue, is now the treatment of choice in resistant cases. It is given by subcutaneous injection and can be given to shrink tumours before definitive treatment or to control symptoms. Bromocriptine is usually reserved for elderly and frail people

THE THYROID AXIS

The thyroid gland secretes predominantly thyroxine (T_4) and only a small amount of the biologically active hormone triiodothyronine (T_3). Most circulating T_3 is produced by peripheral conversion of T_4. Over 99% of T_4 and T_3 circulate bound to plasma proteins, mainly thyroxine-binding globulin (TBG). The feedback pathway that controls secretion of TSH is discussed on pages 389–391. Measurement of plasma TSH is the first-line investigation in patients with suspected thyroid gland dysfunction.

Hypothyroidism

Underactivity of the thyroid gland may be primary from disease of the thyroid gland or, much less commonly, secondary to hypothalamic–pituitary disease.

Aetiology

ATROPHIC (AUTOIMMUNE) HYPOTHYROIDISM. This is the most common cause of hypothyroidism and is associated with microsomal antibodies and lymphoid infiltration of the gland, with eventual fibrosis and atrophy. It is six times more common in females and the incidence increases with age. It is

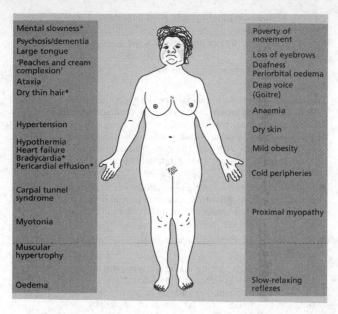

Mental slowness*
Psychosis/dementia
Large tongue
'Peaches and cream complexion'
Ataxia
Dry thin hair*

Hypertension

Hypothermia
Heart failure
Bradycardia*
Pericardial effusion*

Carpal tunnel syndrome

Myotonia

Muscular hypertrophy

Oedema

Poverty of movement

Loss of eyebrows
Deafness
Periorbital oedema
Deap voice
(Goitre)

Anaemia

Dry skin

Mild obesity

Cold peripheries

Proximal myopathy

Slow-relaxing reflexes

Figure 12.5 The symptoms and signs of hypothyroidism. *These indicate signs of greater discriminant value.

associated with other autoimmune conditions such as pernicious anaemia.

HASHIMOTO'S THYROIDITIS. This autoimmune thyroiditis, also associated with thyroid microsomal antibodies, produces atrophic changes with regeneration leading to goitre formation. It is more common in females and in late middle age. Patients may be hypothyroid, euthyroid or go through an initial toxic phase.

IATROGENIC. Forty per cent are hypothyroid by 25 years following radioactive iodine or surgery for hyperthyroidism.

IODINE DEFICIENCY. This still exists in some areas, particularly mountainous areas (Alps, Himalayas, South America). Goitre, occasionally massive, is common. The patients may be euthyroid or hypothyroid depending on the severity of the iodine deficiency.

DYSHORMONOGENESIS. This rare condition is caused by genetic defects in the synthesis of thyroid hormones.

Clinical features

Symptoms and signs of hypothyroidism are illustrated in Figure 12.5. Features are often difficult to distinguish in elderly people and young women. Hypothyroidism should be excluded in all patients with oligomenorrhoea/amenorrhoea, menorrhagia, infertility and hyperprolactinaemia.

Investigations

Measurement of serum TSH is the investigation of choice. A high TSH confirms primary hypothyroidism.

SERUM FREE T_4 LEVELS are low.

THYROID ANTIBODIES and other organ-specific antibodies may be present in the serum.

OTHER FEATURES include anaemia (normocytic or macrocytic), hypercholesterolaemia and hyponatraemia (increased antidiuretic hormone and impaired clearance of free water).

Management

Replacement therapy with thyroxine (100–200 µg/day) is required for life. The starting dose is 100 µg/day (50 µg/day in elderly people) and adequacy of replacement is assessed clinically and by thyroid function tests after at least 6 weeks on a steady dose. In patients with ischaemic heart disease, starting doses should be even lower (25 µg/day) and increased at 2 to 6-week intervals if ischaemic symptoms do not deteriorate.

Myxoedema coma

Severe hypothyroidism may rarely present with confusion and coma, particularly in elderly people. Typical features include hypothermia (page 421), cardiac failure, hypoventilation, hypoglycaemia and hyponatraemia. The optimal treatment is controversial but most would advocate the use of T_3 2.5–5 µg 8-hourly either orally or intravenously. Other measures should include oxygen, intravenous hydrocortisone (in case hypothyroidism is a manifestation of hypopituitarism) and dextrose to prevent hypoglycaemia.

Myxoedema madness

Depression is common but occasionally, with severe hypothyroidism in elderly people, the patient may become frankly demented or psychotic, sometimes with striking delusions. This may occur shortly after starting thyroxine replacement.

Hyperthyroidism

Hyperthyroidism is common affecting 2–5% of all women at some time, mainly between the ages of 20 and 40 years. The most common causes are Graves' disease, a toxic solitary nodule and toxic multinodular goitre. Rarer causes include De Quervain's thyroiditis, thyroiditis factitia (*surreptitious T_4 consumption*), drugs (*amiodarone*), metastatic differentiated thyroid carcinoma and TSH-secreting tumours (e.g. *of the pituitary*).

GRAVES' DISEASE

Graves' disease is the most common cause of hyperthyroidism and is the result of IgG antibodies binding to the TSH receptor and stimulating thyroid hormone production. It is associated with typical eye changes (see below), vitiligo, pretibial myxoedema (skin infiltration) and, rarely, lymphadenopathy and splenomegaly. It is also associated with other autoimmune diseases such as pernicious anaemia and myasthenia gravis.

SOLITARY TOXIC NODULE (PLUMMER'S DISEASE)

This is responsible for about 5% of cases. Prolonged remission is rarely induced by drug therapy.

TOXIC MULTINODULAR GOITRE

This commonly occurs in older women and again drug therapy is rarely successful in inducing a remission.

DE QUERVAIN'S THYROIDITIS

Transient hyperthyroidism sometimes results from acute inflammation of the gland probably as a result of viral infection. It is usually accompanied by fever, malaise and pain in the neck. Treatment is with aspirin, reserving prednisolone for severely symptomatic cases.

Clinical features

Typical symptoms and signs of hyperthyroidism are shown in Figure 12.6.

Clinical features vary with age and underlying aetiology. Eye signs (see below), pretibial myxoedema and thyroid acropachy (*clubbing, swollen fingers* and *periosteal new bone formation*) occur only in Graves' disease. Elderly patients may present with atrial fibrillation and/or heart failure or with a clinical picture resembling hypothyroidism ('apathetic thyrotoxicosis').

Investigations

SERUM TSH is suppressed.

SERUM T_4 AND T_3 are elevated. Occasionally T_3 alone is elevated (*T_3 toxicosis*).

SERUM MICROSOMAL AND THYROGLOBULIN ANTIBODIES are present in most cases of Graves' disease.

Management

- ANTITHYROID DRUGS: carbimazole 10–20 mg 8-hourly inhibits the formation of thyroid hormones and is also an immunosuppressive agent. As clinical benefit may not be apparent for 10–20 days, β-blockers may be used to provide rapid symptomatic control because many manifestations are mediated via the sympathetic system.

Symptoms

Weight loss
Increased appetite
Irritability/behaviour change
Restlessness
Malaise
Muscle weakness
Tremor
Choreoathetosis
Breathlessness
Palpitation
Heat intolerance
Vomiting
Diarrhoea
Eye complaints*
Goitre
Oligomenorrhoea
Loss of libido
Gynaecomastia
Onycholysis
Tall stature (in children)

*Only in Graves' disease

Signs

Irritability
Psychosis
Hyperkinesis
Tremor

Systolic hypertension
Cardiac failure
Tachycardia or atrial fibrillation
Warm vasodilated peripheries

Onycholysis
Palmar erythema

Thyroid acropachy
Pretibial myxoedema

Exophthalmus
Lid lag
Conjunctival oedema
Ophthalmoplegia
Goitre, bruit

Weight loss

Proximal muscle wasting
(shoulder and hips)
Proximal myopathy

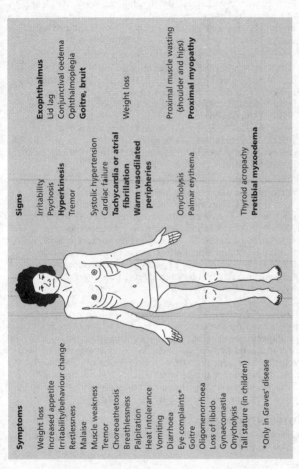

Figure 12.6 The symptoms and signs of hyperthyroidism. The bold type indicates signs of greater discriminatory value.

407

Carbimazole is then reduced according to clinical state over the next 12–18 months. Some physicians prefer the 'block and replace regimen' where full doses of carbimazole 30–45 mg/day are given for 18 months to suppress the thyroid completely, while replacing thyroid activity with thyroxine. Claimed advantages are avoidance of under- or over-treatment and better use of the immunosuppressive action. Fifty per cent of patients with Graves' disease will relapse on discontinuation of drug treatment, mostly within the following 2 years

- RADIOACTIVE IODINE: ^{131}I accumulates in the gland and destroys the gland by local irradiation. The indications for radioactive iodine are similar to those for surgery and include recurrence after drug treatment, poor compliance or side effects with drugs. It is more commonly used in older patients. It is effective in 75% of patients in 4–12 weeks. If hyperthyroidism persists, a further dose of ^{131}I can be given although this increases the rate of subsequent hypothyroidism

- SURGERY: subtotal thyroidectomy should only be performed in patients who have been rendered euthyroid. Anti-thyroid drugs are stopped 10–14 days before the operation and replaced with oral potassium iodide which inhibits thyroid hormone release and reduces the vascularity of the gland. Indications for surgery include those for ^{131}I and large goitres. Risks of surgery include transient hypocalcaemia, hypothyroidism hypopara-thyroidism, recurrent laryngeal nerve palsy and recurrent hyperthyroidism

Thyroid crisis

This is a rare life-threatening condition in which there is a rapid deterioration of thyrotoxicosis with hyperpyrexia, tachycardia and extreme restlessness. It is most commonly precipitated by infection, stress or surgery, or radioactive iodine therapy in an unprepared patient. Treatment is with full dose propranolol together with potassium iodide, anti-thyroid drugs and corticosteroids.

Thyroid eye disease

This is also known as dysthyroid eye disease or ophthalmic Graves' disease.

Aetiology
It is currently believed that the exophthalmos of Graves' disease, which may be unilateral or bilateral, is the result of specific antibodies causing retro-orbital inflammation and subsequent oedema. TSH antibodies are found in the serum although their role in pathogenesis is not clear.

Clinical features
The clinical appearances are characteristic. Proptosis and
limitation of eye movements are direct effects of the
inflammation, whereas conjunctival oedema, lid lag and
corneal scarring are secondary to the proptosis and lack of
eye cover. Eye manifestations do not parallel the clinical
course of Graves' disease, particularly the degree of
thyrotoxicosis. Orbital CT and magnetic resonance imaging
may be necessary to exclude other causes of exophthalmos,
e.g. retro-orbital tumour.

Management
Thyroid status should be normalized and hypothyroidism
avoided because this may exacerbate the eye problem.
Specific treatment includes methyl cellulose eye drops or, if
more severe, high-dose systemic steroids to reduce
inflammation. Lateral tarsorraphy will protect the cornea if
the lids cannot be closed. Occasionally irradiation of the
orbits or surgical decompression is required.

Goitre (thyroid enlargement)

Goitre is more common in women than in men and may be
physiological or pathological in origin (Table 12.7).

Table 12.7 Causes of goitre

Physiological: puberty, pregnancy
Autoimmune: Graves' disease, Hashimoto's disease
Thyroiditis: acute (de Quervain's thyroiditis), chronic fibrotic (Riedel's thyroiditis)
Iodine deficiency (endemic goitre)
Dyshormonogenesis
Multinodular goitre
Diffuse goitre
Benign cysts, lymphoma, carcinoma

Clinical features
It is usually noticed as a cosmetic defect, although discomfort
and pain in the neck can occur and, occasionally, oesophageal
or tracheal compression produces dysphagia or difficulty in
breathing. The gland may be diffusely enlarged, multinodular
or possess a solitary nodule. A bruit may be present and
occasionally lymphadenopathy is present.

Investigations
THYROID FUNCTION TESTS: TSH plus T_4 or T_3.

RADIOGRAPH of chest and thoracic inlet where appropriate to
detect tracheal compression.

FINE NEEDLE ASPIRATION for cytology should be performed for solitary nodules or a dominant nodule in a multinodular goitre because there is a 5% chance of malignancy.

OTHER TESTS are not usually required. Thyroid ultrasonography can delineate nodules and demonstrate whether they are solid or cystic. Thyroid scan (^{125}I or ^{131}I) distinguishes between a functioning ('hot') or non-functioning ('cold') nodule. Hot nodules are rarely malignant whereas cold nodules are malignant in up to 10% of cases.

Management
Treatment is usually not required apart from inducing euthyroidism if necessary. Surgical intervention may be required for cosmetic reasons, pressure effects or if there is a possibility of malignancy.

Thyroid carcinoma

Thyroid cancer is relatively uncommon, being responsible for 400 deaths annually in the UK. Characteristics are listed in Table 12.8. Treatment of follicular and papillary cancers is surgical with total thyroidectomy. Ablative radioactive iodine is subsequently given which will be taken up by remaining thyroid tissue or metastatic lesions. Treatment of anaplastic carcinoma is largely palliative.

Table 12.8 Characteristics of thyroid cancer

Cell type	Frequency (%)	Behaviour	Spread	Prognosis
Papillary	70	Young people, slow growing	Local	Good
Follicular	20	More common in females	Lung/bone	Good if resected
Anaplastic	< 5	Aggressive	Local	Very poor
Lymphoma	< 2	Variable		Variable*
Medullary cell	5	Often familial	Local/metastases	Poor

*Sometimes responsive to radiotherapy.

THE GLUCOCORTICOID AXIS

The adrenal gland consists of an outer cortex producing steroids (cortisol, aldosterone and androgens) and an inner medulla secreting catecholamines. Aldosterone secretion is under the control of the renin–angiotensin system (see later). Corticotrophin-releasing factor (CRF) from the hypothalamus stimulates ACTH (from the anterior pituitary), which stimulates cortisol production by the adrenal cortex. The cortisol secreted feeds back on the hypothalamus and pituitary to inhibit further CRF/ACTH release. CRF release, and hence cortisol release, is in response to a circadian rhythm, stress and other factors. Random 'one-off' cortisol measurements may therefore be misleading in the diagnosis of hypoadrenalism or Cushing's syndrome. Cortisol has many effects particularly on carbohydrate metabolism. It leads to increased protein catabolism, increased deposition of fat and glycogen, sodium retention, increased renal potassium loss and a diminished host response to infection.

Addison's disease – primary hypoadrenalism

This is an uncommon condition in which there is destruction of the adrenal cortex.

Aetiology
Eighty per cent of cases result from antibodies against adrenal cortex antigens. This is associated with other autoimmune conditions, e.g. Hashimoto's thyroiditis, Graves' disease, pernicious anaemia and insulin-dependent diabetes mellitus. Rarer causes are adrenal gland tuberculosis, surgical removal, haemorrhage (in meningococcal septicaemia) and malignant infiltration.

Clinical features
Adrenal insufficiency has an insidious presentation with lethargy, depression, anorexia and weight loss. It may also present as an emergency with vomiting, abdominal pain and hypovolaemic shock. The important signs are hypotension (which may only be postural) caused by salt and water loss and hyperpigmentation (buccal mucosa, pressure points, skin creases and recent scars) resulting from stimulation of melanocytes by excess ACTH. There may be vitiligo and loss of body hair in women because of the dependence on adrenal androgens.

Investigations
SERUM UREA AND ELECTROLYTES may be normal but classically there is hyponatraemia, hyperkalaemia, a raised urea and hypoglycaemia.

BLOOD COUNT shows a neutrophil leucocytosis and eosinophilia.

ADRENAL ANTIBODIES are detected in most cases of autoimmune adrenalitis.

RADIOGRAPHS of the chest and abdomen may show evidence of TB with calcified adrenals.

THE DIAGNOSIS is usually made using the short tetracosactrin (Synacthen or synthetic ACTH) test (Table 12.9). In the acute situation treatment should not be delayed pending this investigation. Intramuscular hydrocortisone 100 mg is given immediately after a sample of blood is taken for measurement of plasma cortisol (which will be inappropriately low) and ACTH (which will be high because of loss of negative feedback).

Management

This is with lifelong steroid replacement taken as tablets.

- HYDROCORTISONE. The usual dose is 20 mg on waking and 10 mg in the evening which mimics the normal diurnal rhythm. The dose is best monitored by measuring a series of cortisol levels throughout the day.

- FLUDROCORTISONE, a synthetic mineralocorticoid, 0.05–0.4 mg daily. The dose is adequate when there is no postural drop in blood pressure and plasma renin levels are suppressed to within the normal range.

  In a normal individual stress of any type, e.g. infection, trauma and surgical operations, causes an immediate and marked increase in ACTH and hence in cortisol. This is a necessary response and therefore it is very important in patients on steroid replacement that the dose is increased when placed in any of these situations. All patients on steroids must carry a 'steroid card' and a MedicAlert bracelet must be worn in case of accidents.

Table 12.9 Tetracosactrin (Synacthen) tests

Short test	Take blood for measurement of plasma cortisol then give tetracosactrin (Synacthen) 250 µg i.m. and take blood specimens for cortisol estimation at 30 and 60 minutes. Adrenal failure is excluded if the basal plasma cortisol exceeds 170 nmol/l and rises by at least 330 nmol/l to 690 nmol/l
Long test	Take blood for measurement of plasma cortisol, then give tetracosactrin (Synacthen) 1 mg i.m. and take blood samples for cortisol at 1, 4, 8 and 24 hours. Patients with normal adrenal function reach a plasma cortisol concentration of over 1000 nmol/l by 4 hours. In patients with Addison's disease the cortisol response is impaired throughout and in secondary adrenal insufficiency a delayed but normal response is seen

Secondary hypoadrenalism

This may arise from hypothalamic–pituitary disease or from long-term steroid therapy leading to hypothalamic–pituitary–adrenal suppression. The clinical features are the same as those of Addison's disease but there is no pigmentation because ACTH levels are low and, in pituitary disease, there are usually features of failure of other pituitary hormones. A long tetracosactrin (Synacthen) test (Table 12.9) will differentiate between primary and secondary adrenal failure. Treatment is with hydrocortisone; fludrocortisone is unnecessary. If adrenal failure is secondary to long-term steroid therapy, the adrenals will recover if steroids are withdrawn very slowly.

Cushing's syndrome

Cushing's syndrome is caused by persistently and inappropriately elevated glucocorticoid levels. Most cases result from administration of steroids for the treatment of medical conditions, e.g. asthma. Spontaneous Cushing's syndrome is rare (Table 12.10). *Cushing's disease* must be distinguished from *Cushing's syndrome*. The latter is a general term which refers to the abnormalities resulting from a chronic excess of glucocorticoids whatever the cause, while Cushing's disease specifically refers to excess glucocorticoids resulting from inappropriate ACTH secretion from the pituitary. Alcohol excess mimics Cushing's syndrome clinically and biochemically (pseudo-Cushing's syndrome). The pathogenesis is incompletely understood but the features resolve when alcohol is stopped.

Table 12.10 Aetiology of spontaneous Cushing's syndrome

	Percentage of cases
ACTH-dependent causes	
Pituitary adenoma (Cushing's disease)	60
Ectopic ACTH-producing tumours	
(small cell lung cancer, carcinoid tumours)	15
Non-ACTH-dependent causes	
Adrenal adenomas	9
Adrenal carcinomas	7
Rare causes, e.g. adrenal hyperplasia	

Clinical features
Patients are obese, fat distribution is typically central affecting the trunk, abdomen and neck (*buffalo-hump*). They have a plethoric complexion with a *moon face*. Many of the features are the result of the protein-catabolic effects of cortisol: the skin is thin and bruises easily, and there are purple striae on the abdomen, breasts and thighs (Figure 12.7). Pigmentation occurs with ACTH-dependent cases.

Investigations
CONFIRM RAISED CORTISOL
The *low-dose dexamethasone suppression test* is the most reliable screening test. Dexamethasone (a potent synthetic glucocorticoid) 0.5 mg 6-hourly is given orally for 48 hours. Normal individuals suppress serum cortisol by 48 hours.

Other tests
● Raised 24-hour urinary free cortisol (normal < 700 nmol/24h)

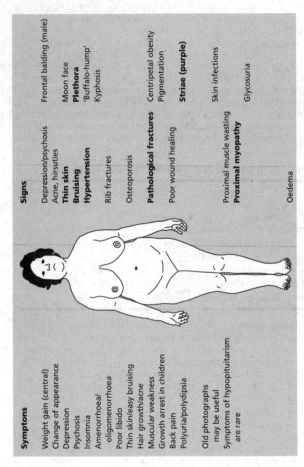

Symptoms

Weight gain (central)
Change of appearance
Depression
Psychosis
Insomnia
Amenorrhoea/
  oligomenorrhoea
Poor libido
Thin skin/easy bruising
Hair growth/acne
Muscular weakness
Growth arrest in children
Back pain
Polyuria/polydipsia

Old photographs
may be useful
Symptoms of hypopituitarism
are rare

Signs

Depression/psychosis   Frontal balding (male)
Acne, hirsuties
Thin skin   Moon face
Bruising   **Plethora**
Hypertension   'Buffalo–hump'
                              Kyphosis
Rib fractures
Osteoporosis

Pathological fractures   Centripetal obesity
                              Pigmentation
Poor wound healing

                              Striae (purple)

                              Skin infections

Proximal muscle wasting
Proximal myopathy

                              Glycosuria

Oedema

Figure 12.7 The signs of Cushing's syndrome. Bold type indicates signs of greater discriminatory value.

- Circadian rhythm studies show loss of the normal circadian fall of cortisol at 24h in patients with Cushing's syndrome

ESTABLISHING THE CAUSE OF CUSHING'S SYNDROME

- High-dose dexamethasone suppression test: dexamethasone 2.0 mg 6-hourly is given orally for 48 hours. Most patients with pituitary-dependent Cushing's disease suppress serum cortisol by 48 hours. Failure of suppression suggests an ectopic source of ACTH or an adrenal tumour.

- Plasma ACTH levels are low or undetectable in non-ACTH-dependent disease.

- Corticotrophin-releasing hormone test. An exaggerated plasma ACTH response to exogenous CRF (bolus given intravenously) suggests pituitary-dependent Cushing's disease.

- Other tests will depend on the probable cause of Cushing's syndrome which has been established from the above tests. Chest radiograph, bronchoscopy and CT of the body may localize ectopic ACTH-producing tumours. Selective venous sampling for ACTH will localize pituitary tumours and an otherwise occult ectopic ACTH-producing tumour.

Management

SURGICAL REMOVAL is indicated for most pituitary (usually a trans-sphenoidal approach) and adrenal tumours and may be appropriate for many cases of ectopic ACTH-producing tumours.

METYRAPONE, an inhibitor of cortisol synthesis, may be useful in cases not amenable to surgery.

IRRADIATION of the pituitary produces a very slow response and is restricted to cases where surgery is unsuccessful, contraindicated or unacceptable to the patient.

Iatrogenic Cushing's syndrome responds to a reduction in steroid dosage when possible. Immunosuppressant drugs such as azathioprine may be used in conjunction with steroids to enable lower doses to be used to control the underlying disease.

Incidental adrenal tumours

With the advent of abdominal CT, unsuspected adrenal masses have been discovered in about 1% of scans. These include primary tumours, metastases and cysts. If found, functional tests to exclude secretory activity should be performed; if none is found then most authorities recommend removal of large (> 4–5 cm) and functional tumours but observation of smaller lesions.

THE THIRST AXIS

Secretion of antidiuretic hormone (ADH, vasopressin) from the posterior pituitary gland is determined principally by the plasma osmolality. ADH secretion is suppressed at levels below 280 mosmol/kg thus allowing maximal water diuresis. Secretion increases to a maximum at a plasma osmolality of 295 mosmol/kg. Large falls in blood pressure or volume also stimulate vasopressin secretion. The major hormonal action is on the collecting tubule of the kidney to cause water reabsorption. At high concentrations vasopressin also causes vasoconstriction.

Syndrome of inappropriate ADH secretion (SIADH)

There is continued ADH secretion in spite of plasma hypotonicity and a normal or expanded plasma volume.

Aetiology
SIADH is caused by ectopic production of ADH, e.g. small cell lung cancer or disordered hypothalamic–pituitary secretion (Table 12.11).

Table 12.11 Causes of SIADH

Cancer	Many tumours of which the most common is small cell cancer of the lung
Brain	Meningitis, cerebral abscess, head injury, tumour
Lung	Pneumonia, tuberculosis, lung abscess
Metabolic	Porphyria, alcohol withdrawal
Drugs	Opiates, chlorpropramide, carbamazepine, vincristine

Clinical features
There is nausea, irritability and headache with mild hyponatraemia (< 125 mmol/l). Fits and coma may occur with severe hyponatraemia (< 115 mmol/l).

Investigations
SIADH must be differentiated from other causes of dilutional hyponatraemia (page 206). The criteria for diagnosis are:

- Low serum sodium (< 125 mmol/l)
- Low plasma osmolality
- Urine osmolality 'inappropriately' higher than plasma osmolality
- Continued urinary sodium excretion (> 30 mmol/l)
- Absence of hypotension and hypovolaemia
- Normal renal, adrenal and thyroid function

Management
Mild asymptomatic cases need no treatment other than that
of the underlying cause. For symptomatic cases the options
are:

● Water restriction – 500 ml in 24 hours

● Dimethylchlorotetracycline inhibits the action of
  vasopressin on the kidney and may be useful if water
  restriction is poorly tolerated or ineffective

● Hypertonic saline (300 mmol/l i.v. slowly), with frusemide
  to prevent circulatory overload, may be necessary in
  severe cases

Diabetes insipidus

This is the result of impaired vasopressin secretion (*cranial
diabetes insipidus, CDI*) or renal resistance to the action of
vasopressin (*nephrogenic diabetes insipidus, NDI*). It must be
distinguished from primary polydipsia which is a psychiatric
distubance characterized by excessive intake of water.

Aetiology
The causes are listed in Table 12.12.

Table 12.12 Causes of diabetes insipidus

Cranial diabetes insipidus	Nephrogenic diabetes insipidus
Familial	Familial
Idiopathic*	Renal tubular acidosis
Head injury*	Metabolic: hypercalcaemia, hypokalaemia*
Surgery: transfrontal, trans-sphenoidal*	Drugs*
	Lithium chloride
Hypothalamic–pituitary tumours	Dimethylchlorotetracycline
	Glibenclamide
Granulomas: sarcoidosis, histiocytosis	
Infections: meningitis, encephalitis	
Vascular: haemorrhage, thrombosis	

* Indicates the most common causes. Diabetes insipidus after surgery may only
be transient.

Clinical features
There is polyuria (as much as 15 litres urine a day) and
polydipsia. Patients depend on a normal thirst mechanism
and access to water to maintain normonatraemia.

Investigations
Urine volume must be measured to confirm polyuria.

PLASMA BIOCHEMISTRY shows high or high–normal sodium concentration and osmolality.

URINE OSMOLALITY is inappropriately low.

A WATER DEPRIVATION TEST with desmopressin (synthetic vasopressin analogue) confirms the diagnosis and will usually distinguish CDI, NDI and primary polydipsia (Table 12.13). Water is restricted for 8 hours during which time blood and urine osmolality are measured hourly. Patients are weighed hourly and the test stopped if body weight drops by 5% as this indicates significant dehydration.

Table 12.13 Response to fluid deprivation and desmopressin in polyuric patients

Urine osmolality (mosmol/kg)		
After 8 h fluid deprivation	After desmopressin	Diagnosis
< 300	> 800	CDI
< 300	< 300	NDI
> 800	> 800	Primary polydipsia

Management
Treatment of the underlying condition seldom improves established CDI. In mild cases (3–4 litres urine per day) no specific treatment is necessary. Desmopressin administered as a nasal spray is useful for more severe cases. Treatment of the cause will usually improve NDI.

ENDOCRINOLOGY OF BLOOD PRESSURE CONTROL

In approximately 90% of cases of hypertension no cause can be found (page 312) and patients are said to have essential hypertension. In the remaining minority an underlying cause can be identified and these include endocrine causes of hypertension (Table 12.14). Young patients (< 35 years), those with abnormal baseline screening tests (page 313) or patients with hypertension resistant to treatment should be screened for secondary causes.

Primary hyperaldosteronism

This is a rare condition (< 1% of all hypertension) where high aldosterone levels exist independent of the renin–angiotensin system. It is caused by an adrenal adenoma (Conn's syndrome, 60% of cases) or by bilateral adrenal hyperplasia.

Clinical features
The major function of aldosterone is to cause an exchange transport of sodium and potassium in the distal renal tubule, that is, absorption of sodium (and hence water) and excretion

of potassium. Therefore hyperaldosteronism causes hypertension resulting from expansion of intravascular volume and hypokalaemia, which is rarely low enough to produce symptoms.

Table 12.14 Endocrine causes of hypertension

Excessive renin production	Renal artery stenosis Renin-secreting tumours
Excessive aldosterone production	Adrenal adenoma Adrenal hyperplasia
Excessive production of other mineralocorticoids	Cushing's syndrome (cortisol is a weak mineralocorticoid)
Excessive production of catecholamines	Phaeochromocytoma
Excessive production of growth hormone	Acromegaly
Oral contraceptive pill (the mechanism is unclear)	

Investigations
UREA AND ELECTROLYTES show a low serum potassium and normal or high sodium.

THE DIAGNOSIS is made by demonstrating increased plasma aldosterone levels, that are not suppressed with saline infusion (300 mmol over 4 h) or fludrocortisone (a mineralocorticoid), associated with suppressed plasma renin levels.

Antihypertensives, except bethanidine and prazosin, interfere with renin activity and should be stopped before these investigations.

CT OR MAGNETIC RESONANCE IMAGING of the adrenals is used to differentiate adenomas from hyperplasia.

Management
An adenoma is removed surgically. Hypertension resulting from hyperplasia is treated with the aldosterone antagonist – spironolactone.

Phaeochromocytoma

This is a rare (0.1% of hypertension) catecholamine-producing tumour (90% benign) of the sympathetic nervous system. Ninety per cent occur in the adrenal medulla. Some are associated with multiple endocrine neoplasia (page 420).

Clinical features
Symptoms may be episodic and include headache, palpitations, sweating, anxiety, nausea and weight loss. The

signs, which may also be intermittent, include hypertension, tachycardia and pallor. There may be hyperglycaemia.

Investigations

A 24-hour urine collection for urinary metanephrines (degradation products of adrenaline) is a useful screening test. Raised levels of plasma catecholamines confirm the diagnosis. The tumour is then localized by CT and scintigraphy using *meta*-[^{131}I]iodobenzylguanidine (MIBG) which is selectively taken up by adrenergic cells.

Management

The treatment of choice is surgical excision of the tumour under α- and β-blockade using phenoxybenzamine and pro-pranolol which is started before the operation. These drugs can also be used long term where operation is not possible.

Multiple endocrine neoplasia

This is the name given to the synchronous or metachronous (occurring at different times) occurrence of tumours involving a number of endocrine glands (Table 12.15). They are inherited in an autosomal dominant manner. Management involves surgical excision of the tumours if possible and biochemical screening of first- and second-degree relatives.

Table 12.15 Multiple endocrine neoplasia (MEN) syndrome

Organ	Clinical features
TYPE 1	
Parathyroid	Hypercalcaemia
Pituitary	Prolactinoma, acromegaly, Cushing's syndrome
Pancreas	Insulinoma, gastrinoma, VIPoma, glucagonoma
Adrenal	Non-functioning adenomas
Thyroid	Multiple or single adenomas
TYPE 2a	
Adrenal	Phaeochromocytoma, Cushing's syndrome
Thyroid	Medullary carcinoma producing calcitonin
Parathyroid	Hypercalcaemia
TYPE 2b	
Type 2a with marfanoid phenotype and intestinal and visceral ganglioneuromas	
Neuromas are also present around the lips and tongue	

VIP, vasoactive intestinal polypeptide.

Hypothermia

Hypothermia is defined as a drop in core (i.e. rectal) temperature to below 35°C. It is frequently fatal when the temperature falls below 32°C.

Aetiology

Very young and elderly individuals are particulary prone to

hypothermia, the latter having a decreased ability to feel the cold. Hypnotics, alcohol or intercurrent illness may contribute. In healthy individuals, prolonged exposure to extremes of temperature or prolonged immersion in cold water are the most common underlying causes.

Clinical features

Mild hypothermia (32–35°C) causes shivering and a feeling of intense cold. More severe hypothermia leads progressively to altered consciousness and coma. This is usually associated with a fall in pulse rate and blood pressure, muscle stiffness and depressed reflexes. As coma ensues, the pupillary and other brain-stem reflexes are lost. Ventricular arrhythmias or asystole is the usual cause of death.

Diagnosis

Measurement of core temperature with a low reading thermometer makes the diagnosis. Alteration in consciousness usually indicates a core temperature of below 32°C: this is a medical emergency. 'J' waves (deflections at the junction of the QRS complex and ST segment) may be seen in severe hypothermia.

Management

The principles of treatment are to rewarm the patient gradually while correcting metabolic abnormalities and treating cardiac arrythmias. Hypothyroidism should always be looked for. In mild to moderate hypothermia (temperature > 32°C), rewarming can be achieved by placing the patient in a warm room, using 'space blankets' and giving warm fluids orally. With more severe hypothermia, warmed intravenous fluids can be given, and direct surface heat from, for example, an electric blanket can be used. If hypothyroidism if suspected, it should be treated with intravenous triiodothyronine.

FINAL MEDICINE EXAMINATION: ENDOCRINOLOGY

1. What are the clinical features of thyrotoxicosis? State the drugs available for treatment and their major side effects.

2. Describe briefly the principal common features of Graves' disease. Discuss briefly three methods of treatment.

3. What are the clinical features of myxoedema? How would you confirm or refute the diagnosis?

4. An 85-year-old lady is found lying on the floor of her unheated flat; hypothermia is suspected:
   (a) How would you confirm the diagnosis?

(b) What abnormality might there be on ECG?

(c) What would be your management? What measures would you avoid?

5. How would you establish a diagnosis of Cushing's syndrome? Indicate how you would determine the cause.

ANSWERS

1. The clinical features of thyrotoxicosis are listed on page 407. The drugs available for treatment are:

   - Carbimazole is most often used in the UK.
   - Methimazole, the active metabolite of carbimazole, is used in the USA.
   - Propylthiouracil is occasionally used.

   Side effects of all these drugs are rash, nausea, vomiting and agranulocytosis. Patients should be warned to report infection, e.g. sore throat, so that a white cell count can be done. β-Blockers are used for *symptomatic* relief but do not alter the course of the disease.

2. The features of Graves' disease are listed on page 406. In addition to symptoms and signs resulting from hyperthyroidism there are important eye signs (page 409). The three treatment options are drugs, radioactive iodine or surgery and these are discussed on page 406.

3. The symptoms and signs of myxoedema are listed on page 404. Almost all cases of hypothyroidism are the result of disease of the thyroid gland; much less commonly it is caused by hypothalamic–pituitary disease. In primary hypothyroidism measurement of serum TSH (which will be high because of loss of feedback inhibition of secretion by T_4) and free T_4 (which will be low) will confirm the diagnosis.

4. The diagnosis and management of hypothermia is discussed on page 421. Hypothermia is diagnosed when the core (rectal) temperature is < 35°C measured with a low reading rectal thermometer. The ECG abnormalities are 'J' waves (pathognomic of hypothermia), a tachycardia with a bradycardia developing at temperatures < 32°C. At very low temperatures there may be ventricular arrhythmias. The treatment is described on page 421. Alcohol must be avoided because it may cause confusion, lead to vasodilatation (and heat loss) and precipitate hypoglycaemia.

5. This question is discussed on page 413.

CHAPTER 13

Diabetes Mellitus and other Disorders of Metabolism

DIABETES MELLITUS

During a meal insulin is released from the beta (β) cells of the pancreatic islets and is the key hormone that facilitates the storage of nutrients in the form of glycogen in liver and muscle, and triglyceride in fat. [CM p. 829]

Diabetes mellitus is a group of metabolic disorders characterized by chronic hyperglycaemia resulting from relative insulin deficiency, insulin resistance or both. Diabetes is usually primary but may be secondary to other conditions which include pancreatic (e.g. total pancreatectomy, chronic pancreatitis, haemochromatosis) and endocrine diseases (e.g. acromegaly and Cushing's disease). It may also be drug induced, most commonly by thiazide diuretics and corticosteroids.

Primary diabetes is divided into insulin-dependent diabetes mellitus (IDDM, type 1 diabetes) and non-insulin-dependent diabetes (NIDDM, type 2 diabetes). In clinical terms these represent two ends of a spectrum (Table 13.1).

Table 13.1 The spectrum of diabetes: a comparison of insulin-dependent diabetes mellitus and non-insulin-dependent diabetes

	IDDM (type 1)	NIDDM (type 2)
Epidemiology	Patients are: Younger, incidence maximal at 10–13 years of age	Patients are: Older, diagnosis usually made after 40 years of age
	Usually lean	Often overweight
	European extraction	All racial groups
Inheritance HLA system	HLA-DR3 or -DR4 in > 90% of patients. (40% in general population)	No HLA links
Risk to identical twin (%)	30–35	> 90
Aetiology	Autoimmune Viral?	No evidence of immune disturbance or viral aetiology
Clinical	Complete insulin deficiency May develop ketoacidosis	Partial insulin deficiency May develop non-ketotic hyperosmolar state
	Always need insulin	Sometimes need insulin

Aetiology and pathogenesis [CM p. 833]

NON-INSULIN-DEPENDENT DIABETES MELLITUS

Studies of identical twins with NIDDM have shown that the disease has a strong genetic basis, but the genetic defects responsible for most cases have yet to be identified. The β-cell mass is reduced to about 50% of normal. Hyperglycaemia is the result of reduced insulin secretion (inappropriately low for the glucose level) and peripheral insulin resistance.

INSULIN-DEPENDENT DIABETES MELLITUS

The genetic contribution to type 1 diabetes is less than to type 2 and non-genetic factors, probably environmental, are involved. Several pieces of evidence suggest that autoimmune processes are important in the pathogenesis of IDDM and it is possible that a viral infection may trigger an autoimmune destructive process in those genetically predisposed. Diabetes presents clinically when almost all the islets have been destroyed. Antibodies directed against islet cell cytoplasmic antigens (e.g. glutamic acid decarboxylase) and insulin have been described.

Clinical features

Diabetes may present:

- With symptoms
- With complications (see later)
- In asymptomatic individuals diagnosed at routine medical examinations, e.g. for insurance purposes

The symptoms of diabetes are thirst, polyuria, weight loss and lethargy. Polyuria is the result of an osmotic diuresis that results when blood glucose levels exceed the renal tubular reabsorptive capacity (the renal threshold). Fluid and electrolyte losses stimulate thirst. Weight loss is caused by fluid depletion and breakdown of fat and muscle as a result of insulin deficiency. In young patients the history is usually brief (2–4 weeks) and ketoacidosis (see later) is the presenting feature if these early symptoms are not recognized and treated.

Older patients may present with the same symptoms, although less marked and extending over several months.

Investigations

The diagnosis is made by demonstrating:

- Fasting venous blood glucose ≥ 6.7 mmol/l or
- Random blood glucose ≥ 10 mmol/l

If fasting glucose is < 5.5 mmol/l or random glucose is < 7.8 mmol/l, diabetes is an unlikely diagnosis. A glucose tolerance test is only necessary where uncertainty exists (Figure 13.1).

	Fasting blood glucose (mmol/l)	2-hour blood glucose (mmol/l)
Normal	<6.7	<6.7
Diabetes	≥6.7	≥10
Impaired glucose tolerance	<6.7	6.7 – 10

Figure 13.1 The oral glucose tolerance test. After an overnight fast 75 g glucose is taken in 300 ml water. Blood samples are taken in the fasting state and 2 hours after the glucose has been given. Impaired glucose tolerance is linked to a propensity to atheroma and some patients (2–4% yearly) go on to develop diabetes.

Other routine investigations include stix testing the urine for proteinuria (page 217), full blood count, serum urea and electrolytes, and a fasting blood sample for cholesterol and triglyceride levels.

Management
The aims of treatment are to alleviate symptoms of hyperglycaemia and to achieve the best possible control of diabetes, with blood glucose concentrations maintained as near normal as possible to minimize long-term complications. Management is a multidisciplinary approach involving, among others, the hospital doctor, the general practitioner, community nurse and dietician.

PRINCIPLES OF TREATMENT. All patients with diabetes require diet therapy. Insulin is always indicated in a patient who presents in ketoacidosis and is usually indicated in patients under 40 years of age. Insulin is also indicated in other patients who do not achieve satisfactory control with oral hypoglycaemics.

- DIET. In older patients, the first approach is by diet alone. The diet is no different from the normal healthy diet recommended for the rest of the population. Fat should be reduced to 30–35% of total energy intake and consist mainly of unsaturated fats. Protein should be 10–15% and carbohydrate 50% of total energy intake. Patients should eat complex carbohydrates (e.g. potato, pasta) which are absorbed relatively slowly from the gastrointestinal tract, thus preventing the rapid fluctuations in blood glucose that occur when simple sugars, such as sucrose or glucose, are eaten. The nutrient load should be spread throughout the day (three main meals with snacks in between times and at bedtime) which reduces swings in blood glucose

- ORAL HYPOGLYCAEMICS. These are used in association with dietary treatment when this alone has failed to control hyperglycaemia

Sulphonylureas increase insulin secretion from pancreatic β-cells and reduce peripheral resistance to insulin action. Glibenclamide (2.5–20 mg daily in one or two divided doses) is the most popular choice but is best avoided in elderly people and in those with renal failure because of its relatively long duration of action (12–20 hours) and renal excretion. Tolbutamide, which is shorter acting and metabolized by the liver, is a better choice in these patient groups. The most common side effect of this group of drugs is hypoglycaemia.

Biguanides. Metformin, the only available biguanide, reduces glucose absorption from the gut and increases insulin sensitivity. It is used in combination with sulphonylureas when a single agent has failed to control diabetes. It may also be used as a first-line agent in very obese diabetic individuals because, unlike sulphonylureas, appetite is not increased. Side effects include anorexia and diarrhoea. Lactic acidosis has occurred in patients with severe hepatic or renal disease in whom its use is contraindicated.

INSULIN

Insulin of three species is available: porcine insulin, beef insulin and human insulin. Most patients receive human insulin which is manufactured biosynthetically using recombinant DNA technology.

There are two main types of insulin:

- Insulins prepared in a clear solution (soluble or crystalline). These insulins have a rapid onset of action (within 15–60 minutes), are short acting (4–6 hours) and are the only insulins to be used in emergencies such as ketoacidosis or for surgical operations.

- Insulins premixed with retarding agents (either protamine or zinc) that precipitate crystals of varying size according to the conditions employed. These insulins are intermediate (12–24 hours) or long acting (more than 24 hours). The protamine insulins are also known as isophane or NPH insulins, and the zinc insulins as lente insulins.

In young patients a reasonable starting regimen is subcutaneous injection of an intermediate-acting insulin, 8–10 units administered half an hour before breakfast and before the evening meal. In many patients who present with acute diabetes there is some recovery of endogenous insulin secretion soon after diagnosis ('the honeymoon period') and the insulin dose may need to be reduced. Requirements rise thereafter and a multiple injection regimen (often using a 'pen injector' device), which may improve control and allows greater meal flexibility, is then appropriate for most younger patients. An example of this is soluble insulin administered before each meal and a long-acting insulin given at bedtime. An alternative is to use a small pump strapped to the waist which delivers a continuous subcutaneous insulin infusion (CSII). Meal-time doses are delivered when the patient presses a button on the side of the pump. This should only be used under the guidance of specialized centres.

In patients with NIDDM who eventually require insulin, a twice daily regimen of premixed soluble and isophane insulin (e.g. Mixtard) is suitable in many patients.

Measuring control

Patients may feel very well and be asymptomatic even if their blood glucose is consistently above the normal range. Self-monitoring at home is therefore necessary because of the immediate risks of hyper- and hypoglycaemia and because it has now been shown that persistently good control (i.e. near normoglycaemia) reduces the risk of progression to retinopathy, nephropathy and neuropathy in IDDM.

HOME TESTING

- Most patients, especially those on insulin, are taught to monitor control by testing finger-prick blood samples with enzyme-impregnated reagent strips which change colour according to the blood glucose level. Patients are asked to take regular profiles (e.g. four times daily samples on 2 days each week) and to note these in a diary or record book

- Urine testing for glucose (using stix) is a crude measure of glycaemic control because glycosuria only appears above the renal threshold for glucose (which varies between a blood glucose of 7 and 13 mmol/l) and because urine glucose lags behind blood glucose. It is usually reserved for the elderly patient in whom tight control is unnecessary

- Urine ketones, also measured with stix (Ketostix), is useful if the patient is unwell because ketonuria indicates potentially serious metabolic derangement

HOSPITAL TESTING

Single random blood glucose measurements, obtained at clinic visits, are of limited value.

- Glycosylated haemoglobin (HbA_{1c}) is produced by the attachment of glucose to Hb and measurement of this Hb fraction (normally 4–8%) is a useful measure of the average glucose concentration over the life of the Hb molecule (approximately 6 weeks)

- Glycosylated plasma proteins (fructosamine) are less reliable than HbA_{1c} but may be useful in certain situations, e.g. thalassaemia where haemoglobin is abnormal

DIABETIC METABOLIC EMERGENCIES

Hypoglycaemia (blood glucose < 2.2 mmol/l)

This is the most common complication of insulin treatment and may also occur in patients taking sulphonylureas.

Clinical features

Increased sympathetic activity causes hunger, sweating, pallor and tachycardia. Hours later there is personality change, fits, occasionally hemiparesis and finally coma. In patients with long-standing diabetes and autonomic neuropathy the early 'adrenergic features' may be absent.

Investigations

Immediate diagnosis and treatment are essential. A blood glucose confirms the diagnosis but treatment should begin immediately (while waiting for the result) if hypoglycaemia is suspected on clinical grounds.

Management

A rapidly absorbed carbohydrate, e.g. sugary water, should be given orally if possible. In unconscious patients, treatment is with intravenous glucose (50 ml of 50% dextrose) or intramuscular glucagon (1 mg) which acts rapidly by mobilizing hepatic glycogen and is particularly useful where intravenous access is difficult.

Diabetic ketoacidosis

Diabetic ketoacidosis results from insulin deficiency and is the result of previously undiagnosed diabetes, the stress of intercurrent illness (e.g. infection or surgery) or interruption of insulin therapy. A common error is for insulin to be reduced or stopped if the patient is ill and feels unable to eat. Insulin should never be stopped and most patients in fact need a larger dose when ill.

Pathogenesis

Ketoacidosis is a state of uncontrolled catabolism associated with insulin deficiency. In the absence of insulin there is an unrestrained increase in hepatic gluconeogenesis. High circulating glucose levels result in an osmotic diuresis by the kidneys and consequent dehydration. In addition peripheral lipolysis leads to an increase in circulating free fatty acids which are converted within the liver to acidic ketones leading to a metabolic acidosis. These processes are accelerated by the 'stress hormones': catecholamines, glucagon and cortisol; these are secreted in response to dehydration and intercurrent illness.

Clinical features

There is profound dehydration secondary to water and electrolyte loss from the kidney. The eyes are sunken, tissue turgor is reduced, the tongue is dry and, in severe cases, the blood pressure is low. Kussmaul's respiration (deep rapid breathing) may be present, as a sign of respiratory compensation for metabolic acidosis, and the breath smells of ketones. Some disturbance of consciousness is common but only 5% present in coma. Body temperature is often subnormal despite intercurrent infection.

Investigations

The diagnosis is based on demonstration of hyperglycaemia in combination with acidosis and ketosis.

BLOOD GLUCOSE shows significant hyperglycaemia, usually > 20 mmol/l.

PLASMA KETONES are easily detected by centrifuging a blood sample and testing the plasma obtained with Ketostix which will usually show ++ or +++.

URINE STIX TESTING shows heavy glycosuria and ketonuria.

ARTERIAL BLOOD GASES show a metabolic acidosis.

SERUM UREA AND ELECTROLYTES. Urea and creatinine are often raised through dehydration. The total body potassium is low as a result of osmotic diuresis, but the serum potassium concentration is often raised because of the absence of the action of insulin, which allows potassium to shift out of cells.

FULL BLOOD COUNT may show an elevated white cell count even in the absence of infection.

FURTHER INVESTIGATIONS are directed towards identifying a precipitating cause: blood cultures, chest radiograph and urine microscopy and culture to look for evidence of infection and an ECG to look for evidence of myocardial infarction.

Management

The aims of treatment are to replace fluid and electrolyte loss (Table 13.2), replace insulin and restore acid–base balance. A treatment regimen for a patient with severe ketoacidosis is set out below.

Table 13.2 Average loss of fluid and electrolytes in an adult with ketoacidosis

Water	6 litres
Sodium	500 mmol
Potassium	400 mmol

- FLUID: physiological saline 0.9%, 2 litres in 1.5 hours, then 1 litre in 2 hours, then 1 litre in 4 hours, then 1 litre in 6 hours
- POTASSIUM: serum potassium falls rapidly with rehydration and insulin treatment. KCl 20 mmol is added to each litre

of saline. More is needed if serum potassium is low (e.g. < 3.5 mmol/l)

- INSULIN: intravenous soluble insulin 6 units immediately and 6 units hourly thereafter by infusion pump. Alternatively insulin is given by intramuscular injection 20 units stat and then 6 units hourly

- ACID–BASE BALANCE: intravenous bicarbonate 1.26% should only be given if the blood pH is less than 7.0

- SPECIAL MEASURES: infection is treated with broad-spectrum antibiotics. A urinary catheter is passed if oliguria persists 2 hours after rehydration begins. In elderly or seriously ill individuals a central venous pressure line may be necessary to monitor fluid replacement accurately. Coma necessitates standard care of the unconscious patient (page 462). It is essential to pass a nasogastric tube to prevent aspiration and the rare but fatal complication of acute gastric dilatation

- MONITOR: blood glucose hourly and serum electrolytes 2-hourly. The pulse, blood pressure, temperature and respiratory rate are measured hourly. Admission to the intensive care unit is necessary in the seriously ill

- SUBSEQUENT MANAGEMENT: once blood glucose falls to 10–12 mmol/l the infusion fluid is changed to 5% dextrose plus 20 mmol KCl, 1 litre 6-hourly. Insulin is continued at 3 units hourly. This is continued until the patient is able to take adequate food and fluid by mouth, when preprandial subcutaneous soluble insulin is given until a maintenance regimen is started

Non-ketotic hyperosmolar state

This condition, in which severe hyperglycaemia develops without significant ketosis, is the metabolic emergency characteristic of uncontrolled NIDDM.

Table 13.3 The main biochemical differences between diabetic ketoacidosis and non-ketotic hyperosmolar coma

Examples of blood values	Severe keto-acidosis	Non-ketotic hyperosmolar coma
Serum Na^+ (mmol/l)	140	155
Serum urea (mmol/l)	8	15
Blood glucose (mmol/l)	30	50
Serum osmolality (mosmol/kg)*	328	385
Arterial pH	7.0	7.35

* See pages 199–200 for definition and discussion of plasma osmolality.

Clinical features
Endogenous insulin levels are reduced, but are still sufficient to inhibit hepatic ketogenesis, whereas glucose production is unrestrained. Patients present with profound dehydration (secondary to an osmotic diuresis) and a decreased level of consciousness which is directly related to the elevation of plasma osmolality. The main biochemical differences between ketoacidosis and hyperosmolar coma are illustrated in Table 13.3.

Management
This is exactly the same as that for ketoacidosis, except that 0.45% (half physiological) saline is given if the serum sodium is more than 170 mmol/l and a lower rate of insulin infusion (3 U/h) is often sufficient as these patients are extremely sensitive to insulin. The hyperosmolar state predisposes to thrombosis and prophylactic subcutaneous heparin is given.

Prognosis
Mortality rate is around 20–30%, mainly because of the advanced age of the patients and the frequency of intercurrent illness. Unlike ketoacidosis, non-ketotic hyperglycaemia is not an absolute indication for subsequent insulin therapy, and survivors may do well on diet and oral agents.

Lactic acidosis

Lactic acidosis is a rare complication in patients taking metformin. Patients present with severe metabolic acidosis without significant hyperglycaemia or ketosis. Treatment is with rehydration and intravenous bicarbonate.

COMPLICATIONS OF DIABETES

Patients with diabetes have a reduced life expectancy. Insulin-treated patients diagnosed before the age of 20 years have only a 60–70% chance of living past the age of 45 years. The excess deaths are mainly the result of diabetic nephropathy. Heart disease, peripheral vascular disease and stroke are the major causes of death in patients over the age of 50 years.

Vascular

Macrovascular complications
Diabetes is a risk factor for atherosclerosis and this is additive with other risk factors for large vessel disease, e.g. smoking, hypertension and hyperlipidaemia. Atherosclerosis results in stroke, ischaemic heart disease and gangrene of the feet.

Microvascular complications

Small vessels throughout the body are affected but the disease process is of particular danger in three sites: the retina, the renal glomerulus and the nerve sheath. Diabetic retinopathy, nephropathy and neuropathy tend to manifest 10–20 years after diagnosis in young patients. They present earlier in older patients, probably because these have had unrecognized diabetes for months or even years before diagnosis.

Diabetic eye disease

BACKGROUND RETINOPATHY is the earliest feature of retinopathy. Capillary microaneurysms appear as tiny red dots, haemorrhages are seen as larger red spots (blot haemorrhages) and capillary leaks of fluid rich in lipid and protein give rise to hard exudates (yellow–white discrete patches). There is no specific treatment for background retinopathy, but patients should undergo regular specialist examination to look for any deterioration. Background retinopathy does not itself constitute a threat to vision but may progress to two other distinct forms of retinopathy: maculopathy or proliferative retinopathy. Both are the consequence of damage to retinal blood vessels and resultant retinal ischaemia.

MACULOPATHY. Macular oedema is the first feature of maculopathy and will result in permanent damage if not treated early. It cannot be detected by standard ophthalmoscopy and the only sign may be deteriorating visual acuity detected by Snellen chart testing. At a later stage there are perimacular haemorrhages and hard exudates.

PRE-PROLIFERATIVE RETINOPATHY is characterized by 'cottonwool spots' which are indistinct pale lesions and represent oedema from retinal infarcts. Venous beading and/or venous loops are other pre-proliferative changes.

PROLIFERATIVE RETINOPATHY. Hypoxia is thought to be the signal for new vessel formation. These are fragile and bleed easily, resulting in loss of vision because of vitreous haemorrhage. Fibrous tissue associated with new vessels may shrink and cause retinal detachment.

Maculopathy and proliferative retinopathy are treated by laser photocoagulation of the retina. Effective early therapy of proliferative retinopathy reduces the risk of visual loss by about 50%.

Other eye complications of diabetes are blurred vision (caused by reversible osmotic changes in the lens in patients with acute hyperglycaemia), cataracts, glaucoma and external ocular palsies.

The diabetic kidney

The kidney may be damaged by diabetes as a result of glomerular disease, ischaemic renal lesions and ascending urinary tract infection.

DIABETIC GLOMERULOSCLEROSIS. Nephropathy secondary to glomerular disease affects 30–40% of patients who are diagnosed before the age of 30 years. On histological investigation there is thickening of the glomerular basement membrane and later glomerulosclerosis which may be diffuse form or nodular form (Kimmelstiel–Wilson lesion). The earliest evidence of glomerular damage is 'microalbuminuria' (defined as an increase above the normal range in urinary albumin excretion but undetectable by stix) which in turn may, after some years, progress to intermittent albuminuria followed by persistent proteinuria, sometimes with a frank nephrotic syndrome. At the stage of persistent proteinuria, the plasma creatinine is normal but the average patient is only some 8–10 years from end-stage renal failure.

The urine of all patients should be checked regularly by stix for the presence of protein. Many centres also screen for microalbuminuria, because meticulous glycaemic control and early antihypertensive treatment at this stage may delay the onset of frank proteinuria. Aggressive control of blood pressure is the most important factor to reduce disease progression in those with established proteinuria; angiotensin-converting enzyme (ACE) inhibitors are the treatment of choice. Many will develop end-stage renal failure and need dialysis and eventually renal transplantation.

ISCHAEMIC LESIONS. Arteriolar lesions with hypertrophy and hyalinization of the vessels affect both afferent and efferent arterioles. The appearances are similar to those of hypertensive disease but are not necessarily related to the blood pressure in patients with diabetes.

INFECTIVE LESIONS. Urinary tract infections are common (page 228). A rare complication is renal papillary necrosis in which renal papillae are shed in the urine and may cause ureteral obstruction.

Diabetic neuropathy (Table 13.4)

Diabetic neuropathy is thought to result from nerve ischaemia or accumulation of fructose and sorbitol (metabolized from glucose in peripheral nerves) which disrupts function and structure of the nerve.

SYMMETRICAL SENSORY NEUROPATHY. This is the most common form of neuropathy and first affects the most distal parts of the longest nerves, i.e. the toes and soles of the feet. Symptoms consist of numbness, tingling and pain which is typically worse at night. Involvement of the hands is less common and results in a 'stocking and glove' sensory loss. Complications include unrecognized trauma, beginning as blistering as a result of an ill-fitting shoe or hot water bottle, and leading to ulceration. Abnormal mechanical stress and repeated minor trauma, usually prevented by pain, may lead to the development of a neuropathic arthropathy (Charcot's joints) in the ankle and knee where the joint is grossly deformed and swollen.

Table 13.4 Diabetic neuropathies

Progressive	Symmetrical sensory polyneuropathy (distal)
	Autonomic neuropathy
Reversible	Acute painful neuropathy
	Mononeuropathy and multiple mononeuropathies
	Cranial nerve lesions
	Isolated peripheral nerve lesions
	Diabetic amyotrophy

AUTONOMIC NEUROPATHY may present with impotence (page 397), postural hypotension, diarrhoea, and nausea and vomiting as a consequence of gastroparesis. In addition bladder involvement may result in a neuropathic bladder with painless urinary retention.

ACUTE PAINFUL NEUROPATHY. The patient describes burning or crawling pains in the lower limbs. These symptoms are typically worse at night, and pressure from bedclothes may be intolerable. There is usually a good response to improved glycaemic control.

DIABETIC MONONEUROPATHY. Individual nerves are affected. In some instances, this relates to local pressure, e.g. carpal tunnel syndrome. In others it results from a localized nerve infarction; commonly the third and sixth cranial nerves are affected resulting in diplopia (page 453). More than one nerve may be affected – *mononeuritis multiplex*.

DIABETIC AMYOTROPHY (PROXIMAL MOTOR NEUROPATHY). This presents with painful wasting, usually asymmetrical, of the quadriceps muscles. The wasting may be very marked and knee reflexes are diminished or absent.

Infections

Poorly controlled diabetes impairs function of polymorpho-nuclear leukocytes and confers an increased risk of infection particularly of the urinary tract and skin, e.g. cellulitis, boils and abscesses. Tuberculosis and mucocutaneous candidiasis are more common in diabetic individuals. Infections may lead to loss of glycaemic control and are a common cause of ketoacidosis. Insulin-treated patients may need to increase their insulin therapy even if they feel nauseated and unable to eat. Non-insulin-treated patients may need insulin for the same reasons.

The skin

Lipohypertrophy is where fat lumps develop at frequently used insulin injection sites and may be avoided by varying the injection site from day to day. Necrobiosis lipoidica diabeticorum is an unusual complication of diabetes, characterized by erythematous plaques, often over the shins, which gradually develop a brown waxy discoloration. Other skin lesions are vitiligo (symmetrical white patches seen in organ-specific autoimmune diseases) and granuloma annulare which presents as flesh-coloured rings and nodules, principally over the extensor surfaces of the fingers.

SPECIAL SITUATIONS

Surgery

Smooth control of diabetes minimizes the risk of infection and balances the catabolic response to anaesthesia and surgery. If possible diabetic patients should be first on the operating list. In insulin-treated patients, longer-acting insulins are stopped the day before surgery and substituted with soluble insulin. During surgery an infusion of 5% glucose/insulin/potassium is given and glucose levels checked hourly. This is maintained postoperatively until the patient is able to eat normally.

Non-insulin-treated patients must stop oral hypoglycaemics 2 days before major surgery. The intravenous regimen, described above, is only necessary in patients with a high blood glucose on the morning of surgery.

Pregnancy and diabetes

Poorly controlled diabetes is associated with congenital malformations, macrosomia (large babies), hydramnios, pre-eclampsia and intrauterine death. In the neonatal period there is an increased risk of hyaline membrane disease and neonatal hypoglycaemia (unlike insulin, maternal glucose crosses the placenta and causes hypersecretion of insulin from the fetal islets which continues when the umbilical cord is cut). Meticulous control of blood glucose levels achieves results comparable to those with non-diabetic pregnancies.

Gestational diabetes refers to diabetes that develops in the course of pregnancy and remits following delivery. Treatment is with diet in the first instance, but most patients require insulin cover during pregnancy. It is likely to recur in subsequent pregnancies and non-insulin-dependent diabetes may develop later in life.

Brittle diabetes

There is no precise definition for this term, which is used to describe patients with recurrent ketoacidosis and/or recurrent hypoglycaemic coma. Of these, the largest group is made up of those who experience recurrent severe hypoglycaemia.

HYPOGLYCAEMIA

The causes and mechanism of hypoglycaemia are listed in Table 13.5. Insulin or sulphonylurea therapy for diabetes accounts for the vast majority of cases of severe hypoglycaemia encountered in an accident and emergency department.

Table 13.5 Causes of hypoglycaemia

	Mechanism of hypoglycaemia
Drug induced: insulin, sulphonylureas, quinine, pentamidine and salicylates in overdose	Variety of mechanisms
Islet cell tumour of the pancreas (insulinoma)	Inappropriately high circulating insulin levels
Non-pancreatic tumours, e.g. sarcoma, hepatoma	Secretion of IGF-1 by some tumours
Endocrine causes: ACTH deficiency, Addison's disease	Impaired counterregulation to the action of insulin
Fulminant liver failure	Failure of hepatic gluconeogenesis
End-stage renal failure	Failure of renal cortical gluconeogenesis
Excess alcohol	Enhanced insulin response to carbohydrate Inhibition of hepatic gluconeogenesis by alcohol
After gastric surgery	Rapid gastric emptying and mismatching of food and insulin
Factitious hypoglycaemia	Surreptitious self-administration of insulin or sulphonylureas often in a non-diabetic

Insulinomas

These are pancreatic islet cell tumours (usually benign) that secrete insulin. They may be part of the multiple endocrine neoplasia syndrome (page 420).

Clinical features

The classic presentation is with fasting hypoglycaemia. Hypoglycaemia produces symptoms as a result of neuroglycopenia and stimulation of the sympathetic nervous system. These include, sweating, palpitations, diplopia and weakness, progressing to confusion, abnormal behaviour, fits and coma.

Investigations

The diagnosis is made by demonstrating hypoglycaemia in association with inappropriate and excessive insulin secretion:

- Measurement of overnight fasting glucose and plasma insulin levels on three occasions

- Performing a prolonged 72-h supervised fast if overnight testing is inconclusive and symptoms persist

Further investigations are used to localize the tumour before surgery and include CT, angiography and venous sampling (measurement of insulin in blood sampled from different levels of the pancreatic vein).

Treatment

The treatment of choice is surgical excision of the tumour. Diazoxide which inhibits insulin release from islet cells is useful when the tumour is malignant, in patients in whom a tumour is very small and cannot be located, or in elderly patients with mild symptoms.

DISORDERS OF LIPID METABOLISM

[CM p. 854]

Fats are transported in the blood stream as lipoprotein particles composed of lipids (principally triglycerides, cholesterol and cholesterol esters), phospholipids and proteins, called apoproteins. These proteins exert a stabilizing function and allow the particles to be recognized by receptors in the liver and peripheral tissues.

Five principal types of lipoprotein particles exist.

CHYLOMICRONS are synthesized in the small intestine and serve to transport *exogenous* dietary fat (mainly triglycerides, small amounts of cholesterol) to the liver and peripheral tissues.

VERY-LOW-DENSITY LIPOPROTEINS (VLDLs) are synthesized and secreted by the liver and transport *endogenous* triglycerides (formed in the liver from plasma free fatty acids) to the periphery. In fat and muscle, triglycerides are removed from chylomicrons and VLDLs by the tissue enzyme lipoprotein lipase and the essential cofactor apoprotein C-II.

INTERMEDIATE-DENSITY LIPOPROTEINS (IDLs), derived from the peripheral breakdown of VLDLs, are transported back to the liver and metabolized to yield the cholesterol rich particles – low-density-lipoproteins (LDLs).

LOW-DENSITY LIPOPROTEINS (LDLs) deliver most cholesterol to the periphery and liver by binding to LDL receptors in these tissues.

HIGH-DENSITY LIPOPROTEINS (HDLs) transport cholesterol from peripheral tissues to the liver. HDL particles carry 20–30% of the total quantity of cholesterol in the blood.

The major clinical significance of hypercholesterolaemia (both total plasma and LDL concentration) is as a risk factor for atheroma and hence ischaemic heart disease. The risk is greatest in those with other risk factors, e.g. smoking. There is a weak independent link between raised concentrations of (triglyceride-rich) VLDL particles and cardiovascular risk. In addition, severe hypertriglyceridaemia may induce acute pancreatitis. In contrast, HDL particles, which transport cholesterol away from the periphery, appear to protect against atheroma.

Measurement of plasma lipids

Most patients with hyperlipidaemia are asymptomatic, with no clinical signs, and they are discovered through routine screening. A single fasting blood sample is necessary for measurement of total plasma cholesterol, total triglyceride and HDL cholesterol levels. Specific diagnosis of the defect (see below) requires measurement of individual lipoproteins by electrophoresis but this is not usually necessary. If a lipid disorder has been detected, it is vital to carry out a clinical history, examination and simple special investigations (i.e. blood glucose, urea and electrolytes, liver biochemistry and thyroid function tests) to detect causes of secondary hyperlipidaemia (Table 13.6).

Table 13.6 Causes of secondary hyperlipidaemia

Hypothyroidism
Poorly controlled diabetes mellitus
Alcohol
Obesity
Renal impairment
Nephrotic syndrome
Dysglobulinaemia
Hepatic dysfunction
Drugs: oral contraceptives in susceptible individuals, thiazide diuretics, corticosteroids

The primary hyperlipidaemias

Hypertriglyceridaemia alone

- POLYGENIC HYPERTRIGLYCERIDAEMIA accounts for most cases, in which there are many genes acting together, and interacting with environmental factors, to produce a modest elevation in serum triglyceride levels

- FAMILIAL HYPERTRIGLYCERIDAEMIA is inherited in an autosomal dominant fashion. The exact defect is not known and the only clinical feature is a history of pancreatitis or retinal vein thrombosis in some individuals

- LIPOPROTEIN LIPASE DEFICIENCY and APOPROTEIN C-II DEFICIENCY are rare diseases which usually present in childhood with severe hypertriglyceridaemia complicated by pancreatitis, retinal vein thrombosis and eruptive xanthomas – crops of small yellow lipid deposits in the skin

Hypercholesterolaemia alone

- FAMILIAL HYPERCHOLESTEROLAEMIA is the result of underproduction of the LDL cholesterol receptor in the liver which results in high plasma concentrations of LDL cholesterol. Heterozygotes may be asymptomatic or develop coronary artery disease in their forties. Typical clinical features include tendon xanthomas (lipid nodules in the tendons, especially extensor tendons of hands and Achilles tendon) and xanthelasmas. Homozygotes have a total absence of LDL receptors in the liver. They have grossly elevated plasma cholesterol levels (> 16 mmol/l) and, without treatment, die in their teens from coronary artery disease

- POLYGENIC HYPERCHOLESTEROLAEMIA accounts for those patients with a modest elevation in cholesterol who do not have familial hypercholesterolaemia. The precise nature of the polygenic variation in plasma cholesterol remains unknown

Combined hyperlipidaemia (hypercholesterolaemia and hyperlipidaemia)

POLYGENIC COMBINED HYPERLIPIDAEMIA and FAMILIAL COMBINED HYPERLIPIDAEMIA account for the vast majority of patients in this group. A small minority are the result of the rare condition, *remnant hyperlipidaemia.*

Management of hyperlipidaemia

The aim of treatment is to reduce serum cholesterol to at least < 6.5 mmol/l which is the upper limit of the normal range. A serum triglyceride concentration below 2.0 mmol/l is normal. In the range 2.0–6.0 mmol/l no specific intervention will be needed, unless there are other cardiovascular risk factors, particularly hypercholesterolaemia, when the aim is to reduce serum triglycerides into the normal range.

GUIDELINES TO THERAPY

The initial treatment in all cases of hyperlipidaemia is dietary modification. Patients with familial hypercholesterolaemia will probably need drug treatment. Secondary hyperlipidaemia should be managed by treatment of the underlying condition wherever possible.

LIPID-LOWERING DIET

- Dairy products and meat are the principal sources of fat in the diet. Chicken and poultry should be substituted for red meats and the food grilled rather than fried. Low fat cheeses and skimmed milk should be substituted for the full fat varieties

- Polyunsaturated fats, e.g. corn and soya oil, should be used instead of saturated fats

- Reduction of cholesterol intake from liver, offal and fish roe

- Increased intake of soluble fibres, e.g. pulses and legumes, which reduce circulating cholesterol

- Avoid excess alcohol and obesity, both causes of secondary hyperlipidaemias

LIPID-LOWERING DRUGS

Table 13.7 shows the drugs used in the management of hyperlipidaemia. They may be used singly or sometimes in combination. The exact mechanism of action for some of these drugs is not known. Bile acid-binding resins (e.g. cholestyramine and colestipol) bind bile acids in the gut preventing the enterohepatic circulation. This promotes liver to convert cholesterol to bile acids. They also stimulate formation of hepatic LDL receptors which take up more cholesterol from the circulation. Hydroxymethylglutaryl-coenzyme A (HMG-CoA) reductase inhibitors, e.g. simvastatin and pravastatin, inhibit cholesterol synthesis. Side effects include hepatitis and myositis.

The fibric acid derivatives (gemfibrozil, bezafibrate) are useful drugs for all types of hyperlipidaemia.

Table 13.7 Drugs used in the management of hyperlipidaemias (listed in the order that they are usually selected for treatment)

Hypertriglyceridaemia	Hypercholesterolaemia	Combined
Fibric acid derivatives	HMG-CoA reductase inhibitors	Fibric acid derivatives
Nicotinic acid	Fibric acid derivatives	Nicotinic acid
Fish oil capsules (ω-3 marine triglycerides)	Bile acid-binding resins	

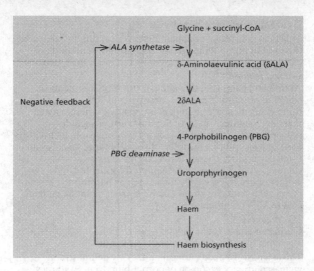

Figure 13.2 Pathways in porphyrin metabolism.

THE PORPHYRIAS

The porphyrias are a rare group of inherited heterogeneous disorders resulting from abnormalities of a number of enzymes involved in the biosynthesis of haem. This leads to an overproduction of the intermediate compounds called porphyrins (Figure 13.2).

In porphyrias the excess production of porphyrins occurs within the liver (hepatic porphyria) or in the bone marrow (erythropoietic porphyria) but porphyrias can also be classified in terms of clinical presentation as acute or non-acute (Table 13.8). Acute porphyrias usually produce neuropsychiatric problems and are associated with excess production and urinary excretion of δ-aminolaevulinic acid. These metabolites are not increased in the non-acute porphyrias.

Table 13.8 The classification of porphyrias

	Hepatic	Erythropoietic
Acute	Acute intermittent porphyria Variegate porphyria Hereditary coproporphyria	
Non-acute	Porphyria cutanea tarda	Congenital porphyria Erythropoietic protoporphyria

Acute intermittent porphyria

This is an autosomal dominant disorder caused by a defect at the level of porphobilinogen deaminase. Presentation is in early adult life, and women are affected more than men.

Clinical features

Abdominal pain, vomiting and constipation are the most common presenting features, occurring in 90% of patients (mimicking an acute abdomen, especially as there may be fever and leukocytosis). Additional features include polyneuropathy (especially motor), hypertension, tachycardia and neuropsychiatric disorder (fits, depression, anxiety and frank psychosis). The urine may turn red or brown on standing. Attacks may be precipitated by alcohol and a variety of drugs, especially those such as barbiturates which are enzyme-inducing drugs and increase δ-aminolaevulinic acid (δALA) synthetase activity.

Investigations

During an attack there may be a neutrophil leucocytosis, abnormal liver biochemistry and a raised urea.

The diagnosis is made during an attack by demonstrating increased urinary excretion of porphobilinogen. Erythrocyte porphobilinogen deaminase may be measured between attacks or, in some cases, urinary porphobilinogen remains high.

Management

This is largely supportive. A high carbohydrate intake must be maintained because this depresses δALA synthetase activity as does an intravenous haematin infusion which is used in some cases.

Other porphyrias

Variegate porphyria and hereditary coproporphyria present with features similar to those of acute intermittent porphyria, together with the cutaneous features of porphyria cutanea tarda. Porphyria cutanea tarda has a genetic predisposition and presents with a bullous eruption on exposure to light. The eruption heals with scarring. Most patients give a history of alcohol abuse.

The erythropoietic porphyrias are very rare and present with photosensitive skin lesions.

AMYLOIDOSIS

This is a heterogeneous group of disorders characterized by intracellular deposition of an insoluble fibrillar protein called amyloid. Amyloidosis is acquired or hereditary (e.g. in familial Mediterranean fever) and may be localized or systemic. Clinical features are the result of amyloid deposits affecting the normal structure and function of the affected tissue. The diagnosis of amyloidosis is made with Congo red staining of affected tissues. In systemic amyloid a simple rectal biopsy may be used for histological diagnosis. Amyloid deposits stain red and show green fluorescence in polarized light. The features of some amyloid types are shown in Table 13.9.

Table 13.9 Classification of the more common types of amyloid and amyloidosis

Type	Fibril protein precursor	Clinical syndrome
AA	Protein A, a precursor of serum amyloid A (an acute phase reactant)	Occurs with chronic infections (e.g. TB), inflammation (e.g. rheumatoid arthritis) and malignancy (e.g. Hodgkin's disease). Presents with proteinuria and hepatosplenomegaly
AL	Monoclonal immunoglobulin light chains	Associated with myeloma, Waldenström's macroglobulinaemia and non-Hodgkin's lymphoma. Presents with cardiac failure, nephrotic syndrome, carpal tunnel syndrome and macroglossia (large tongue)
Aβ	β Protein (also known as A4 protein)	Cerebral amyloid occurring in patients with Alzheimer's disease
Aβ$_2$M	β$_2$-Microglobulin	Periarticular amyloid in patients with renal failure and long-term dialysis

Inborn errors of metabolism
[CM pp. 862–865]
Most of the inborn errors of metabolism are rare and tend to present early in childhood.

FINAL MEDICINE EXAMINATION: DIABETES AND METABOLISM

1. A 45-year-old West Indian woman weighing 95 kg and 160 cm (5 feet 4 inches) tall, is found, on routine examination, to have glycosuria without ketonuria, and a random blood glucose of 17 mmol/l. Outline your management.
2. What are the common, long-term complications of diabetes mellitus? Describe the aetiology, natural history and treatment of two of these.

---

3. A man of 56 has been diabetic since the age of 20. He now complains of bilateral ankle swelling. Discuss the differential diagnosis and how you would investigate and manage this patient.

4. Outline your assessment and management of an 18-year-old man presenting with diabetic ketoacidosis.

5. A 20-year-old woman complains of being very thirsty and passing large quantities of urine. What are the likely causes and how would you establish the diagnosis?

6. What are the features of an attack of hypoglycaemia? Suggest the mechanism of each manifestation and what causes of a series of proven attacks ought to be considered.

7. Describe the changes on serum cholesterol of changes in:
   (a) dietary saturated fat
   (b) dietary unsaturated fat
   (c) dietary cholesterol
   (d) sugar.

ANSWERS

1. The random blood sugar confirms the presence of diabetes mellitus. Her age, obesity (body mass index > 30) and absence of symptoms and ketosis suggest that this is NIDDM. Initial management involves patient education and weight reduction achieved with a 1000–1600 kcal diet, planned in conjunction with a dietician. Diabetic complications must be sought by physical examination, blood tests and urinalysis (page 431). Oral hypoglycaemics (page 425) are necessary if blood glucose remains high in spite of weight loss having been achieved.

2. The long-term complications of diabetes are described on page 431.

3. The most probable causes of leg oedema in this patient are complications resulting from long-standing diabetes, i.e. nephrotic syndrome (page 433) or heart failure (secondary to ischaemic heart disease). These will be distinguished by physical examination, chest radiograph, urinalysis and measurement of the serum albumin. Further management depends on the cause and is described on page 433.

4. The management of diabetic ketoacidosis is described on page 429.

5. Frequency of micturition must not be confused with polyuria (usually > 3 l/day); a 24-hour urine output chart is helpful if there is doubt. The first and most simple test to perform is a random blood sugar which will be high if polyuria is secondary to diabetes mellitus. Other causes are primary or hysterical polydipsia (a relatively common cause of polyuria and polydipsia in young women), cranial diabetes insipidus (CDI), nephrogenic DI (page 417) and chronic renal failure. A full history and examination must include a drug history (e.g. lithium causes nephrogenic DI). Investigations, other than a blood glucose, include serum osmolality, urine osmolality, serum urea, electrolytes and calcium. A water deprivation test may be necessary (page 418).

6. Symptoms are the result of secretion of counterregulatory hormones (catecholamines cause hunger, sweating, pallor and tachycardia) and neuroglycopenia (e.g. confusion, drowsiness, fits and eventually coma). The causes of hypoglycaemia are listed on page 436. In an otherwise healthy person (e.g. in the absence of cancer, severe liver or renal failure), the most likely causes of recurrent hypoglycaemia are drugs, factitious hypoglycaemia, alcoholic binges and insulinoma. Often the cause will be apparent from the history, physical examination and measurement of blood glucose and plasma insulin during a hypoglycaemic episode. A supervised fast with measurement of glucose and insulin may be needed (page 437).

7. Serum cholesterol is mainly derived from *endogenous* synthesis (page 437) and thus any dietary modification will have only a moderate effect. Hypercholesterolaemia is reduced by restricting the intake of cholesterol and saturated fat (both found in animal fat) and replacing with vegetable fat (containing unsaturated fats). Carbohydrate restriction reduces serum triglyceride levels.

CHAPTER **14**

Neurology

THE CRANIAL NERVES

The 12 cranial nerves and their nuclei are approximately equally distributed between the three brain-stem segments (Figure 14.1). The exceptions are the first and second cranial nerves (nerves I and II) whose neurons project to the cerebral cortex. In addition, the sensory nucleus of nerve V extends from midbrain to spinal cord and the nuclei of nerves VII and VIII lie not only in the pons but also in the medulla.

The olfactory nerve (first cranial nerve)

The olfactory nerve subserves the sense of smell. The most common cause of anosmia (loss of the sense of smell) is simply nasal congestion. Neurological causes include tumours on the floor of the anterior fossa and head injury.

The optic nerve (second cranial nerve) and the visual system

The optic nerves enter the cranial cavity through the optic foramina and unite to form the optic chiasm, beyond which they are continued as the optic tracts. Fibres of the optic tract project to the visual cortex (via the lateral geniculate body) and the third nerve nucleus for pupillary light reflexes (Figure 14.2 and 14.3).

The assessment of optic nerve function includes measurement of visual acuity (using a Snellen test chart), colour vision (using Ishihara colour plates), the visual fields (by confrontation and perimetry) and examination of the fundi with the ophthalmoscope. In addition the pupillary responses, mediated by both the optic and oculomotor nerve (third cranial nerve), must be tested.

Visual field defects

There are three main types of visual field defects (Figure 14.2):

- Monocular defects caused by damage to the eye or nerve.
- Bitemporal defects resulting from lesions at the chiasm.
- Homonymous hemianopia caused by lesions in the tract, radiation or lesion in the visual cortex.

OPTIC NERVE LESIONS

Unilateral visual loss, starting as a central or paracentral scotoma (an area of depressed vision within the visual field),

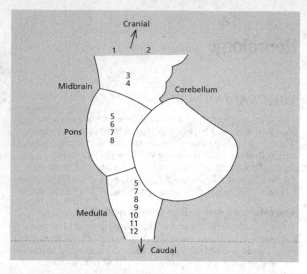

Figure 14.1 The location of the cranial nerves and their nuclei within the midbrain, pons and medulla as seen laterally.

is characteristic of optic nerve lesions. Complete destruction of one optic nerve results in blindness in that eye and loss of the pupillary light reflex (direct and consensual). Optic nerve lesions result from demyelination (e.g. multiple sclerosis), nerve compression and occlusion of the retinal artery (e.g. in giant cell arteritis). Other causes include trauma, papilloedema, severe anaemia and drugs or toxins, e.g. ethambutol, quinine, tobacco and methyl alcohol.

DEFECTS OF THE OPTIC CHIASM
The most common cause of bitemporal hemianopia (i.e. blindness in the outer half of each visual field) is a pituitary adenoma which compresses the decussating fibres from the nasal half of each eye. Other causes are craniopharyngioma and secondary neoplasm.

DEFECTS OF THE OPTIC TRACT AND RADIATION
Damage to the tracts or radiation, usually by tumours or vascular accidents, produces a homonymous hemianopia (blindness affecting either the right or left half of each visual field) in one half of the visual field contralateral to the lesion.

DEFECTS OF THE OCCIPITAL CORTEX
Homonymous hemianopic defects are caused by unilateral posterior cerebral artery infarction. The macular region may be spared in ischaemic lesions as a result of the dual blood

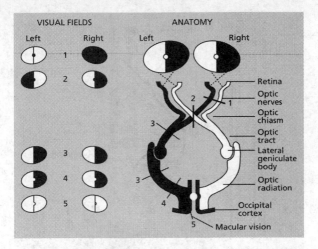

Figure 14.2 Diagram of the visual pathways demonstrating the main field defects. At the optic chiasm, fibres derived from the nasal half of the retina (the temporal visual field) decussate whereas the fibres from the temporal half of the retina remain uncrossed. Thus, the right optic tract is composed of fibres from the right half of each retina which 'see' the left half of both visual fields. Lesion at 1 produces blindness in the right eye with loss of direct light reflex. Lesion at 2 produces bitemporal hemianopia. Lesion at 3 produces homonymous hemianopia with macular involvement. Lesion at 4 produces homonymous hemianopia with macular sparing and a lesion at 5 produces a macular defect. (Adapted from Swash, 1989, *Hutchison's Clinical Methods,* 19th edn, London, Baillière Tindall.)

supply of this area from middle and posterior cerebral arteries. In contrast injury to one occipital pole produces a bilateral macular (central) field defect.

Optic disc oedema (papilloedema) and optic atrophy

The principal pathological appearances of the visible part of the nerve, the disc, are:

- Disc swelling (papilloedema)
- Disc pallor (optic atrophy)

PAPILLOEDEMA

Papilloedema produces few visual symptoms in the early stages. As disc oedema develops there is enlargement of the blind spot and blurring of vision. The exception is optic neuritis in which there is early and severe visual loss. The common causes of papilloedema are:

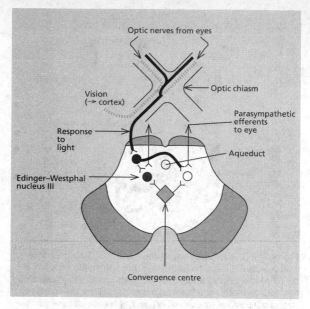

Figure 14.3 Midbrain control of response to light, accommodation and convergence. Afferent impulses in the optic nerve are distributed bilaterally; thus, when a light is shone in one eye both pupils will constrict (*direct and consensual* reflex). The reflex arc for the pupillary response to light is complete within the brain stem and thus the pupils of a patient rendered blind by damage to the occipital lobe will still react when illuminated.

- Raised intracranial pressure, e.g. from a tumour, an abscess or meningitis
- Retinal vein obstruction (thrombosis or compression)
- Optic neuritis (inflammation of the optic nerve often caused by demyelination)
- Accelerated hypertension

OPTIC ATROPHY
Optic atrophy is the end result of many processes that damage the nerve (see Optic nerve lesions above). The degree of visual loss depends upon the underlying cause.

The pupils

The pupils constrict in response to a bright light and convergence (when the centre of focus shifts from a distant to a near object). The parasympathetic efferents that control the constrictor muscle of the pupil arise in the Edinger–Westphal nucleus in the midbrain and run with the oculomotor (third) nerve to the eye. The Edinger–Westphal nucleus receives afferents from the optic nerve (for the light reflex) and from the convergence centre in the midbrain (Figure 14.3).

Sympathetic fibres which arise in the hypothalamus produce pupillary dilatation. They run from the hypothalamus through the brain stem and cervical cord and emerge from the spinal cord at T1. They then ascend in the neck as the cervical sympathetic chain and travel with the carotid artery into the head.

The main causes of persistent pupillary dilatation are:

- A third cranial nerve palsy (see later)

- Antimuscarinic eye drops (instilled to facilitate examination of the fundus)

- The myotonic pupil (Holmes Adie pupil): this is a dilated pupil seen most commonly in young women. There is absent, or very delayed, reaction to light and convergence. It is of no pathological significance and may be associated with absent tendon reflexes

The main causes of persistent pupillary constriction are:

- Parasympatheticomimetic eye drops used in the treatment of glaucoma

- Horner's syndrome, resulting from interruption of sympathetic fibres to one eye. There is unilateral pupillary constriction, slight ptosis (sympathetic fibres innervate the levator palpebrae superioris), enophthalmos (backward displacement of the eyeball in the orbit) and loss of sweating on the ipsilateral side of the face. A lesion affecting any part of the sympathetic pathway to the eye results in a Horner's syndrome. Causes include diseases of the cervical cord, e.g syringomyelia, involvement of the T1 root by apical lung cancer (Pancoast's tumour) and lesions in the neck, such as trauma, surgical resection or malignant lymph nodes

- The Argyll Robertson pupil: this is the pupillary abnormality seen mainly in neurosyphilis (page 489). There is a small irregular pupil which is fixed to light but constricts on convergence

Cranial nerves III–XII

The cranial nerves III–XII may be damaged by lesions in the brain stem or during their intracranial and extracranial course. The causes are listed in Table 14.1. The site of a lesion may be suggested if clinical examination shows involvement of other cranial nerves at that site, e.g. a seventh nerve palsy together with cerebellar signs and involvement of the fifth,

Table 14.1 The structural causes of lesions of cranial nerves III–XII

Nerve	Brain stem (UMNL)	Intracranial course (LMNL)	Extracranial course (LMNL)
III	Infarction	Posterior communicating artery aneurysm (III)	
IV	Tumour	'Coning' of the temporal lobe (III)	Orbital trauma
	MS	Cavernous sinus lesions, e.g. internal carotid artery aneurysm	
V	Infarction	Cerebellopontine angle tumours	
VI	Tumour	Cavernous sinus lesions (V and VI)	Neoplastic infiltration of skull base
VII	MS	Petrous temporal bone lesions (VII and VIII)	Parotid gland tumour (VII)
VIII	MND		
IX	Infarction		
X	Tumour	Infiltrating nasopharyngeal carcinoma	
XI	MS	Skull base trauma	Tumours and trauma in the neck
XII	MND		
	Syringobulbia		

MS, multiple sclerosis; MND, motor neuron disease; UMNL, upper motor neuron lesion; LMNL, lower motor neuron lesion. The nerves may also be involved by any of the causes of mononeuritis multiplex (page 500). Diabetes mellitus particularly affects the third and sixth nerves.

sixth and eighth cranial nerves suggest a lesion of the cerebellopontine angle, commonly a meningioma or acoustic neuroma. In contrast, an isolated seventh nerve palsy in a patient with a parotid tumour suggests involvement during its extracranial course in the parotid.

The ocular movements and the third, fourth and sixth cranial nerves

These three cranial nerves supply the six external ocular muscles which move the eye in the orbit (Figure 14.4). The abducens nerve (sixth cranial nerve) supplies the lateral rectus muscle and the trochlear (fourth cranial nerve) supplies the superior oblique muscle. All the other extraocular muscles, the sphincter pupillae (parasympathetic fibres) and the levator palpebrae superioris are supplied by the oculomotor nerve (third cranial nerve). Normally the brain stem (with in-put from the cortex, cerebellum and vestibular nucleus) coordinates the functions of these three cranial nerves so that eye movement is symmetrical (conjugate gaze). Thus *infranuclear (lower motor neuron)* lesions of the third, fourth and sixth cranial nerves lead to paralysis of individual muscles or muscle groups. *Supranuclear (upper motor neuron)* lesions, e.g. brain-stem involvement by multiple sclerosis, leads to paralysis of conjugate movements of the eyes.

A lesion of the oculomotor nerve causes unilateral complete ptosis, the eye faces 'down and out', and the pupil is dilated and fixed to light and accommodation. This is the picture of a complete third nerve palsy of which the most common cause is a 'berry' aneurysm arising in the posterior communicating artery which runs alongside the nerve. Frequently the lesion is partial, particularly in diabetes mellitus, when parasympathetic fibres are spared and the pupil reacts normally. Less common causes are listed in Table 14.1.

In a sixth nerve lesion the eye cannot be abducted beyond the midline. The unopposed pull of the medial rectus muscle causes the eye to turn inward, thereby producing a squint (squint or *strabismus* is the appearance of the eyes when the visual axes do not meet at the point of fixation). The patient complains of diplopia or double vision which worsens when they attempt to gaze to the side of the lesion.

Isolated lesions of the trochlear nerve are rare. The patient complains of diplopia when attempting to look down and away from the affected side.

Disordered ocular movements may also result from disease of the ocular muscles (e.g. muscular dystrophy, dystrophia myotonica) or of the neuromuscular junction (e.g. myasthenia gravis). In these conditions all the muscles tend to be affected equally, presenting a generalized restriction of eye movements.

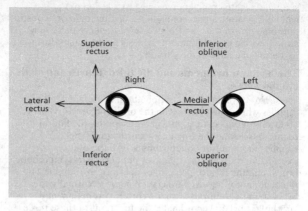

Figure 14.4 The action of the external ocular muscles. (Adapted from Swash, 1989, *Hutchison's Clinical Methods*, London, Baillière Tindall.)

The trigeminal nerve (fifth cranial nerve)

The trigeminal nerve supplies, through its three divisions, sensation to the face and scalp as far back as the vertex (Figure 14.5). It also supplies the mucous membranes of the sinuses, the nose, mouth, tongue and the teeth. The motor root travels with the mandibular division and supplies the muscles of mastication.

Diminution of the corneal reflex is often the first sign of a fifth nerve lesion. A complete fifth nerve lesion on one side causes unilateral sensory loss on the face, tongue and buccal mucosa. The jaw deviates to the side of the lesion when the mouth is opened. A brisk jaw jerk is seen with upper motor neuron lesions, i.e. above the motor nucleus in the pons.

The facial nerve (seventh cranial nerve)

The facial nerve is largely motor in function, supplying the muscles of facial expression. It has, in addition, two major branches: the chorda tympani which carries taste from the anterior two-thirds of the tongue and the nerve to the stapedius muscle (this has a damping effect to protect the ear from loud noise). These two branches arise from the facial nerve during its intracranial course through the facial canal of the petrous temporal bone. Therefore damage to the facial nerve in the temporal bone (e.g. Bell's palsy, trauma, herpes zoster, middle-ear infection) may be associated with undue

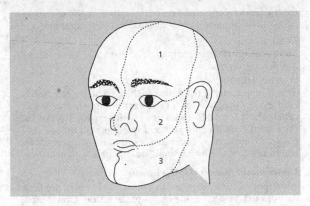

Figure 14.5 Cutaneous distribution of the trigeminal nerve.
1, ophthalmic or first division; 2, maxillary or second division;
3, mandibular or third division.

sensitivity to sounds (hyperacusis) and loss of taste to the anterior two-thirds of the tongue.

Lower motor neuron (LMN) lesions

A unilateral LMN lesion causes weakness of *all* the muscles of facial expression on the same side as the lesion. The face, especially the angle of the mouth, falls and dribbling occurs from the corner of the mouth. There is weakness of frontalis, the eye will not close and the exposed cornea is at risk of ulceration. The causes of a lower motor neuron lesion are outlined in Table 14.1, the most common being Bell's palsy (see below). In addition the nerve may also be affected in polyneuritis (e.g. Guillain–Barré syndrome) when there may be bilateral involvement.

BELL'S PALSY

Bell's palsy is a common, acute, isolated facial palsy believed to be the result of a viral infection that causes swelling of the nerve within the petrous temporal bone.

Clinical features

There is lower motor neuron weakness of the facial muscles, sometimes with loss of taste on the anterior two-thirds of the tongue.

Investigations

The diagnosis is clinical.

Management

The eyelid must be closed to protect the cornea from ulceration (either adhesive tape or surgery in prolonged cases). Oral prednisolone reduces the proportion of patients with a severe deficit if given at the onset of symptoms.

Prognosis

Most patients recover completely, although 15% are left with a severe permanent weakness.

RAMSAY HUNT SYNDROME

This is herpes zoster (shingles) of the geniculate ganglion (the sensory ganglion for taste fibres) situated in the facial canal. There is a LMN facial palsy with herpetic vesicles in the external auditory meatus and sometimes in the soft palate. Deafness may occur as a result of involvement of the eighth nerve in the facial canal. Treatment is with acyclovir.

Upper motor neuron (UMN) lesions

An upper motor neuron lesion causes weakness of the lower part of the face on the side opposite the lesion. Upper facial muscles are spared because of the bilateral cortical innervation of neurons supplying the upper face. Wrinkling of the forehead (frontalis muscle) and eye closure are normal. The most common cause is a stroke when there is an associated hemiparesis.

The vestibulocochlear nerve (eighth cranial nerve)

The eighth cranial nerve has two components: cochlear and vestibular, subserving hearing and equilibrium respectively. The clinical features of a cochlear nerve lesion are sensorineural deafness and tinnitus. The causes of a cochlear nerve lesion are outlined in Table 14.1; however, deafness is very rare in pontine lesions. Sensorineural deafness may also be the result of disease of the cochlear itself: Ménière's disease (see below), drugs (e.g. gentamicin) and presbyacusis (deafness of old age).

The main symptom of a vestibular nerve lesion is vertigo which may be accompanied by vomiting. Nystagmus is the principal physical sign, often with ataxia (loss of balance).

Table 14.2 Principal causes of vertigo

Labyrinth	Ménière's disease, vestibular neuronitis, benign positional vertigo
Eighth nerve	Cerebellopontine angle lesions, drugs (e.g. gentamicin)
Brain stem	Tumours, ischaemia/infarction, multiple sclerosis, migraine
Cerebellum	Acute cerebellar lesions

Vertigo

Vertigo is the definite illusion of movement – a sensation as if the external world were revolving around the patient. It results from disease of the inner ear, the eighth nerve or its central connections (Table 14.2).

Nystagmus

Nystagmus is a rhythmic oscillation of the eyes which must be sustained for more than a few beats to be significant. It is a sign of disease of either the ocular or the vestibular system and its connections. Nystagmus is described as either pendular or jerk.

PENDULAR NYSTAGMUS

A pendular movement of the eye occurs; there is no rapid phase. It occurs where there is poor visual fixation (i.e. long-standing severe visual impairment) or a congenital lesion.

JERK NYSTAGMUS

Jerk nystagmus has a fast and a slow component to the rhythmic movement.

- Horizontal or rotary nystagmus may be either peripheral (middle ear) or central (brain stem and cerebellum) in origin. In peripheral lesions it is usually transient (minutes or hours); in central lesions it is long lasting (weeks, months or more)
- Vertical nystagmus is caused only by central lesions

Ménière's disease

Ménière's disease is a disorder of the inner ear in which there is dilatation of the membranous labyrinth because of accumulation of endolymph. The aetiology is unknown and symptoms rarely start before middle age. It is characterized by recurrent attacks, lasting minutes to hours, of vertigo, tinnitus and deafness. Vomiting and nystagmus may accompany an attack. Ultimately deafness develops and the vertigo ceases. Betahistine, a histamine analogue, is useful in some cases. Recurrent severe attacks may require surgery (ultrasonic destruction of the labyrinth or vestibular nerve section).

Vestibular neuronitis

Vestibular neuronitis is believed to be caused by a viral infection affecting the labyrinth. There is sudden onset of severe vertigo, nystagmus and vomiting but no deafness. The attack lasts several days or weeks and treatment is symptomatic with vestibular sedatives (e.g. prochlor-perazine).

Benign positional vertigo

Vertigo occurs with turning and moving. It may follow vestibular neuronitis, head injury or ear infection and usually lasts for some months; treatment is with vestibular sedatives.

Glossopharyngeal, vagus, accessory and hypoglossal nerves (ninth to twelfth cranial nerves)

The lower four cranial nerves (ninth to twelfth) which lie in the medulla (the 'bulb') are usually affected together; isolated lesions are rare. A *bulbar palsy* describes weakness of the lower motor neuron type of the muscles supplied by these cranial nerves. There is dysarthria, dysphagia and nasal regurgitation. The tongue is weak, wasted and fasciculating. The most common causes of a bulbar palsy are motor neuron disease (page 499), syringobulbia (page 497) and Guillain–Barré syndrome (page 502). Poliomyelitis is now a rare cause in developed countries. *Pseudobulbar palsy* is an upper motor neuron weakness of the same muscle groups. There is also dysarthria, dysphagia and nasal regurgitation, but the tongue is small and spastic and there is no fasciculation. The jaw jerk is exaggerated and the patient is emotionally labile. In many patients there is a partial palsy with only some of these features. The most common cause of pseudobulbar palsy is a stroke, but it may also occur in motor neuron disease and multiple sclerosis.

THE MOTOR SYSTEM

The corticospinal tracts

The upper motor neuron

The corticospinal tracts originate from neurons of the motor cortex and terminate on the motor nuclei of the cranial nerves and the anterior horn cells. The clinically important pathways cross over in the medulla and pass to the contralateral halves of the spinal cord as the crossed lateral corticospinal tracts (Figure 14.6), which then synapse with the anterior horn cells. This is known as the pyramidal system, disease of which results in upper motor neuron (UMN) lesions with characteristic clinical features (Table 14.3).

Two main patterns of clinical features occur in UMN disorders: hemiparesis and paraparesis.

HEMIPARESIS means weakness of the limbs of one side and is usually caused by a lesion within the brain, e.g. a stroke.

PARAPARESIS (weak legs) indicates bilateral damage to the corticospinal tracts and is most often caused by lesions in the spinal cord below the arms (page 496). Tetraparesis (weakness of the arms and legs) indicates high cervical cord damage often from trauma.

The lower motor neuron

The lower motor neuron (LMN) is the motor pathway from the anterior horn cell or cranial nerve via a peripheral nerve to the motor end plate. Physical signs (Table 14.3) follow rapidly if the LMN is interrupted at any point in its course.

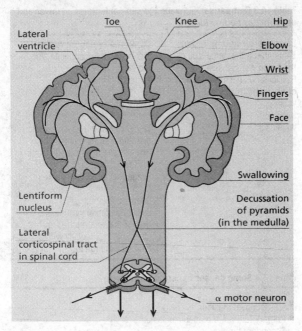

Figure 14.6 The crossed corticospinal ('pyramidal') tracts showing cortical representation of various parts of the body.

Muscle disease may give a similar clinical picture but reflexes are usually preserved.

LMN lesions are most commonly caused by the following:

● Anterior horn cell lesions, e.g. motor neuron disease, poliomyelitis

● Spinal root lesions, e.g. cervical and lumbar disc lesions

● Peripheral nerve lesions, e.g. trauma, compression or polyneuropathy

The extrapyramidal system

The extrapyramidal system is described on page 479.

The cerebellum

Each lateral lobe of the cerebellum is responsible for coordinating movement of the ipsilateral limb. The midline vermis is concerned with maintenance of axial (midline) balance and posture. Causes of cerebellar disease are listed in Table 14.4.

Table 14.3 Comparison between the clinical features of lower and upper motor neuron lesions

Lower motor neuron lesion	Upper motor neuron lesion
Signs are on the same side of the lesion	Signs are on the opposite side of the lesion
Fasciculation (visible contraction of single motor units)	No fasciculation
Wasting	No muscle wasting
Hypotonia	Spasticity
Weakness	Weakness with a characteristic distribution (predominantly extensors in the arms, flexors in the legs)
Loss of tendon reflexes	Exaggerated tendon reflexes
	Extensor plantar response
	Sustained clonus
	Loss of abdominal reflexes
	Drift of the outstretched arm (downwards, medially with a tendency to pronate)

Table 14.4 Some causes of cerebellar disease

Multiple sclerosis
Space-occupying lesion
  Primary tumour, e.g. medulloblastoma
  Secondary tumour
  Abscess
  Haemorrhage
Chronic alcohol abuse
Anticonvulsant drugs
Non-metastatic manifestation of malignancy

A lesion within one cerebellar lobe causes one or all of the following:

● An ataxic gait with a broad base; the patient falters to the side of the lesion

● An 'intention tremor' (compare Parkinson's disease) with past-pointing

● Clumsy rapid alternating movements, e.g. tapping one hand on the back of the other (dysdiadochokinesis)

● Horizontal nystagmus with the fast component towards the side of the lesion (page 457)

● Dysarthria usually with bilateral lesions. The speech has a halting jerking quality, 'scanning speech'

● Titubation (rhythmic tremor of the head), hypotonia and depressed reflexes. There is no muscle weakness

Lesions of the cerebellar vermis cause a characteristic ataxia of the trunk so that the patient has difficulty sitting up or standing.

THE SENSORY SYSTEM

The peripheral nerves carry all the modalities of sensation from nerve endings to the dorsal root ganglia and thus to the cord. These then ascend to the thalamus and cerebral cortex in two principal pathways:

- Posterior columns which carry sensory modalities for vibration, joint position sense, two-point discrimination and light touch. These fibres ascend uncrossed to the gracile and cuneate nuclei in the medulla. Axons from the second order neurons cross the midline to form the medial lemniscus and pass to the thalamus

- Spinothalamic tracts which carry sensations of pain and temperature. These fibres synapse in the dorsal horn of the cord, cross the midline and ascend as the spinothalamic tracts to the thalamus (Figure 14.7)

Paraesthesiae (pins and needles), numbness and pain are the principal symptoms of lesions of the sensory pathways below the level of the thalamus. The quality and distribution of the symptoms may suggest the site of the lesion.

PERIPHERAL NERVE LESIONS
Symptoms are felt in the distribution of the affected peripheral nerve.

SPINAL ROOT LESIONS
Symptoms are referred to the myotome supplied by that root, often with a tingling discomfort in that dermatome.

SPINAL CORD LESIONS
Symptoms (e.g. loss of sensation) are usually evident below the level of the lesion. Spinothalamic tract lesions result in isolated contralateral loss of pain and temperature with preservation of light touch (dissociated sensory loss).

PONTINE LESIONS
Pontine lesions lie above the decussation of the posterior columns. As the medial lemniscus and spinothalamic tracts are close together, there is loss of all forms of sensation on the side opposite the lesion.

THALAMIC LESIONS
A thalamic lesion is a rare cause of complete contralateral sensory loss. Spontaneous pain may also occur most commonly as the result of a thalamic infarct.

CORTICAL LESIONS
Sensory loss, neglect of one side of the body and subtle disorders of sensation may occur with lesions of the parietal cortex. Pain is not a feature of cortical lesions.

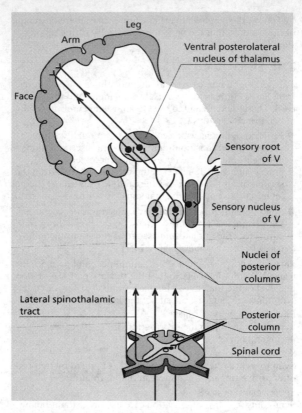

Figure 14.7 The principal sensory pathways.

UNCONSCIOUSNESS AND COMA

The central reticular formation, which extends from the brain stem to the thalamus, influences the state of arousal. It consists of clusters of interconnected neurons throughout the brain stem, with projections to the spinal cord, the hypothalamus, the cerebellum and the cerebral cortex.

Coma is a state of unconsciousness from which the patient cannot be roused. A *stuporous* patient is sleepy but will respond to vigorous stimulation. The Glasgow Coma Scale (Table 14.5) is a simple grading system used to assess the level of consciousness. It is easy to perform and provides an objective assessment of the patient. Serial measurements are particularly useful to monitor the conscious level and thus

detect a deterioration which may indicate the need for
further investigation or treatment.

Table 14.5 Glasgow Coma Scale

Category	Score
Eye opening	
Spontaneous	4
To speech	3
To pain	2
None	1
Best verbal response	
Oriented	5
Confused	4
Inappropriate	3
Incomprehensible	2
None	1
Best motor response	
Obeys commands	6
Localises	5
Withdraws	4
Flexing	3
Extending	2
None	1

The scores in each category are added up to give an overall score which may vary
from 3 (in the deeply comatose patient) to 14.

Aetiology
Altered consciousness is produced by three types of
processes:

● DIFFUSE METABOLIC, TOXIC OR NEUROLOGICAL
  DISTURBANCE.

● BRAIN-STEM LESIONS which damage the reticular formation.

● CORTICAL AND CEREBELLAR LESIONS. These will only cause
  coma if there is raised intracranial pressure and secondary
  brain-stem compression, i.e. an indirect effect

The principal causes of coma and stupor are shown in Table
14.6. A common cause of coma is self-poisoning (page 375).

Assessment
IMMEDIATE ASSESSMENT, which takes only seconds, is essential:

● Clear the airway and intubate if ventilation is inadequate

● Check the pulse; if absent and rescuscitation appropriate,
  perform cardiopulmonary resuscitation

● Check for head injury and, if present, anticipate
  deterioration

In all patients presenting in coma a history should be
obtained from any witnesses and relatives (e.g. speed of onset

of coma, diabetes, drug or alcohol abuser, past medical history, medication and drug abuse).

Table 14.6 Causes of coma and stupor

Toxins	Drug overdose, alcohol, anaesthetic gases
	Carbon monoxide poisoning
Metabolic	Hypo- or hyperglycaemia
	Severe hypo- or hypercalcaemia
	Severe hypo- or hypernatraemia
	Hypoxic/ischaemic brain injury
	Hypoadrenalism
	Hypothyroidism
	Renal failure
	Hepatic failure
	Respiratory failure with CO_2 retention
Diffuse neurological disease	Subarachnoid haemorrhage
	Hypertensive encephalopathy
	Encephalitis, cerebral malaria
Brain-stem lesions	Tumour
	Haemorrhage/infarction
	Demyelination, e.g. multiple sclerosis
	Trauma
	Wernicke–Korsakoff syndrome (page 385)
Cortical/cerebellar lesions	Tumour
	Haemorrhage/infarction
	Abscess
	Encephalitis

FURTHER ASSESSMENT. The depth of coma should be noted (Table 14.5) and a full general examination carried out. Clues to the cause of coma should be looked for, for example, the smell of alcohol or ketones (in diabetic ketoacidosis) on the breath, needle track marks of a drug abuser, Medic-Alert bracelet carried by some diabetic people and patients on steroid replacement therapy. The neurological examination must include:

● The head and neck: the patient should be examined for evidence of trauma and neck stiffness (indicating meningitis or subarachnoid haemorrhage)

● The pupils: the size of the pupils and their reaction to light must be recorded

A fixed dilated pupil indicates herniation of the temporal lobe ('coning') through the tentorial hiatus and compression of the third cranial nerve (page 451). This indicates the need for urgent neurosurgical intervention.

Bilateral fixed dilated pupils are a cardinal sign of brain death. They also occur in deep coma of any cause, but particularly coma caused by barbiturate intoxication or hypothermia.

Pinpoint pupils are seen with opiate overdose or with pontine lesions that interrupt the sympathetic pathways to the dilator muscle of the pupil.

Midpoint pupils that react to light are characteristic in coma of metabolic origin and coma caused by most CNS depressant drugs.

- The fundi: these should be examined for papilloedema which indicates raised intracranial pressure

- Eye movements: cerebral hemisphere lesions may produce conjugate deviation of the eyes towards the side of the lesion ('the eyes look *towards the normal limbs*'). In a pontine brain-stem lesion, sustained conjugate lateral gaze occurs away from the site of the lesion (*towards the paralysed limbs*)

  Passive head rotation normally causes conjugate ocular deviation in the direction opposite to the induced head movement (doll's head reflex). This reflex is lost in very deep coma and is absent in brain-stem lesions.

- Motor responses: asymmetry of spontaneous limb movements, tone and reflexes indicates a unilateral cerebral hemisphere or brain-stem lesion. The plantar responses are often both extensor in coma of any cause

Investigations

In many cases the cause of coma will be evident from the history and examination and appropriate investigations should then be carried out. However, if the cause is still unclear further investigations will be necessary.

BLOOD AND URINE TESTS

- Serum and urine for drug analysis, e.g salicylates
- Serum for urea and electrolytes, liver biochemistry and calcium
- Blood glucose
- Arterial blood gases
- Thyroid function tests and serum cortisol
- Blood cultures

RADIOLOGY. CT of the head may indicate an otherwise unsuspected mass lesion or intracranial haemorrhage.

CSF EXAMINATION. Lumbar puncture is performed if subarachnoid haemorrhage or meningoencephalitis is suspected and a mass lesion is excluded on CT.

Management
The immediate management consists of treatment of the cause, careful nursing, meticulous attention to the airway and frequent observation to detect any change in vital function.

Prognosis
The outlook depends upon the cause of coma. A cause must be established before decisions are made about withdrawing supportive care.

Brain death

Brain death means the irreversible loss of the capacity for consciousness combined with the irreversible loss of the capacity to breathe. Two independent senior medical opinions are required for the diagnosis to be made. The three main criteria for diagnosis are the following.

IRREMEDIAL STRUCTURAL BRAIN DAMAGE. A disorder that can cause brain-stem death, e.g. intracranial haemorrhage, must have been diagnosed with certainty. Patients with hypothermia, significant electrolyte imbalance or drug overdose are excluded but may be reassessed when these are corrected.

ABSENT MOTOR RESPONSES to any stimulus. Spinal reflexes may be present.

ABSENT BRAIN-STEM FUNCTION, demonstrated by:

● Pupils fixed and unresponsive to light

● Absent corneal, gag and cough reflexes

● Absent doll's head reflex (page 465)

● Absent caloric responses: ice-cold water run into the external auditory meatus causes nystagmus with normal brain-stem function

● Lack of spontaneous respiration

In suitable cases and provided the patient was carrying a donor card and/or the consent of relatives has been obtained, the organs of those in whom brain-stem death has been established may be used for transplantation.

CEREBROVASCULAR DISEASE

Stroke

Definitions
STROKE is a focal neurological deficit (e.g. hemiplegia) lasting longer than 24 hours which is the result of a vascular lesion.

A COMPLETED STROKE is when the neurological deficit has reached its maximum (usually within 6 hours).

A STROKE 'IN EVOLUTION' is when the symptoms and signs are getting worse (usually within 24 hours of onset).

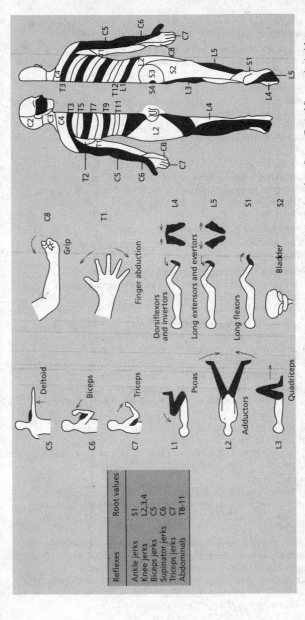

Reflexes	Root values
Ankle jerks	S1
Knee jerks	L2,3,4
Biceps jerks	C5
Supinator jerks	C6
Triceps jerks	C7
Abdominals	T8-11

Figure 14.8 Simple scheme depicting motor and sensory innervation of arms and legs and root values for reflexes. (Part of figure adapted from Malcolm Parsons, *A Colour Atlas of Clinical Neurology*, Mosby-Wolfe, an imprint of Times Mirror International Publishers Ltd, London, UK, 1993.)

A MINOR STROKE is one in which the patient recovers without a significant neurological deficit usually within 1 week.

TRANSIENT ISCHAEMIC ATTACK is a focal deficit lasting less than 24 hours and from which there is complete neurological recovery.

Epidemiology

Stroke is the third most common cause of death in the UK and the most common cause of physical disability in adults. The incidence rises steeply with age; it is uncommon in those under 40 years. It is slightly more common in men.

Pathogenesis

A stroke is caused by cerebral infarction or cerebral haemorrhage. The clinical picture of 'stroke' may also be caused by a space-occupying lesion in the brain, e.g. tumour or abscess, although onset of symptoms and signs is usually much slower.

CEREBRAL INFARCTION may be the result of:

- Thrombosis at the site of an atheromatous plaque in a major cerebral vessel
- Emboli arising from atheromatous plaques in the carotid/vertebrobasilar arteries or from cardiac mural thrombi (e.g. following myocardial infarction) or from the left atrium in atrial fibrillation

Rarely cerebral infarction is the result of severe hypotension (e.g. systolic blood pressure < 75 mmHg), vasculitis, meningovascular syphilis or emboli from vegetations in infective endocarditis.

CEREBRAL HAEMORRHAGE (15% OF STROKES)

In most cases this is the result of rupture of a microaneurysm (Charcot–Bouchard aneurysms) in a hypertensive patient.

Risk factors

The major risk factors for stroke are those for atheroma, i.e. hypertension, diabetes mellitus, cigarette smoking and hyperlipidaemia. Others are obesity, oestrogen-containing oral contraceptives, alcohol and polycythaemia.

Clinical features

The history and physical examination in all stroke patients must include a search for risk factors (see above) and source of emboli (?atrial fibrillation, valve lesion, carotid bruits in the neck).

In most patients symptoms and signs develop over a few minutes and reach maximum disability within 1–2 hours. It is usually impossible to distinguish clinically between haemorrhage and infarction; cerebral haemorrhage tends, however, to be accompanied by a severe headache and produce a more diffuse neurological deficit.

The neurological deficit produced by occlusion of a vessel may be predicted by a knowledge of neuroanatomy and vascular supply (Figures 14.6, 14.9 and 14.10). In practice it is less clear-cut because of collateral supply to brain areas.

CEREBRAL HEMISPHERE INFARCTS

The most common stroke is the hemiplegia caused by infarction of the internal capsule (the narrow zone of motor and sensory fibres that converges on the brain stem from the cerebral cortex – Figure 14.6) following occlusion of a branch of the middle cerebral artery. The signs are contralateral to the lesion: hemiplegia (arm > leg), hemisensory loss, upper motor neuron facial weakness and hemianopia. Initially the patient has a hypotonic hemiplegia with decreased reflexes; within days this develops into a spastic hemiplegia with increased reflexes and an extensor plantar response. Weakness may recover gradually over days or months.

Occlusion of the main trunk of the middle cerebral artery produces contralateral hemiplegia, hemisensory loss and aphasia (if located in the dominant hemisphere). Lacunar infarcts are small infarcts which produce localized deficits, e.g. pure motor stroke, pure sensory stroke.

BRAIN-STEM INFARCTION

Brain-stem infarction causes complex patterns of dysfunction depending on the sites involved:

● The lateral medullary syndrome, the most common of the brain-stem vascular syndromes, is caused by occlusion of the posterior inferior cerebellar artery. It presents with sudden vomiting and vertigo, ipsilateral Horner's syndrome, facial numbness, cerebellar signs and palatal paralysis with a diminished gag reflex. On the side opposite the lesion, there is loss of pain and temperature.

● Coma as a result of involvement of the reticular formation

● Pseudobulbar palsy may be caused by brain-stem infarction

MULTI-INFARCT DEMENTIA is a syndrome caused by multiple small cortical infarcts, resulting in generalized intellectual loss; there is a stepwise progression with each infarct. The final picture is of dementia, pseudobulbar palsy and a shuffling gait resembling Parkinson's disease.

Investigations

Stroke is usually a straightforward clinical diagnosis. The purpose of the investigation is to differentiate between haemorrhage and infarction, and to identify aetiological or risk factors which can be eliminated or reduced.

CT OR MAGNETIC RESONANCE IMAGING can distinguish between infarction and haemorrhage, and is indicated in virtually all patients.

FURTHER INVESTIGATIONS

- BLOOD GLUCOSE to identify patients with diabetes mellitus
- HAEMOGLOBIN to identify patients with polycythaemia
- ESR which will be raised in the few cases of endocarditis, giant cell arteritis and vasculitis that present with stroke
- ECG may show evidence of a recent myocardial infarction or atrial fibrillation
- SYPHILIS SEROLOGY will identify the rare cases of meningovascular syphilis

CAROTID DOPPLER AND DUPLEX SCANNING are indicated in patients with a cerebral infarct, who may be suitable for surgery (see below), to look for carotid atheroma and stenosis.

ANGIOGRAPHY of the carotid territory may be considered in younger patients to define stenotic lesions more accurately before surgery.

Management

Many mild strokes may be managed at home if social circumstances allow.

Immediate therapy is supportive with maintenance of hydration, frequent turning to avoid pressure sores and other measures as for the unconscious patient (page 463). An expanding intracerebral haematoma causing deepening coma (with eventual coning) should be considered for urgent neurosurgical removal.

SECONDARY PREVENTION

This involves advice and treatment to reverse risk factors. Control of hypertension is the single most important factor in the prevention of stroke.

- Long-term anticoagulation is indicated in cerebral infarction when there is atrial fibrillation, with some valvular lesions (uninfected) or cardiomyopathy
- Internal carotid endarterectomy reduces the risk of recurrent stroke (by 75%) in patients who have had an infarct and who have internal carotid artery stenosis which narrows the arterial lumen by more than 70%. It is considered in patients with a non-disabling stroke who are likely to have some recoverable function

In all stroke patients rehabilitation plays an important part of management. Physiotherapy is particularly useful in the first few months in reducing spasticity, relieving contractures and teaching patients to use walking aids. Following recovery, the occupational therapist plays a valuable role in assessing the requirement and arranging the provision of various aids and modifications in the home, such as stair rails, hoists, wheel chairs, etc.

Prognosis

Between 30% and 50% of patients will die in the first month following a stroke although prognosis is much worse for bleeds than for infarction. About 10% of patients will suffer a recurrent stroke within 1 year and of initial survivors only about 30–40% are alive after 3 years.

Transient ischaemic attacks

Transient ischaemic attacks (TIAs) are less common than stroke but they are an important predictive factor for stroke and myocardial infarction.

Aetiology

The risk factors and causes of TIAs are the same as those for thromboembolic stroke. Most are the result of emboli (which subsequently lyse) arising from internal carotid artery atheromas.

Clinical features

There is a sudden loss of function in one region of the brain which by definition resolves in 24 hours. Symptoms and signs depend on the site of the brain involved (Table 14.7). The history and physical examination must include a search for risk factors and possible sources of emboli.

Table 14.7 Features of TIAs in different arterial territories

Carotid system	Vertebrobasilar system
Amaurosis fugax	Diplopia, vertigo, vomiting
Aphasia	Choking and dysarthria
Hemiparesis	Ataxia
Hemisensory loss	Hemisensory loss
Hemianopic visual loss	Hemianopic visual loss
	Transient global amnesia
	Tetraparesis
	Loss of consciousness (rare)

Amaurosis fugax is a sudden loss of vision in one eye as a result of the passage of emboli through the retinal arteries. Transient global amnesia describes a condition in which there are sudden episodes of amnesia associated with confusion, probably caused by ischaemia in the posterior circulation.

The investigation and management of TIAs is similar to that of stroke. Aspirin (300 mg daily) reduces the incidence of stroke and is given to most patients. The exact dose is under review.

Primary intracranial haemorrhage

Intracerebral haemorrhage

This is discussed under Stroke above.

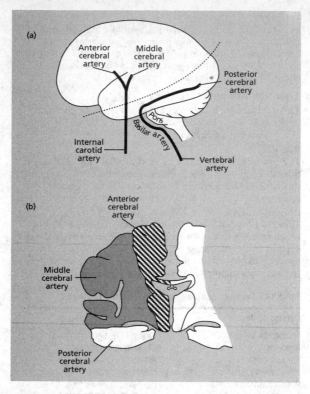

Figure 14.9 The arterial supply to the brain. (a) The area above the dotted line is supplied by the internal carotid artery and the area below the line is supplied by the vertebral artery. (b) A coronal section through the brain. The anterior cerebral artery supplies the medial surface of the hemisphere and the middle cerebral artery supplies the lateral surface of the hemisphere including the internal capsule.

Subarachnoid haemorrhage

The term 'subarachnoid haemorrhage' (SAH) describes spontaneous rather than traumatic arterial bleeding into the subarachnoid space.

Incidence

SAH accounts for 10% of cerebrovascular disease and has an annual incidence of 15 per 100 000.

Aetiology

SAH is caused by rupture of:

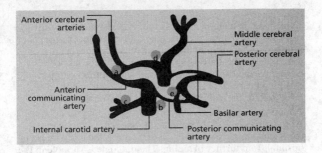

Figure 14.10 The main cerebral arteries showing the circle of Willis and the most common sites for berry aneurysms (shaded). Frequency of occurrence, a–e (decreasing order). a, anterior communicating artery; b, origin of the posterior communicating artery; c, trifurcation of the middle cerebral artery; d, termination of the internal carotid artery; e, basilar artery.

- Saccular ('berry') aneurysms (in 70%) which form on the circle of Willis and adjacent branches. Common sites for aneurysm formation are shown in Figure 14.10
- Congenital arteriovenous malformations in 10%

In 20% of cases no lesion can be found.

Clinical features
The onset is sudden with a devastating headache, often occipital. This is followed by vomiting and often loss of consciousness. Examination reveals neck stiffness and a positive Kernig's sign (irritation of the sciatic nerve roots causes pain on extending the knee with the hip flexed). Papilloedema may be present, sometimes accompanied by retinal and subhyaloid haemorrhages. Some patients have experienced small warning headaches a few days before the major bleed.

Investigation
COMPUTERIZED TOMOGRAPHY shows subarachnoid or intraventricular blood in 95%.

LUMBAR PUNCTURE is indicated only if there is diagnostic difficulty after CT. The CSF is uniformly blood-stained in the early stages and, after some days, develops a yellow discoloration (xanthochromia).

Patients who are potentially fit for surgery should be referred urgently to a neurosurgical unit for cerebral angiography to establish the source of bleeding.

Management

Immediate management consists of bed rest and supportive measures with cautious control of hypertension. Oral or intravenous nimodipine (a calcium channel blocker) is given to reduce cerebral artery spasm, an important cause of ischaemia and further neurological deterioration. Surgery (clipping the neck of the aneurysm at craniotomy) is indicated for patients likely to make a reasonable recovery.

Prognosis

Approximately 50% of patients die suddenly or soon after the haemorrhage. A further 10–20% die in the early weeks in hospital from further bleeding. The outcome is variable in the survivors; some patients are left with a severe neurological deficit.

Subdural haematoma

Subdural haematoma (SDH) occurs when blood accumulates in the subdural space following rupture of a vein running from the hemisphere to the sagittal sinus. It is almost always the result of head injury, often minor, and the latent interval between injury and symptoms may be weeks or months. Elderly patients and alcoholics are particularly susceptible because they are accident prone and their atrophic brains make the connecting veins more susceptible to rupture. The main clinical symptoms are headache, drowsiness and confusion which may fluctuate. The diagnosis is usually made on CT and treatment is by surgical removal of the haematoma.

Extradural haemorrhage

Extradural haematomas are caused by injuries that fracture the temporal bone and rupture the underlying middle meningeal artery. Clinically there is the picture of a head injury with a brief period of unconsciousness followed by a lucid interval of recovery. This is then followed by rapid deterioration with focal neurological signs and a deterioration in conscious level if surgical drainage is not carried out.

EPILEPSY AND OTHER CAUSES OF RECURRENT LOSS OF CONSCIOUSNESS

Epilepsy

An epileptic seizure is a convulsion or transient abnormal event experienced by the subject as a result of a paroxysmal discharge of cerebral neurons. Epilepsy by definition is the continuing tendency to have such seizures.

Epidemiology

Epilepsy is a common condition with 3% of the UK population having two or more seizures during their lives.

Classification
Epilepsy is classified according to the clinical type of seizure (Table 14.8). They are broadly divided into generalized seizures in which abnormal electrical activity is widespread in the brain, and partial seizures in which the electrical abnormality is focal (e.g. temporal lobe), although these may later become generalized.

TONIC–CLONIC: there is a sudden onset of a rigid tonic phase followed by a convulsion (clonic phase) in which the muscles jerk rhythmically. The episode lasts typically for seconds to minutes, may be associated with tongue biting and incontinence, and is followed by a period of drowsiness or coma.

Table 14.8 The classification of epilepsy

Generalized seizures
Tonic–clonic seizures (*grand mal*)
Absence seizures (*petit mal*)
Myoclonic seizures (rare form of epilepsy with involuntary muscle jerks)

Partial seizures
Simple partial seizures (no impairment of consciousness),
e.g. jacksonian seizures
Complex partial seizures (with impairment of consciousness),
e.g. temporal lobe epilepsy

TYPICAL ABSENCES (PETIT MAL): this is usually a disorder of childhood in which the child ceases activity, stares and pales for a only few seconds. It is characterized by 3-Hz spike and wave activity on the electroencephalogram (EEG).

JACKSONIAN (MOTOR) SEIZURES: these simple partial seizures originate in the motor cortex and result in jerking movements, typically beginning in the corner of the mouth or thumb and index finger and spreading to involve the limbs on the opposite side of the epileptic focus. Paralysis of the involved limbs may follow for several hours (Todd's paralysis).

TEMPORAL LOBE SEIZURES: these complex partial seizures are associated with olfactory and visual hallucinations, feelings of unreality (*jamais-vu*) or undue familiarity (*déjà-vu*) with the surroundings.

Precipitating factors
Flashing lights or a flickering television screen may provoke an attack in susceptible patients.

Aetiology
No cause for epilepsy is found in over 75% of patients. About 30% of patients have a first-degree relative with epilepsy although the exact mode of inheritance is unknown. Head

injury, brain surgery, cerebral tumours and infarction are common predisposing factors. Inflammatory conditions of the brain such as encephalitis, chronic meningitis (e.g. TB) and cerebral abscess may sometimes present initially with seizures. Drug overdose, alcohol withdrawal and metabolic disturbances, e.g. hypoglycaemia, hypoxia, hypocalcaemia and hyponatraemia, are other causes.

Investigations
The diagnosis is often made clinically; a detailed description of the attack from an eye witness is invaluable.

The ELECTROENCEPHALOGRAM (EEG) is the single most useful test in the diagnosis of epilepsy but the recording is frequently normal between attacks. During a seizure, the EEG is almost always abnormal and is shown typically by a cortical spike focus (e.g. in a temporal lobe) or by generalized spike and wave activity.

CT OR MAGNETIC RESONANCE IMAGING should be performed in all patients other than children to exclude an underlying lesion. Even in adults, however, the pick-up rate for treatable lesions is very low.

Management
The emergency treatment is to ensure that the patient harms him- or herself as little as possible and that the airway remains patent.

Table 14.9 A typical scheme for anticonvulsant treatment

Seizure type	Drug	Major side effects of drug treatment
Generalized tonic–clonic seizures	Phenytoin	Rashes, blood dyscrasias, lymphadenopathy
Generalized absence seizures	Sodium valproate	Anorexia, hair loss, liver damage
Partial seizures	Carbamazepine Sodium valproate	Rashes, leukopenia See above

Anticonvulsant drugs are indicated in recurrent seizures; some authorities will treat after a single seizure. Phenytoin, carbamazepine and sodium valproate are generally the most effective drugs prescribed, although phenobarbitone, primidone and clonazepam are also used. Table 14.9 gives a suggested scheme for treatment and lists the idiosyncratic side effects (i.e. non-dose related) which tend to be more common than dose-related effects. Intoxication with all anticonvulsants causes a syndrome of ataxia, nystagmus and dysarthria. Side effects of chronic administration of phenytoin (gum hypertrophy, hypertrichosis, osteomalacia and folate deficiency) are reduced by maintaining serum levels within the therapeutic range. Phenytoin is a potent hepatic enzyme inducer and will reduce efficacy of the contraceptive pill.

Vigabatrin and lamotrigine are new drugs used in patients not satisfactorily controlled with other antiepileptics.

The question of withdrawal of drug therapy is often raised by patients. Gradual withdrawal of drugs should only be considered when the patient has been seizure-free for at least 2 years. Many patients will have further fits resulting in a threat to employment and driving (see below).

NEUROSURGICAL TREATMENT (e.g. amputation of the anterior temporal lobe) may be of value in those with poorly controlled epilepsy with a clearly defined focus of abnormal electrical activity.

ADVICE TO PATIENTS
Patients should restrict their lives as little as possible but follow simple advice, e.g. avoid swimming alone, avoid dangerous sports, e.g. rock climbing, leave the door open when taking a bath. In the UK patients with epilepsy (whether on or off treatment) may drive a motor vehicle (but not a heavy goods or public service vehicle), provided that they have had a seizure-free period of 2 years or seizures have only occurred at night for the last 3 years.

Status epilepticus

Status epilepticus is a medical emergency which exists when seizures follow each other without recovery of consciousness. When grand mal seizures follow one another, there is a significant risk of death from cardiorespiratory failure. Management is summarized in Table 14.10.

Table 14.10 Management and investigation of status epilepticus

GENERAL MEASURES
Remove false teeth, insert oropharyngeal tube, give 60% oxygen; 50 ml of 50% glucose i.v. if hypoglycaemia a possibility

DIAZEPAM
Intravenous injection (10 mg) followed by infusion 200 mg/l over 24 hours
Rectal solution (10 mg) if intravenous access difficult

START REGULAR ANTICONVULSANT THERAPY, e.g. oral phenytoin

IF SEIZURES CONTINUE
Chlormethiazole (0.8%) or phenytoin infusion
Consider transfer to ITU, paralyse and ventilate

INVESTIGATIONS
Serum anticonvulsant levels, blood glucose, serum electrolytes and calcium. Consider urgent CT if new presentation of epilepsy

Other causes of recurrent attacks of disturbed consciousness

Episodes of transient disturbance of consciousness are common clinical problems (Table 14.11). Differentiation of seizures from other disorders often depends entirely on the medical history. An eye witness account is invaluable.

A simple faint occurs as a result of reflex bradycardia and peripheral and splanchnic vasodilatation. Fear, pain and prolonged standing are the principal causes. Fainting almost never occurs in the recumbent position. Rapid recovery from the attack and absence of jerking movements or incontinence of urine suggest a faint. Syncope may occur after micturition in men (particularly at night) and when the venous return to the heart is obstructed by breath holding and severe coughing. Carotid sinus syncope is thought to be the result of excessive sensitivity of the sinus to external pressure. It may occur in elderly patients who lose consciousness on touching the neck.

Table 14.11 Common causes of attacks of altered consciousness and falls in adults

Syncope
   'Simple faint'
   Cough
   Effort
   Micturition
   Carotid sinus

Epilepsy
   Narcolepsy and cataplexy

Transient ischaemic attacks

Psychogenic attacks
   Panic attacks
   Hyperventilation

Cardiac arrhythmias

Postural hypotension

Hypoglycaemia

Postural hypotension occurs on standing in those with impaired autonomic reflexes, e.g. elderly people, in autonomic neuropathy and with some drugs (phenothiazines, tricyclic antidepressants).

Narcolepsy is characterized by periods of irresistible sleep in inappropriate circumstances. Cataplexy is a related condition in which sudden loss of tone develops in the lower limbs with preservation of consciousness. Attacks are set off by sudden surprise or emotion.

EXTRAPYRAMIDAL DISEASE – PARKINSON'S DISEASE AND OTHER MOVEMENT DISORDERS

The extrapyramidal system is a general term for the basal ganglia and their connections with other brain areas, particularly those concerned with movement. The overall function of this system is the initiation and modulation of movement. Clinically, extrapyramidal disorders are broadly classified into the akinetic–rigid syndromes, where there is loss of movement with increase in muscle tone, and dyskinesias where there are added movements outside voluntary control (Table 14.12). Parkinson's disease is the most common of these movement disorders.

Table 14.12 A classification of movement disorders

Akinetic–rigid syndromes
Idiopathic Parkinson's disease
Drug-induced parkinsonism, e.g. phenothiazines
MPTP-induced parkinsonism
Postencephalitic parkinsonism
'Parkinsonism plus'
Childhood akinetic–rigid syndromes, e.g.Wilson's disease and athetoid cerebral palsy

Dyskinesias
Benign essential tremor
Chorea
Hemiballismus
Myoclonus
Tick or 'habit spasms'
Torsion dystonias

MPTP, methylphenyl tetrahydropyridine.

Akinetic rigid syndromes

Idiopathic Parkinson's disease

The clinical features of Parkinson's disease principally result from depletion of dopamine-containing neurons in the substantia nigra of the basal ganglia and relative excess of acetylcholine stimulation.

Epidemiology

The disease usually presents in elderly people, the prevalence rising to 1 in 200 in those over 70 years.

Aetiology

The cause of the disease is unknown. MPTP (methylphenyl tetrahydropyridine, an impurity produced during illegal synthesis of opiates) produces severe and irreversible parkinsonism. Survivors of an encephalitis epidemic (encephalitis lethargica 1918–1930), which was presumed to be a viral disease, developed parkinsonism. There is no evidence, however, that idiopathic Parkinson's disease is caused by an environmental toxin or an infective agent.

Clinical features
There is a combination of tremor, rigidity and akinesia (slow movements), together with changes in posture. The features of Parkinson's disease may be unilateral initially but the disease subsequently progresses to involve both sides of the body.

- TREMOR. This is a characteristic 4–7 Hz rest tremor (compare cerebellar disease), usually most obvious in the hands ('pill rolling' of the thumb and fingers), improved by voluntary movement and made worse by anxiety

- RIGIDITY refers to the increase in tone in the limbs and trunk. The limbs resist passive extension throughout movement (*lead-pipe rigidity* or *cog-wheel* when combined with tremor), in contrast to the hypertonia of an upper motor neuron lesion (page 460) where resistance falls away as the movement continues (*clasp-knife*)

- AKINESIA. There is difficulty in initiating movement (starting to walk or rising from a chair). The face is expressionless and unblinking and may give the appearance of depression. Speech is slow and monotonous. The writing becomes small (micrographia) and tends to tail off at the end of a line

- POSTURAL CHANGES. A stoop is characteristic and the gait is shuffling, festinant and with poor arm swinging. The posture is sometimes called 'simian' to describe the forward flexion, immobility of the arms and lack of facial expression. Balance is poor with a tendency to fall

Other features include dribbling of saliva, dysphagia, constipation, depression and dementia in the later stages. There is gradual progression of the disease over 10–15 years with death resulting most commonly from bronchopneumonia.

Investigations
The diagnosis is clinical. Investigations for other akinetic–rigid syndromes are only necessary in an atypical case, e.g. a young patient.

Management
LEVODOPA
The treatment of choice is the dopamine precursor, levodopa (L-dopa) in combination with a peripheral decarboxylase inhibitor, e.g. Madopar (L-dopa plus benserazide) or Sinemet (L-dopa plus carbidopa). This combined therapy reduces the peripheral side effects, principally nausea, of L-dopa and its metabolites. Over the years therapy may become less

effective even with increasing doses. Patients may also switch between periods of dopamine-induced dyskinesias (choreas and dystonic movements) and periods of immobility ('on–off' syndrome). This problem may be ameliorated by: slow release L-dopa, frequent small doses of L-dopa or the addition of other anti-parkinsonian drugs.

OTHER TREATMENTS

● Bromocriptine, a dopamine agonist

● Selegiline – a type B monoamine oxidase inhibitor – inhibits the catabolism of dopamine in the brain

● Amantadine increases synthesis and release of dopamine and has a weak antiparkinsonian effect

● Anticholinergic drugs, e.g. benzhexol have most effect on tremor and little effect on akinesia. They often cause mental confusion

SURGICAL TREATMENT

Surgery to transplant dopamine-producing cells (fetal or autologous adrenal medulla) has not produced significant clinical improvement.

Other akinetic–rigid syndromes

DRUG-INDUCED PARKINSONISM

Reserpine, phenothiazines and butyrophenones block dopamine receptors and may induce a parkinsonian syndrome with slowness and rigidity, but usually with little tremor. These syndromes tend not to progress, they respond poorly to L-dopa and the correct management is to stop the drug.

'PARKINSONISM PLUS'

This describes rare disorders in which there is parkinsonism and evidence of a separate pathology. Progressive supranuclear palsy is the most common disorder and consists of axial rigidity, dementia and signs of parkinsonism, together with a striking inability to move the eyes vertically or laterally. There is a poor response to L-dopa.

Dyskinesias

Benign essential tremor

This is usually a familial (autosomal dominant) tremor of the arms and head (titubation) which occurs most frequently in elderly people. Unlike the tremor of Parkinson's disease, it is not usually present at rest but is most obvious when the hands adopt a posture such as holding a glass or a spoon. It is made worse by anxiety and improved by alcohol and propranolol.

Chorea

Chorea is a continuous flow of jerky quasi-purposive movements, flitting from one part of the body to another. They may interfere with voluntary movements but cease during sleep. The causes of chorea are listed in Table 14.13. Treatment is with phenothiazines or tetrabenazine.

Table 14.13 Causes of chorea

Huntington's disease
Sydenham's chorea (see Rheumatic fever)
Benign hereditary chorea in elderly people
Drug induced
    Phenytoin
    L-Dopa
    Alcohol
Systemic disease
    Thyrotoxicosis
    Systemic lupus erythematosus
    Pregnancy (chorea gravidarum)
Other CNS diseases
    Stroke
    Trauma
    Tumour

HUNTINGTON'S DISEASE

Huntington's disease is a rare autosomal dominant condition with full penetrance; the abnormal gene is on the short arm of chromosome 4. There is loss of neurons within the basal ganglia leading to depletion of GABA (γ-aminobutyric acid) and acetylcholine but sparing dopamine. Symptoms begin in middle age and there is then a relentlessly progressive course with chorea and personality change preceding dementia and death. There is no treatment which arrests progression of the disease, and the management is symptomatic treatment of chorea and genetic counselling of family members.

Hemiballismus

Hemiballismus (also called hemiballism) describes violent swinging movements of one side of the body, usually caused by infarction or haemorrhage in the contralateral subthalamic nucleus. Treatment is with tetrabenazine.

Myoclonus

Myoclonus is the sudden, involuntary jerking of a single muscle or a group of muscles. The most common example is benign essential myoclonus which refers to the sudden jerking of a limb or the body on falling asleep. Myoclonus may also occur with epilepsy and some encephalopathies.

Tics

Tics are brief, repeated stereotypical movements usually involving the face and shoulders. Unlike other involuntary movements it is usually possible for the patient to control tics.

Dystonias

Dystonias are prolonged spasms of muscle contraction. They may occasionally occur as a symptom of neurological disease, e.g. Wilson's disease, but are usually of unknown cause and occur without other neurological problems, e.g. blepharospasm (spasms of forced blinking) or spasmodic torticollis (the head is turned and held to one side or drawn backwards or forwards). The treatment of choice for many dystonias is the injection of minute amounts of botulinum toxin into the muscle. Acute dystonic reactions are seen with phenothiazines, butyrophenones and metoclopramide and can occur after a single dose of the drug. Spasmodic torticollis, trismus and oculogyric crises (i.e. episodes of sustained upward gaze) may occur. Acute dystonias respond promptly to the intravenous injection of an anticholinergic drug (benztropine 1–2 mg).

MULTIPLE SCLEROSIS

Multiple sclerosis (MS) is a common disease of unknown cause in which there are multiple areas of demyelination within the brain and spinal cord. These are 'disseminated in time and place' (hence the old name 'disseminated sclerosis').

Epidemiology

The most common age of onset is between 20 and 35 years, the disease being more common in women. The prevalence varies widely (6 per 10 000 in England); it is rare in tropical countries.

Aetiology

The aetiology is unknown; viruses and autoimmune mechanisms have been implicated. The disease is more common in family members, although there is no clear-cut pattern of inheritance.

Pathology

The essential features are perivenular plaques of demyelination which have a predilection for the following sites within the brain:

- Optic nerves
- Brain stem and cerebellar connections
- Cervical cord
- Periventricular region

The peripheral nerves are never affected.

Clinical features

Symptoms are variable and characteristically appear suddenly before resolving partially or completely. Inflammation of the optic nerve produces blurred vision and pain in and around the eye. A lesion in the optic nerve head produces disc swelling (optic neuritis) and pallor (optic atrophy) following the attack. When inflammation occurs in the optic nerve further away from the eye (retrobulbar neuritis) there are often no ophthalmoscopic features. Brainstem demyelination produces diplopia, vertigo, dysphagia and nystagmus.

In some patients there will only be one or two attacks with little residual neurological deficit and they remain very well for years. At the other extreme, in some patients, an increasing neurological deficit accumulates and the final stages are characterized by spastic tetraparesis, ataxia, brainstem signs, blindness, incontinence and dementia. Death follows from recurrent urinary tract infection, uraemia and bronchopneumonia.

Differential diagnosis

Initially individual plaques (e.g. in the optic nerve, brain stem or cord) may cause diagnostic difficulty and must be distinguished from compressive, inflammatory, mass or vascular lesions. In young patients with a relapsing and remitting course, the diagnosis is straightforward as few other diseases produce this clinical picture.

Investigations

The diagnosis is made on the basis of clinical findings taken in combination with the findings on investigation.

RADIOLOGY. MRI is the first-line investigation and shows plaques, particularly in the periventricular area and brain stem.

ELECTROPHYSIOLOGICAL TESTS. Visual, auditory and somatosensory evoked potentials may be prolonged even in the absence of any past or present visual symptoms.

CSF is not usually obtained as the diagnosis is made with MRI or evoked potentials. Protein concentration and white cell count are raised. The IgG portion of the total protein is increased and electrophoresis reveals oligoclonal bands which indicate the production of immunoglobulin (to unknown antigens) within the CNS.

Management

Treatment of MS is largely supportive. Short courses of ACTH or corticosteroids may promote remission in relapse, but do not influence the outlook in the long term. Physiotherapy and occupational therapy maintain mobility of joints and muscle relaxants (e.g baclofen, dantrolene and benzodiazepines) reduce the discomfort and pain of spasticity. Urinary catheterization is eventually needed for those with bladder involvement.

Subcutaneous administration of β-interferon has recently been shown to reduce frequency of exacerbations of MRI lesions in some patients. Further studies are in progress to define its role in treatment.

INFECTIVE AND INFLAMMATORY DISEASE

Meningitis ND

Meningitis (inflammation of the meninges) can be caused by infection, drugs and contrast media, malignant cells and blood (following subarachnoid haemorrhage). The term is, however, usually reserved for inflammation caused by infective agents (Table 14.14).

Table 14.14 Infective causes of meningitis in the UK

Bacteria	*Neisseria meningitidis**
	Steptococcus pneumoniae*
	Haemophilus influenzae
	Staphylococcus aureus
	Listeria monocytogenes
	Gram-negative bacilli
	Mycobacterium tuberculosis
	Treponema pallidum
	Leptospira spp.
Viruses	Enteroviruses (echo, Coxsackie, polio)
	Mumps
	Herpes simplex virus
	HIV
	Epstein–Barr virus
Fungi	*Cryptococcus neoformans*
	Candida spp.

*These organisms account for most cases of pyogenic meningitis in otherwise healthy adults.

Clinical features
There is usually a rapid onset of severe headache, photophobia (intolerance of light) and vomiting with malaise, fever and rigors. Neck stiffness and Kernig's sign are usually present. Consciousness is usually not impaired, although the patient may be delirious with a high fever. Papilloedema may occur. The presence of drowsiness, lateralizing signs and cranial nerve lesions indicate the presence of a complication, e.g. venous sinus thrombosis, severe cerebral oedema or cerebral abscess.

ACUTE BACTERIAL MENINGITIS. Most cases in adults are caused by meningococci. The organism is carried asymptomatically in the nasopharynx and spread from person to person by respiratory droplets or direct spread. Meningitis occurs after the organism invades the blood stream from the nasopharynx, to reach the meninges. Characteristically, there is a sudden onset of the disease with high fever and a petechial/purpuric skin rash is often present. In patients with fulminant meningococcal septicaemia, there are often large ecchymoses and gangrenous skin lesions.

The pneumococcus is the most common cause of meningitis in elderly people and may complicate pneumonia or other respiratory tract infection. Direct spread of the organism may occur from an infected middle ear or via a skull fracture. The features of meningitis appear rapidly and the mortality rate may be as high as 30%.

VIRAL MENINGITIS is usually a benign self-limiting condition lasting for about 4–10 days. There are no serious sequelae.

TUBERCULOUS MENINGITIS is often a chronic illness with vague symptoms of headache, lassitude, anorexia and vomiting. Signs of meningism may be absent or appear late in the course of the disease.

Investigations

The diagnosis is confirmed by lumbar puncture and urgent CSF microscopy and analysis for protein and glucose concentration. Typical changes are shown in Table 14.15. However, if there are focal neurological signs or loss of consciousness, CT of the brain is the initial investigation to rule out an intracranial mass lesion, e.g. abscess. Additional investigations include blood cultures, blood glucose and viral serology.

Table 14.15 Typical changes in the CSF in meningitis

	Normal	Viral	Pyogenic	Tuberculous
Appearance	Clear	Clear/turbid	Turbid/purulent	Turbid/viscous
Mononuclear (*cells/mm^3*)	< 5	10–100	< 50	100–300
Polymorph (*cells/mm^3*)	Nil	Nil	200–3000	0–200
Protein (g/l)	0.2–0.4	0.4–0.8	0.5–2.0	0.5–3.0
Glucose (*% blood glucose*)	> 50	> 50	< 50	< 30

Management

Bacterial meningitis is an emergency with a high mortality rate (15%), even with treatment. If the diagnosis is suspected clinically, antibiotics must be given immediately with subsequent urgent investigations. As a result of the emergence of resistant organisms, cefotaxime is replacing penicillins and chloramphenicol for the initial treatment of bacterial meningitis. Subsequent treatment is given depending on the results of culture and the antibiotic sensitivies of the organism. In children with haemophilus meningitis, dexamethasone reduces meningeal inflammation and limits sensorineural hearing loss in survivors. There are few data in adults and it is not recommended.

Tuberculous meningitis is treated for at least 9 months with triple antituberculous therapy (page 344).

NOTIFICATION
All cases of meningitis must be notified (by law) to the local Public Health Authority; this allows contact tracing and provides data for epidemiological studies.

MENINGOCOCCAL PROPHYLAXIS
Oral rifampicin is given to patients and close (usually household) contacts to eradicate nasopharyngeal carriage of the organism.

Encephalitis

Encephalitis is inflammation of the brain parenchyma. It is caused by a wide variety of viruses and may also occur in bacterial and other infections. In certain groups (e.g. homosexuals, intravenous drug abusers) HIV infection and opportunistic organisms (e.g. *Toxoplasma gondii* in patients with full-blown AIDS) are important causes.

Acute viral encephalitis

A viral aetiology is often presumed, although not confirmed serologically or by culture. In the UK the common organisms are Echo, Coxsackie, mumps and herpes simplex viruses.

Clinical features
Many of these infections cause a mild self-limiting illness with headache and drowsiness. Less commonly the illness is severe with focal signs (e.g. hemiparesis, dysphasia), seizures and coma. Severe encephalitis is most commonly caused by herpes simplex virus (HSV1) which has a mortality rate of about 20% even with treatment.

Investigations
VIRAL SEROLOGY of blood and CSF may identify the causative virus.

COMPUTERIZED TOMOGRAPHY may show areas of oedema.

EEG often shows slow-wave activity.

Treatment
Suspected herpes simplex encephalitis is immediately treated with intravenous acyclovir. If the patient is in a coma the prognosis is poor whether or not treatment is given.

Intracranial abscesses

An abscess may develop in the epidural, subdural or intracerebral sites. Epidural abscesses are uncommon, subdural abscess presents similarly to intracerebral abscess (see below).

Cerebral abscess

Cerebral abscess may follow direct spread of organisms from a skull fracture or a focus of infection in the paranasal sinuses or middle ear. Alternatively haematogenous spread of infection may occur from the lung (e.g. bronchiectasis), heart (e.g. endocarditis) or bone (e.g. osteomyelitis). Frequently no cause is found. The most common organisms are streptococci, *Bacteroides* spp., staphylococci and enterobacteria. Infection with tubercle bacilli may result in chronic caseating granulomata (*tuberculomas*) presenting as intracranial mass lesions.

Clinical features

Presenting features include fever, seizures, focal neurological signs, and symptoms and signs of raised intracranial pressure (page 490).

Investigations

CT or MRI will usually outline the abscess. Lumbar puncture is not performed if an abscess is suspected because of the danger of coning in the presence of raised intracranial pressure (page 490).

Management

Treatment involves a combination of intravenous antibiotics and surgical drainage.

Neurosyphilis

Syphilis is described on page 19. Neurosyphilis occurs late in the course of untreated infection. It is now rarely seen in the UK because most cases of syphilis are recognized in the early stages and treated with penicillin. The different clinical syndromes (summarized in Table 14.16) may occur alone or in combination.

Management

Treatment is with parenteral benzylpenicillin for 3 weeks which may arrest, but not reverse, neurological disease. High-dose steroid cover is usually given to reduce the severity of a Jarisch–Herxheimer reaction (page 20).

INTRACRANIAL TUMOURS

Primary intracranial tumours account for 10% of all neoplasms and about one-quarter of all intracranial tumours are metastatic. Primary intracranial tumours may be derived from the skull itself, from any of the structures lying within it

Table 14.16 The clinical syndromes of neurosyphilis

Asymptomatic neurosyphilis	Positive CSF serology without symptoms or signs
Meningovascular syphilis 3–4 years after primary infection	Subacute meningitis with cranial nerve palsies and papilloedema Raised intracranial pressure and focal deficits caused by an expanding intracranial mass (gumma) Paraparesis caused by spinal meningovasculitis
General paralysis of the insane 10–15 years after primary infection	Progressive dementia Brisk reflexes Extensor plantar responses Tremor
Tabes dorsalis 10–35 years after primary infection (caused by demyelination in the dorsal roots)	Lightning pains – short, sharp stabbing pains in the legs Ataxia, loss of reflexes and sensory loss Neuropathic joints (Charcot's joints) Argyll Robertson pupils (page 451) Ptosis and optic atrophy

or from their tissue precursors. They may be malignant on histological investigation but rarely metastasize outside the brain. The most common intracranial tumours occurring in adults are listed in Table 14.17.

Table 14.17 Relative frequency of intracranial tumours in adults on the basis of clinical presentation

Tumour	Relative frequency (%)

Primary malignant
   Astrocytoma
   Oligodendroglioma
	40

Benign
   Meningioma
   Neurofibroma
	30

Metastases
   Bronchus
   Breast
   Stomach
   Prostate
   Thyroid
   Kidney
	25

Clinical features

The clinical features of a cerebral tumour are the result of the following:

- Progressive focal neurological deficit
- Raised intracranial pressure
- Focal or generalized epilepsy

NEUROLOGICAL DEFICIT is the result of a mass effect of the tumour and surrounding cerebral oedema. The deficit depends on the site of the tumour, e.g. a frontal lobe tumour will initially cause personality change, apathy and intellectual deterioration. Subsequent involvement of the frontal speech area and motor cortex produce expressive aphasia and hemiparesis. Rapidly growing tumours destroy cerebral tissue and loss of function is an early feature.

RAISED INTRACRANIAL PRESSURE produces headache, vomiting and papilloedema. The headache is typically most severe on waking and decreases as the patient stands up, thus lowering intracranial pressure. It is made worse by coughing, straining and sneezing.

As the tumour grows there is downward displacement of the brain and pressure on the brain stem, causing drowsiness which progresses eventually to respiratory depression, bradycardia, coma and death.

Distortion of normal structures at a distance from the growing tumour leads to focal neurological signs (false localizing signs). The most common are a third and sixth cranial nerve palsy (page 453) resulting from stretching of the nerves by downward displacement of the temporal lobes.

EPILEPSY. Fits may be generalized or partial in nature. The site of origin of a partial seizure is frequently of value in localization.

Differential diagnosis

The main differential is from other intracranial mass lesions (cerebral abscess, tuberculoma, subdural haematoma and intracranial haematoma) and a stroke which may have an identical clinical presentation.

Investigations

RADIOLOGY. CT with contrast enhancement is the investigation of choice when a tumour is suspected. MRI is of particular value in investigation of tumours of the posterior fossa and brain stem. Cerebral angiography is sometimes necessary to define the site or blood supply of a mass, particularly if surgery is planned. Plain skull radiographs are rarely of diagnostic value, with the exception of pituitary tumours.

OTHER INVESTIGATIONS. These include routine tests, e.g. chest radiograph if metastatic disease is suspected. Lumbar puncture and examination of the CSF are rarely helpful and are contraindicated in this situation. The danger is of immediate herniation of the cerebellar tonsils, impaction within the foramen magnum and compression of the brain stem ('coning').

Management
SURGERY. Surgical exploration and either biopsy or removal of the mass is usually carried out to ascertain its nature. Some benign tumours, e.g. meningiomas, can be removed in their entirety without unacceptable damage to surrounding structures.

RADIOTHERAPY is usually recommended for gliomas and radiosensitive metastases.

MEDICAL TREATMENT. This is palliative to reduce symptoms related to cerebral oedema and raised intracranial pressure. Dexamethasone (either orally or intravenously), a very potent corticosteroid, may produce dramatic improvement in symptoms. Prognosis is very poor in patients with malignant tumours with only 50% surviving 1 year.

HYDROCEPHALUS

Hydrocephalus is a condition marked by an excessive amount of CSF within the cranium. CSF is produced in the cerebral ventricles and normally flows downwards into the central canal of the spinal cord and then out into the subarachnoid space, from where it is reabsorbed. Hydrocephalus occurs when there is obstruction to the outflow of CSF; rarely it is the result of increased production of CSF.

Aetiology
In children, hydrocephalus may be caused by a congenital malformation of the brain (e.g. Arnold–Chiari malformation), meningitis or haemorrhage causing obstruction to the flow of CSF. In adults hydrocephalus is caused by:

- A late presentation of a congenital malformation
- Cerebral tumours in the posterior fossa or brain stem which obstruct the aqueduct or fourth ventricle outflow
- Subarachnoid haemorrhage, head injury and meningitis
- Normal-pressure hydrocephalus in which there is dilatation of the cerebral ventricles without signs of raised intracranial pressure. It presents in elderly people with dementia, urinary incontinence and ataxia

Clinical features
The features are of headache, vomiting and papilloedema caused by raised intracranial pressure. There may be ataxia and bilateral pyramidal signs.

Management
Treatment is by the surgical insertion of a shunt between the ventricles and the right atrium or peritoneum (ventriculo-atrial or ventriculoperitoneal).

HEADACHE

Headache is a common symptom and usually of little clinical significance. In most patients presenting with headache, there are no abnormal physical signs so the diagnosis depends entirely upon an accurate history. The causes of headache can be broadly divided depending on their onset and subsequent course (Table 14.18).

Table 14.18 Causes of headache

Acute severe (onset in hours)	Subarachnoid haemorrhage Migraine Meningitis Head injury Drugs, e.g. alcohol, glyceryl trinitrate
Subacute onset (onset in days to weeks)	Intracranial mass lesion Encephalitis Viral meningitis Giant cell arteritis
Recurrent/chronic	Migraine Tension headache Sinusitis Migranous neuralgia

Tension headaches
Tension headaches are the most common cause of chronic headache.

Clinical features
Pain is described as a pressure behind the eyes, a throbbing headache or a tight band around the head. Headaches may be precipitated by stress, noise, concentrated visual effort and depression.

Aetiology
There is no underlying pathology and the basis for the pain is unclear. Similar headaches may occur after head injury (often minor) when they can be associated with dizziness, malaise and depression.

Management
This involves reassurance, avoiding precipitating events and antidepressants if indicated.

Migraine

Migraine is the term used for recurrent headache associated with both visual and gastrointestinal disturbance; in spite of the origin of the word, it does not invariably mean unilateral headache.

Epidemiology
The prevalence of migraine is approximately 10%; some patients have a strong family history. Onset is usually before the age of 30 years.

Pathogenesis
The cause of migraine remains controversial. The headache is believed, by some, to result from vasodilatation or oedema of blood vessels with stimulation of nerve endings near affected extracranial meningeal arteries. The prodromal symptoms are the result of vasospasm and cerebral ischaemia. There is some evidence that the neurotransmitter serotonin is important in pathogenesis.

Clinical features
The classical symptoms of migraine are of transient prodromal symptoms followed after 15–60 minutes by a throbbing headache accompanied by nausea, vomiting and photophobia. Prodromal symptoms are usually visual: scotomata, unilateral blindness, hemianopic field loss, flashes and fortification spectra. Other prodromal symptoms include aphasia, tingling, numbness and weakness of one side of the body. Migraine may also occur without these prodromal symptoms. The most common way in which a migraine attack resolves is through sleep.

Differential diagnosis
The sudden onset of headache may be similar to meningitis or subarachnoid haemorrhage. The hemiplegic, visual and hemisensory symptoms must be distinguished from thromboembolic TIAs. In TIAs the maximum deficit is present immediately and headache is unusual (page 471).

Management
GENERAL MEASURES. Patients should avoid precipitating factors (chocolate, cheese, too much or too little sleep). Women on the oral contraceptive pill may be helped by stopping the drug or changing the brand.

TREATMENT OF THE ACUTE ATTACK
- Simple analgesia, e.g. paracetamol, and an antiemetic, e.g. metoclopramide, may be all that is necessary for many patients

- Sumatriptan is a serotonin or 5-hydroxytryptamine (5-HT1) agonist which constricts cranial arteries. It is used in patients not responding to simple analgesia and may be given orally or by subcutaneous injection. Occasionally patients have developed cardiac-like chest pain and rarely myocardial infarction after using sumatriptan. Its use is contraindicated in patients with ischaemic heart disease

- Ergotamine is less commonly used since the introduction of sumatriptan. It may be given orally, rectally, intravenously or by nasal inhalation. Its use is absolutely contraindicated in patients with ischaemic heart disease and peripheral vascular disease

PROPHYLAXIS. Prophylaxis is indicated for frequent attacks (> two per month) which do not respond rapidly to treatment. The options are:

- β-blockers, e.g. propranolol

- Serotonin antagonists – pizotifen and methysergide. An occasional side effect of methysergide is retroperitoneal fibrosis which precludes its use for more than 6 months

Giant cell arteritis (cranial arteritis, temporal arteritis)

This is a granulomatous arteritis of unknown aetiology occurring chiefly in those over the age of 60 years and affecting in particular the extradural arteries. Giant cell arteritis is closely related to polymyalgia rheumatica (page 179) and these can occur in the same patient.

Clinical features
There is headache, scalp tenderness (e.g. on combing the hair) and occasionally pain in the jaw and mouth which is characteristically worse on eating (jaw claudication). The superficial temporal artery is tender to touch, pulsation is soon lost and the artery becomes hard, tortuous and thickened. The great danger is sudden and irreversible blindness, caused by inflammation and occlusion of the ciliary and/or central retinal artery, which occurs in 25% of untreated cases. Systemic features include weight loss, malaise and a low-grade fever.

Investigations
ESR is almost always elevated > 50 mm/h.
FULL BLOOD COUNT may show a normochromic/normocytic anaemia.
HISTOLOGY. A temporal artery biopsy which can be performed under local anaesthetic usually confirms the diagnosis. However, the granulomatous changes may be patchy and therefore missed.

Management
High doses of steroids (oral prednisolone, initially 60–100 mg daily) should be started immediately in a patient with typical features and a temporal artery biopsy obtained as soon as possible (the histological changes remain for up to a week after starting treatment). The steroid dose is gradually reduced, guided by symptoms and the ESR, and can usually be stopped after some months to several years.

FACIAL PAIN

The face is richly supplied with pain-sensitive structures – the teeth, gums, sinuses, temporomandibular joints, jaws and eyes – disease of which causes facial pain. Trigeminal nerve lesions (see Table 14.1) may also present with facial pain and this is suggested by the presence of trigeminal sensory or motor loss on physical examination.

Trigeminal neuralgia
Trigeminal neuralgia (tic doloureux) is a condition of unknown cause, seen most commonly in old age.

Clinical features
Severe paroxysms of knife-like pain occur in one or more divisions of the trigeminal nerve (page 454), although rarely in the ophthalmic division. Each paroxysm is stereotyped, brought on by stimulation of a specific 'trigger zone' in the face. The stimuli may be minimal and include washing, shaving and eating. There are no objective physical signs and the diagnosis is based on the history.

Management
The anticonvulsant carbamazepine suppresses attacks in most patients. If this fails thermocoagulation of the trigeminal ganglion or section of the sensory division may be necessary.

Differential diagnosis
Similar pain may occur with structural lesions involving the trigeminal nerve. These lesions are often accompanied by physical signs, e.g. a depressed corneal reflex.

DISEASES OF THE SPINAL CORD

The spinal cord extends from C1 (its junction with the medulla) to the vertebral body of L1. The spinal canal below L1 is occupied by lumbar and sacral nerve roots which group together to form the cauda equina and ultimately extend into the pelvis and thigh (Figure 14.11). Paraplegia (weakness of both legs) is almost always caused by a spinal cord lesion as opposed to hemiplegia (weakness of one side of the body) which is usually the result of a lesion in the brain.

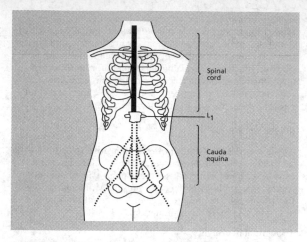

Figure 14.11 The spinal cord and cauda equina. (From Malcolm Parsons, *A Colour Atlas of Clinical Neurology*, Mosby-Wolfe, an imprint of Times Mirror International Publishers Ltd, London, UK, 1993.)

Spinal cord compression

Clinical features

Patients present with spastic paraparesis: there is upper motor neuron weakness in the legs (page 460), loss of sphincter control and sensory loss below the level of the lesion. The onset may be acute (hours to days) or chronic (weeks to months) depending on the cause.

Aetiology

The causes of spinal cord compression are listed in Table 14.19; the most common causes in developed countries are

Table 14.19 Causes of spinal cord compression

Vertebral body neoplasms	Metastases, e.g. from lung, breast, prostate
	Myeloma
Disc and vertebral lesions	Trauma
	Chronic degenerative disease
Inflammatory	Epidural abcess
	Tuberculosis (Pott's paraplegia)
	Granuloma
Spinal cord neoplasms	Primary cord neoplasm, e.g. glioma, neurofibroma
	Metastases
Rarities	Paget's disease, bone cysts, osteoporosis
	Epidural haemorrhage

highlighted. Spinal tuberculosis is a frequent cause in areas where TB is common, e.g. India, Asia, Africa.

Investigations

Urgent investigation is essential in a patient with suspected cord compression, especially with acute or subacute onset, because irreversible paraplegia may follow if the cord is not decompressed.

SPINAL RADIOGRAPHS may show degenerative bone disease and destruction of vertebrae by infection or neoplasm.

MRI identifies the cause and site of cord compression.

MYELOGRAPHY, sometimes with CT is an alternative to MRI.

Management

The treatment depends on the cause but in most cases initial treatment involves surgical decompression of the cord and stabilization of the spine.

Differential diagnosis

The differential diagnosis is from intrinsic lesions of the cord causing paraparesis. Transverse myelitis (acute inflammation of the cord resulting from viral infection, syphilis or radiation therapy), anterior spinal artery occlusion and multiple sclerosis may present with a rapid onset of paraparesis. A more insidious onset occurs with motor neuron disease, subacute combined degeneration of the cord and as a non-metastatic manifestation of malignancy.

Very rarely a parasagittal cortical lesion, e.g. meningioma may cause paraplegia.

Syringomyelia and syringobulbia

Fluid-filled cavities within the spinal cord (myelia) and brain stem (bulbia) are the essential features of these conditions.

Aetiology

The most frequent cause is blockage of CSF flow from the fourth ventricle in association with an Arnold–Chiari malformation (congenital herniation of the cerebellar tonsils through the foramen magnum). The normal pulsatile CSF pressure waves are transmitted to the delicate tissues of the cervical cord and brain stem, with secondary cavity formation. Hydrocephalus may also occur as a result of disturbed CSF flow.

Clinical features

Patients usually present in the third or fourth decade with pain and sensory loss (pain and temperature) in the upper limbs. The clinical features are demonstrated in Figure 14.12.

Investigation

MRI is the investigation of choice and demonstrates the intrinsic cavities.

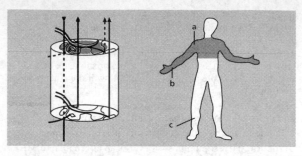

Figure 14.12 Production of physical signs in syringomyelia. Expanding cavities distend the cord. Pain and temperature (a) fibres crossing at that level are destroyed, but sensory fibres in the posterior columns (other sensory modalities) and those that enter the spinothalamic tract at a lower level are spared. Sensory loss is therefore 'dissociated' and confined to the upper trunk and limbs. Further extension damages the anterior horn cells (b), the pyramidal tracts (c) and the medulla, causing wasting in the hands, a spastic paraplegia, nystagmus and a bulbar palsy. (From Malcolm Parsons, *A Colour Atlas of Clinical Neurology*, Mosby-Wolfe, an imprint of Times Mirror International Publishers Ltd, London, UK, 1993.)

Treatment
Surgical decompression of the foramen magnum sometimes reduces the rate of deterioration.

Friedrich's ataxia

This is the most common of the hereditary spinocerebellar degenerations. There is a progressive degeneration of the spinocerebellar tracts and cerebellum causing cerebellar ataxia, dysarthria and nystagmus. Degeneration of the corticospinal tracts causes weakness and extensor plantars. The tendon reflexes are absent as a result of peripheral nerve damage. Loss of the dorsal columns causes absent joint position and vibration sense. Other features are pes cavus, optic atrophy, cardiomyopathy and death by middle age.

Cauda equina lesion

Spinal damage at or distal to L1 (a common cause is central prolapse of an intervertebral disc at the lumbosacral junction) injures the cauda equina which is formed by the lumbar and sacral nerve roots. This produces various mixtures of flaccid paralysis (compare spastic paralysis of a cord lesion above L1), sacral numbness, urinary retention and impotence.

Management of the paraplegic patient

Regular turning, ripple mattresses and water beds will help to prevent pressure sores. In the initial stages patients may need urinary catheterization and manual evacuation of faeces. This may become unnecessary as reflex emptying of the bladder and rectum develops. Passive physiotherapy is helpful in preventing limb contractures. Severe spasticity may be helped by dantrolene sodium, baclofen or diazepam. Many patients graduate to a wheelchair and maintain some degree of independence.

DEGENERATIVE DISEASES

Motor neuron disease

The symptoms of motor neuron disease (MND) are caused by a relentless and unexplained destruction of upper motor neurons and anterior horn cells in the brain and spinal cord which is usually fatal within 3 years.

It presents in middle age and is more common in men.

Clinical features
Three clinical patterns may be identified at diagnosis; however, as the disease progresses most patients develop a mixed picture.

- Progressive muscular atrophy is a predominantly lower motor neuron lesion of the cord causing weakness, wasting and fasciculation in the hands and arms
- Amyotrophic lateral sclerosis is a combination of disease of the lateral corticospinal tracts and anterior horn cells producing a progressive spastic tetraparesis or paraparesis with added lower motor neuron signs (wasting and fasciculation)
- Progressive bulbar palsy results from destruction of upper (*pseudobulbar palsy*) and lower (*bulbar palsy*) motor neurons in the lower cranial nerves. There is dysarthria, dysphagia with wasting and fasciculation of the tongue

There is no involvement of the sensory system or motor nerves to the eye and sphincters.

Investigations
The diagnosis is clinical. An EMG shows muscle denervation but this is not a specific finding.

Differential diagnosis
The most important differential is a cervical spine lesion which may present with upper and lower motor neuron signs in the arms and legs. It is often distinguished by the presence of sensory signs.

Management
There is no specific treatment and management is supportive.

Spinal muscular atrophies

This is a group of rare disorders which destroy the anterior horn cell of the spinal cord. Two forms present in adult life, causing a slowly progressive wasting and weakness of the limbs.

DISEASES OF THE PERIPHERAL NERVES

Mononeuropathies

Mononeuropathy is a process affecting a single nerve and multiple mononeuropathy (or mononeuritis multiplex) is a process affecting several or multiple nerves. Mono-neuropathy may be the result of acute compression particularly where the nerves are exposed anatomically (e.g. common peroneal nerve at the head of the fibula) or entrapment where the nerve passes through a relatively tight anatomical passage (e.g. the carpal tunnel). It may also be caused by direct damage, e.g. major trauma, surgery, penetrating injuries.

Carpal tunnel syndrome

Carpal tunnel syndrome is the most common entrapment neuropathy. It results from pressure on the median nerve as it passes through the carpal tunnel.

Aetiology
It is usually idiopathic but may be associated with hypothyroidism, diabetes mellitus, pregnancy, obesity, rheumatoid arthritis and acromegaly.

Clinical features
The history is of pain and paraesthesiae in the hand, typically worse at night which may wake the patient. On examination there may be no physical signs or weakness and wasting of the thenar muscles, and sensory loss of the palm and palmar aspects of the radial three and a half fingers. Tapping on the carpal tunnel may reproduce the pain (*Tinnel's sign*).

Management
Treatment with nocturnal splints or local steroid injections gives temporary relief. Surgical decompression is the definitive treatment unless the condition is likely to resolve (e.g. with pregnancy, obesity).

Compression neuropathies may also affect the ulnar nerve (at the elbow), the radial nerve (caused by pressure against the humerus) and the common peroneal nerve (resulting from pressure at the head of the fibula).

Mononeuritis multiplex

Mononeuritis multiplex often indicates a systemic disorder (Table 14.20); treatment is that of the underlying disease.

Table 14.20 Causes of mononeuritis multiplex

Diabetes mellitus
Leprosy (the most common cause worldwide)
Connective tissue disease
    Rheumatoid arthritis
    Systemic lupus erythematosus
    Polyarteritis nodosa
Sarcoidosis
Non-metastatic manifestation of malignancy
Amyloidosis
Neurofibromatosis
AIDS

Polyneuropathy

Polyneuropathy describes a diffuse, usually symmetrical, disease process which may be acute or chronic and may involve motor, sensory and autonomic nerves either alone or in combination. Sensory symptoms include numbness, tingling, 'pins and needles', pain in the extremities and unsteadiness on the feet. Numbness typically affects the distal arms and legs in a 'glove and stocking' distribution. Motor symptoms are usually those of weakness. Autonomic neuropathy causes postural hypotension, urinary retention, impotence, diarrhoea (or occasionally constipation), diminished sweating, impaired pupillary responses and cardiac arrhythmias.

Many varieties of neuropathy affect autonomic function to some degree but occasionally autonomic features predominate. This occurs in diabetes mellitus, amyloidosis and the Guillain–Barré syndrome. A classification of polyneuropathy is given in Table 14.21.

Table 14.21 Classification of polyneuropathy

Idiopathic (the majority of cases)

Postinfective (Guillain–Barré syndrome)

Drugs: isoniazid, nitrofurantoin, metronidazole, vincristine

Toxins: excess alcohol, lead poisoning

Metabolic: diabetes mellitus, uraemia, liver disease, amyloidosis

Vitamin deficiency: B_1 , B_6 , B_{12}

Non-metastatic manifestation of malignancy

Autonomic neuropathies

Neuropathies in connective tissue disease

Hereditary sensorimotor neuropathy

Peroneal muscular atrophy

Peroneal muscular atrophy (Charcot–Marie–Tooth disease) is a common clinical syndrome in which there is distal limb wasting and weakness that progresses over many years, mostly in the legs, with variable loss of sensation and reflexes. In advanced cases the distal wasting below the knees is so marked that the legs resemble 'inverted champagne bottles'. The most common form is inherited in an autosomal dominant fashion.

Postinfective polyneuropathy (Guillain–Barré syndrome)

This is the most common recognizable acute neuropathy and follows a viral infection in about 60% of cases.

Clinical features
There is weakness and numbness in the distal limbs which ascends over days or weeks. Disability ranges from mild to very severe with involvement of the respiratory and facial muscles. Autonomic features are sometimes seen.

Pathogenesis
It is thought to be caused by a cell-mediated immune response directed at normal peripheral myelin and this may be provoked in some cases by viral infection.

Investigations
The diagnosis is usually based on clinical grounds.

CSF PROTEIN is typically elevated with a normal sugar and cell count.

NERVE CONDUCTION STUDIES show slowing of motor conduction consistent with segmental demyelination.

Treatment
Treatment is generally supportive and ventilation may be required if the respiratory muscles are involved. Plasmapheresis or intravenous γ-globulin accelerates recovery and both are indicated in more severe disease. Corticosteroids are not of proven benefit.

Prognosis
Gradual recovery over months is the norm. Mortality rate as a result of respiratory, cardiac and autonomic complications is about 5–10%.

Vitamin deficiency neuropathies

THIAMINE (VITAMIN B$_1$)
Alcohol abuse is the most common cause of thiamine deficiency in the West. Presentation is with the Wernicke–Korsakoff syndrome (page 385). Severe deficiency causes the clinical syndrome of beri-beri (polyneuropathy, Wernicke's encephalopathy and cardiac failure), rarely seen in Western countries.

PYRIDOXINE (VITAMIN B$_6$)

Deficiency causes mainly a sensory neuropathy. It may be precipitated during isoniazid therapy (which complexes with pyridoxal phosphate) for tuberculosis in those who acetylate the drug slowly.

VITAMIN B$_{12}$

Deficiency causes the syndrome of subacute combined degeneration of the cord. This comprises distal sensory loss (particularly posterior column), absent ankle jerks (as a result of the neuropathy) and evidence of cord disease (exaggerated knee jerk reflexes, extensor plantar responses). Treatment is with intramuscular vitamin B$_{12}$ which reverses the peripheral nerve damage but has little effect on the CNS (cord and brain signs).

DISEASES OF VOLUNTARY MUSCLE

Myopathies

Weakness is the predominant feature of a myopathy. The myopathies are divided into those that are inherited (muscular dystrophies), inflammatory lesions (the most common is polymyositis, page 177) and those associated with drugs, toxins and endocrine disease (Table 14.22). The second group usually produces weakness of the limb girdles (proximal myopathy); however, severe hypokalaemia may produce a generalized flaccid weakness.

Table 14.22 Causes of a proximal myopathy

Prolonged high-dose steroid therapy
Cushing's syndrome
Thyrotoxicosis
Hypothyroidism (occasionally)
Osteomalacia
Hypokalaemia
Prolonged alcohol abuse
Other drugs, e.g. diamorphine, lithium, quinine, chloroquine

Muscular dystrophies

Muscular dystrophies are progressive genetically determined disorders of skeletal and sometimes cardiac muscle. The most common is Duchenne muscular dystrophy which presents in early childhood and progresses to severe disability with death in the late teens. The milder dystrophies present later in life and are summarized in Table 14.23.

Myasthenia gravis

Myasthenia gravis is an acquired condition characterized by weakness and fatiguability of proximal limb, ocular and bulbar muscles. The heart is not affected. It occurs most

Table 14.23 Limb girdle and facio-scapulo-humeral dystrophies

	Limb girdle	Facio-scapulo-humeral
Inheritance	Autosomal recessive	Autosomal dominant
Onset	10–20 years	10–40 years
Muscle affected	Shoulder and pelvic girdle	Face, shoulder and pelvic girdle
Progress	Severe disability in 20–25 years	Normal life expectancy
Pseudohypertrophy	Rare	Very rare
Serum CPK levels	Slightly raised	Slightly raised or normal

CPK, creatinine phosphate kinase.

commonly in the third decade and is twice as common in women as in men.

Aetiology
The cause is unknown. Serum IgG antibodies to acetylcholine receptors, in the postsynaptic membrane of the neuromuscular junction, cause receptor loss. Myasthenia gravis is associated with thymic hyperplasia in about 70% of patients under 40 years of age, and in about 10% a thymic tumour is found.

Clinical features
Fatiguability is the most important feature with the proximal limb muscles, extraocular muscles, and muscles of mastication, speech and facial expression being most commonly involved. The ocular muscles are the first to be involved in about 65% of patients, resulting in ptosis and complex ocular palsies.

Investigations
ACETYLCHOLINE RECEPTOR ANTIBODIES are specific for myasthenia gravis and found in the serum in 90% of cases of generalized myasthenia gravis.

TENSILON TEST is positive. (Injection of 10 mg edrophonium, an anticholinesterase, results in rapid temporary improvement in weakness).

NERVE STIMULATION TESTS show a characteristic decrement in evoked potential following stimulation of the motor nerve.

Management
Anticholinesterases (pyridostigmine, neostigmine) form the mainstay of treatment and the dose is determined by the patient's response.

IN PATIENTS WITHOUT THYMOMA
Anticholinesterase medication alone is given in mild disease. In patients under 45 years of age, with more severe disease, thymectomy is usually indicated. This results in improvement in about 65% of cases. Immunosuppresive treatment with

steroids and/or azathioprine should be considered in those who fail to respond to thymectomy.

IN PATIENTS WITH THYMOMA

Thymectomy is indicated in these patients because of the ability of the tumour to invade locally. It is unusual for myasthenia to improve following surgery and immunosuppressive treatment is usually required.

Myotonias

These conditions are characterized by myotonia, i.e. continued muscle contraction after cessation of voluntary effort. They are important because the patients tolerate general anaesthetics poorly. The two most common forms are dystrophia myotonica and myotonia congenita, described below.

Dystrophia myotonica

Dystrophia myotonica is an autosomal dominant condition characterized by progressive distal muscle weakness with myotonia, ptosis, facial muscle weakness and thinning. Other features commonly present are cataracts, frontal baldness, cardiomyopathy, mild mental handicap, glucose intolerance and hypogonadism.

Myotonia congenita

Myotonia congenita is also an autosomal dominant disorder characterized by mild isolated myotonia occurring in childhood and persisting throughout life. The myotonia is often accentuated by rest and cold.

DEMENTIA AND DELIRIUM

Delirium (toxic confusional state)

Delirium is an acute or subacute condition in which impairment of consciousness is accompanied by abnormalities of perception and mood. Impairment of consciousness can vary in severity and often fluctuates (compare with dementia). Confusion is usually worse at night and may be accompanied by hallucinations, delusions, restlessness and aggression. Many diseases (Table 14.24) can be accompanied by delirium, particularly in the elderly patient.

Management

Investigation and treatment of the underlying disease should be undertaken. General measures include withdrawing all drugs where possible, rehydration, and adequate pain relief and sedation. Benzodiazepines are usually the drugs of choice although, in severe delirium, intramuscular haloperidol may be preferred.

Table 14.24 Some causes of delirium

Systemic infection	
Drug/alcohol withdrawal	
Metabolic disturbance	Hepatic failure
	Renal failure
	Disorders of electrolyte balance
	Hypoxia
	Hypoglycaemia
Vitamin deficiency	Vitamin B_{12}
	Vitamin B_1 (Wernicke–Korsakoff syndrome)
Brain damage	Trauma
	Tumour
	Abscess
	Subarachnoid haemorrhage
Drug intoxication	Anticonvulsants
	Anticholinergics
	Anxiolytics/hypnotics
	Opiates

Dementia

Dementia is characterized by a disturbance of multiple higher cortical functions, including memory, thinking, orientation, comprehension, calculation, learning capacity, language and judgement. Consciousness is not, however, clouded. Dementia affects about 10% of those aged 65 years and over, and 20% of those over 80 years of age. There are numerous causes of dementia (Table 14.25), although by far the most common is Alzheimer's disease which accounts for 70%.

Table 14.25 Some common causes of dementia

Alzheimer's disease
Multiple cerebral infarction
Alcohol (Wernicke–Korsakoff syndrome)
Hypothyroidism
Intracranial mass, subdural haematoma, hydrocephalus
Chronic traumatic encephalopathy
Sub acute combined degeneration of the cord
General paralysis of the insane

Alzheimer's disease

Alzheimer's disease is a primary degenerative cerebral disease of unknown aetiology. A relationship with the ingestion or accumulation of aluminium has been suggested though not proven.

Clinical features

There is an insidious onset with steady progression over years. Memory loss is usually the most prominent early symptom, but subsequently there is slow disintegration of the personality and intellect, eventually affecting all aspects of cortical function. There are characteristic pathological features which include neuronal reduction in several areas of the brain, neurofibrillary tangles, argentophile plaques, consisting largely of amyloid protein, and granulovacuolar bodies.

Investigations

The presence of dementia is usually diagnosed clinically, although secondary causes should be excluded by the appropriate investigations (see Table 14.25). CT or MRI will confirm the presence of cortical atrophy and exclude lesions such as brain tumours.

Management

In most cases there is no specific treatment, although associated anxiety and depression often need treatment. Patients should be managed in the community as much as possible with appropriate support and help for carers.

Vascular (multi-infarct) dementia

This is the second most common cause of dementia and can be distinguished by its history of onset, clinical features and subsequent course. There is usually a history of transient ischaemic attacks although the dementia may follow a succession of acute cerebrovascular accidents or, less commonly, a single major stroke.

DICTIONARY OF TERMS: NEUROLOGY

APRAXIA is loss of the ability to carry out familiar purposeful movements in the absence of paralysis or other motor or sensory impairment.

Constructional apraxia is inability to copy simple drawings and is often seen in hepatic encephalopathy (page 85) when the patient is unable to copy a five-pointed star.

ATAXIA is due to failure of coordination of complex muscular movements despite intact individual movements and sensation.

APHASIA (dysphasia) means a disturbance of the ability to use language whether in speaking, writing or comprehending. It is caused by left frontoparietal lesions, often a stroke.

Broca's aphasia (expressive aphasia) is due to a lesion in the left frontal lobe. There is reduced fluency of speech with comprehension relatively preserved. The patient knows what he/she wants to say but cannot get the words out.

Wernicke's aphasia (receptive aphasia) is due to a left temperoparietal lesion. The patient speaks fluently but words are put together in the wrong order and in the most severe forms the patient speaks complete rubbish with the insertion of non-existent words. Comprehension is severely impaired.

Global aphasia is due to widespread damage to the areas concerned with speech. The patient shows combined expressive and receptive dysphasia.

DYSARTHRIA is disordered articulation. Any lesion that produces paralysis, slowing or incoordination of the muscles of articulation, or local discomfort will cause dysarthria. Examples are upper and lower motor lesions of the lower cranial nerves (page 458), cerebellar lesions (page 460), Parkinson's disease and local lesions in the mouth, larynx, pharynx and tongue.

LUMBAR PUNCTURE (LP) is used for obtaining samples of cerebrospinal fluid (CSF). Under aseptic conditions a long hollow needle is inserted between the spines of two lumbar vertebrae (usually third and fourth) into the spinal cavity and a few mls of CSF is allowed to drip into specimen containers. Normal CSF is clear and colourless. Specimens of CSF are always sent for microscopy and culture, protein content and glucose concentration (interpreted in relation to plasma concentration). Additional optional investigations are oligoclonal bands (?MS), syphilis serology, cytology, microscopy and culture for acid fast bacilli. LP is contraindicated in the presence of raised intracranial pressure.

ELECTROENCEPHALOGRAM (EEG). Electrodes applied to the patient's scalp pick up small changes in electrical potential which after amplification are recorded on paper or displayed on a video monitor. It is used in the investigation of epilepsy and diffuse brain disorders.

ELECTROMYOGRAPHY (EMG). A needle electrode is inserted percutaneously into voluntary muscle. The amplified recording of action potentials is recorded on an oscilloscope. Normal resting muscle shows no activity and during increasing muscle contractions progressively larger numbers of motor units are recruited. EMG is useful in the diagnosis of primary muscle disease (myopathies and dystrophies, individual motor unit potentials are small) and of lower motor neuron lesions (denervation, spontaneous activity appears at rest).

FINAL MEDICINE EXAMINATION: NEUROLOGY

All aspects of neurology are covered in the final examination; the most common questions cover the causes and management of stroke/transient ischaemic attacks, coma, dementia, delerium and epilepsy. The differential diagnosis of a patient presenting with weak legs also occurs commonly.

1. A lady of seventy wakes one morning with weakness in the right arm and some difficulty in speaking. The symptoms are present the following day and her family bring her to the Accident and Emergency Department. What are the likely causes? How would you manage this patient and what information would you give to the patient and relatives?

2. A man of 65 years suddenly develops weakness and numbness of the left arm, which gradually passes off after 15 minutes. What are the likely causes? How might they be investigated?

3. A 40-year-old man is brought into accident and emergency unconscious and smelling of alcohol. Describe your management.

4. Outline some potentially treatable or reversible causes of apparent dementia. What features of the history and clinical findings might arouse your suspicions?

5. Describe the clinical features of grand mal epilepsy and the investigations which may help to confirm the diagnosis.

6. A 23-year-old woman was admitted on Christmas Eve with a two day history of symmetrical leg weakness and paraesthesiae. Later she was unable to sit up in bed and reported difficulty in coughing and stiffness of the face.

   (a) What is the likely diagnosis?

   (b) What confirmatory tests are possible?

   (c) What complications may arise?

   (d) What is the prognosis?

7. Describe the symptoms, signs and causes of spinal cord compression.

Other questions which occur commonly are:

8. Describe the **three** main clinical features of idiopathic Parkinson's disease. Discuss briefly **three**

different types of pharmacological treatment used in this condition.

9. What are the features of Horner's syndrome? Briefly describe the anatomical pathways involved. What underlying causes may be responsible?

10. Give **three** common causes of ptosis and mention the associated features in each case.

ANSWERS

1. The history is of sudden onset of right-sided weakness and dysphasia which is almost certainly due to a vascular lesion (i.e. stroke). The causes of stroke are discussed on page 468; in a lady of this age it is most likely to be due to thrombosis at the site of atheromatous degeneration in the middle cerebral artery (page 472). The investigations and treatment of stroke are discussed on pages 469–470. A brain CT will differentiate between infarction and haemorrhage. Aspirin is given to patients with infarction to reduce the risk of further attacks. The family must be told that some recovery of function is expected. Any recovery of speech is likely to be within the first few days.

2. This is a transient ischaemic attack (TIA) probably in the territory of the right middle cerebral artery. The causes and investigation of a TIA are listed on page 471.

3. Coma must never be ascribed to excess alcohol until a thorough history (from relatives, ambulance staff), physical examination and investigation have ruled out other causes. The initial management consists of emergency resuscitation to stabilize the patient (page 463). Intravenous glucose and thiamine (see later) are given. Further assessment (page 464) and investigations (page 465) are performed to find the cause of coma. The most likely causes (Table 14.6) in this case are alcohol, drug overdose (with alcohol as a second agent), hypoglycaemia, intracerebral haemorrhage, infarction and Wernicke–Korsakoff syndrome (page 385). Further management consists of treatment of the underlying cause and care of the unconscious patient (page 464).

4. The causes of dementia are listed in Table 14.25. Treatable causes include hypothyroidism, vitamin

B_{12} deficiency, uraemia, hepatic failure, operable cerebral tumour, subdural haematoma and normal pressure hydrocephalus (page 491). Depression may produce a clinical picture that is indistinguishable from dementia (*pseudodementia*) and resolves with treatment. Neurosyphilis (page 488) and Wernicke–Korsakoff syndrome (page 385) may cause dementia; treatment should always be given as the disease process may be arrested but rarely reversed. Young age, focal neurological signs, a history of head injury and evidence of anaemia or hypothyroidism should arouse suspicion that this is not Alzheimer's disease (the usual cause of dementia).

5. The clinical features and investigation of grand mal epilepsy are discussed on pages 475–476.

6. The distal weakness progressing proximally is the typical picture of Guillain–Barré syndrome or acute inflammatory neuropathy (page 502). The difficulty in coughing and facial stiffness is due to early respiratory and facial muscle weakness. Diagnosis is made clinically, by nerve conduction studies and examination of the CSF obtained at lumbar puncture (page 508). Most patients make a complete recovery eventually but during the illness some patients develop respiratory failure and require ventilation. Other complications include those which occur in bed-bound patients, e.g. hypostatic pneumonia, bed sores and infections.

7. This is discussed on page 496.

8. The clinical features and treatment of Parkinson's disease are described on page 480.

9. The features and causes of Horner's syndrome are described on page 451.

10. The causes of ptosis are third nerve lesions (usually complete unilateral ptosis with other eye signs, page 453), sympathetic paralysis (partial unilateral ptosis with other features of a Horner's syndrome, page 451), myopathy (partial bilateral), congenital (present since birth, usually partial, no other neurological signs) and syphilis (tabes dorsalis, page 489).

CHAPTER 15

Dermatology

Introduction

Skin diseases are extremely common although their exact prevalence is unknown. There are over 1000 different entities described but two-thirds of all cases are the result of fewer than ten conditions. The most common conditions include acne, eczema, psoriasis, warts and infections caused by bacteria, fungi and viruses. Some conditions may be part of normal development, e.g. acne, others may be inherited, e.g. Ehlers–Danlos syndrome, whereas others are part of a systemic disease, e.g. the rash of systemic lupus erythematosus (page 172).

Only the most common skin conditions will be described in the following sections.

For description of other skin diseases please see [CM p. 993].

ACNE VULGARIS

Acne vulgaris is a common condition affecting almost 90% of adolescents. It is thought to result from hyperactivity of the sebaceous glands leading to increased production of sebum with blockage of the follicular openings and formation of comedones (blackheads), inflammatory papules, nodules and cysts. Normal skin bacteria, principally *Propionibacterium acnes*, within the blocked follicle are capable of producing pro-inflammatory mediators and lipolytic enzymes which may be responsible for producing the clinical lesions.

Clinical features

The 'blackhead' or comedo is the common first-stage lesion, the pigmentation being provided by melanin from the hair. Closed comedones or 'whiteheads' are flesh-coloured lesions which represent obstructed follicles. They are often the forerunners of the more severe manifestations such as papules, pustules, nodules and cysts. Lesions are most commonly seen on the face, chest and back.

Management

Acne should be actively treated to avoid unnecessary scarring and psychological distress. There are a variety of approaches to treatment, the choice of which depends on the severity of the disease.

LOCAL APPLICATIONS such as abrasives, astringents or exfoliatives are useful in mild disease.

ANTIBIOTICS either given topically for mild disease or orally for inflammatory disease are often successful. Tetracyclines or erythromycin are most commonly used and treatment over several months is often necessary.

HORMONES may be useful in women, particularly the oral contraceptive pill or an antiandrogen such as cyproterone acetate.

ISOTRETINOIN (a vitamin A analogue given orally) is used in severe cystic disease that is unresponsive to other treatments. This drug is highly teratogenic and absolutely contraindicated during pregnancy.

PSORIASIS

Psoriasis is a chronic hyperproliferative disorder, characterized by the presence of well-demarcated silvery scaled plaques over extensor surfaces such as the elbows and knees, and in the scalp. It can affect any group with equal sex incidence and occurs in about 2% of people in temperate zones.

Aetiology
The cause of the condition is unknown although genetic factors are felt to be important. It is associated with several HLA-specific antigens, particularly HLA-CW6. Trigger factors in genetically susceptible individuals include infections (particularly streptococcal infections), local trauma, drugs such as lithium carbonate and β-blockers, and probably also stress.

Clinical features
Several clinical patterns are recognized:

- Plaque psoriasis is the most common, occurring as well-demarcated, salmon-pink, silvery, scaling lesions on the extensor surfaces of the limbs, particularly the elbows and knees. Scalp involvement is common, and is most often seen at the hair margin or over the occiput. Nail involvement, which can occur alone or in association with psoriasis elsewhere, is manifest as pitting and onycholysis (separation of the nail from the underlying vascular bed). The arthropathy associated with psoriasis is described on page 170

- Flexural psoriasis presents as pinkish glazed lesions which are well demarcated and non-scaly. The groin, perianal and genital skin are most commonly involved

- Pustular psoriasis affects the palms or soles most commonly. There are areas of well-demarcated scaling and erythema associated with white, yellow or green pustule formation. Identical features are seen as one of the cutaneous features of Reiter's syndrome (keratoderma blenorrhagica, page 169)

- Erythrodermic psoriasis is a severe and potentially life-threatening condition. The trunk and limbs may be involved by an almost universal scaling, sometimes associated with generalized pustule formation. This disease occurs classically following corticosteroid therapy

Management

The approach to treatment depends on the severity of the disease. As no treatment is universally effective, simple local treatment is used for mild disease with systemic therapy reserved for severe or pustular psoriasis.

LOCAL THERAPY: coal tar, dithranol (inhibits DNA synthesis), topical corticosteroids, or calcipotriol (topical vitamin D_3) may all be useful for relatively mild disease and are suitable for use on an outpatient basis.

PUVA: psoralens (photosensitizing agents taken by mouth) and high intensity ultraviolet (UV) A light are usually highly effective for treating extensive psoriasis. Repeated treatments, however, carry the risk of UV-induced skin cancer.

SYSTEMIC THERAPY: oral retinoic acid derivatives, e.g. acitretin, are useful in severe or pustular psoriasis, although these agents are potentially toxic and also teratogenic. They should not therefore be used in women of child-bearing years. Immunosuppressive and cytotoxic agents, e.g. methotrexate, azathioprine, and cyclosporin are useful in severe intractable disease although toxicity often limits their long-term use.

ECZEMA

Eczema is characterized by superficial skin inflammation with vesicles (when acute), redness, oedema, oozing, scaling and usually pruritus. The terms 'dermatitis' and 'eczema' are usually used interchangeably as both conditions show similar inflammatory changes in the skin.

Eczema may arise from several different stimuli but most commonly it is classified as:

- Endogenous (atopic) eczema
- Exogenous eczema from allergy or chemical irritation

Atopic eczema

Aetiology

The cause of this condition is unknown, although there is a capacity to hyperreact to many environmental factors. There are high levels of serum IgE antibodies although their significance in contributing to the pathogenesis is unclear. There is also a significant hereditary predisposition.

Clinical features

The disease may start in the first few weeks of life with erythema, weeping, itching and scaling. In adults, the flexures at the neck, elbow, wrist and knee are commonly involved.

Management

The offending agents should be removed if possible. Regular use of emollients such as aqueous cream or emulsifying ointments is useful in hydrating the skin. Corticosteroid creams, e.g. 1% hydrocortisone, form the mainstay of treatment.

Exogenous eczema (contact dermatitis)

In this condition there is acute or chronic skin inflammation, often sharply demarcated, produced by substances in contact with the skin. The dermatitis may be caused by a primary chemical irritant, or may be the result of a type IV hypersensitivity reaction. Common chemical irritants are industrial solvents used in the workplace or cleaning and detergent solutions used in the home. With allergic dermatitis there is sensitization of T lymphocytes over a period of time which results in itching and dermatitis upon re-exposure to the antigen.

Clinical features

An unusual pattern of rash with clear-cut demarcation or odd shaped areas of erythema and scaling should arouse suspicion and, in combination with a careful history, should indicate a cause. Patch testing, where the suspected allergen is placed in contact with the skin, is often useful in identifying a suspected allergen.

Management

Causative agents should be removed where possible. Steroid creams are useful for short periods in severe disease. Antipruritic agents are used for symptomatic relief of itching.

ERYTHEMA NODOSUM

Erythema nodosum is an acute and sometimes recurrent paniculitis which produces painful nodules or plaques on the shins with occasional spread to the thighs or arms. Adult females are most commonly affected. Histological features suggest that this is an immunological reaction with immune complex deposition within dermal vessels. In 50% no obvious cause is found. Other causes are listed in Table 15.1.

Clinical features

Painful nodules or plaques up to 5 cm in diameter appear in crops over 2 weeks and slowly fade to leave bruising and staining of the skin. Systemic upset is common with malaise, fever and arthralgia.

Table 15.1 Some causes of erythema nodosum

Drugs	Sulphonamides
	Oral contraceptive pill
	Penicillin
Systemic diseases	Sarcoidosis
	Inflammatory bowel disease
Infection	Bacteria and viruses
	Streptococcal
	Tuberculosis
	Leprosy
	Cat scratch disease
	Tularaemia
	Chlamydia spp.
	Psittacosis
	Lymphogranuloma venereum
	Fungal
	Histoplasmosis
	Coccidioidomycosis
	Blastomycosis
Pregnancy	

The most common causes are highlighted.

Management
NSAIDs such as indomethacin should be given to lessen the pain associated with cutaneous and joint symptoms. Recovery may take weeks and recurrent attacks can occur.

ERYTHEMA MULTIFORME

This is an acute self-limiting condition affecting the skin and mucosal surfaces which is probably related to the deposition of immune complexes. Children and young adults are most commonly affected. The disease is commonly associated with:

● Herpes simplex infection

● *Mycoplasma pneumoniae*

● Drugs, e.g. sulphonamides, sulphonylureas and barbiturates

● Connective tissue diseases

Clinical features
Symmetrically distributed erythematous papules occur most commonly on the back of the hands, palms and forearms. The lesions may show central pallor associated with oedema, bullae formation and peripheral erythema. Severe mucosal

disease may predominate in, for example, infection with *Mycoplasma pneumoniae*. Eye changes include conjunctivitis, corneal ulceration and uveitis.

The Stevens–Johnson syndrome describes a severe erythema multiforme with oral and genital ulceration and marked constitutional symptoms.

Management

The disease is usually self-limiting although the Stevens–Johnson syndrome can be fatal. Offending drugs should be withdrawn and the underlying disease treated. In severe cases, intravenous fluids and feeding may be required.

OTHER DISEASES AFFECTING THE SKIN

Marfan's syndrome

Marfan's syndrome is an autosomal dominant disorder of collagen synthesis. Fragility of the skin may lead to bruising. The most obvious abnormalities are skeletal: tall stature, arm span greater than height, arachnodactyly (long spidery fingers), sternal depression, lax joints and high arched palate. There is often upward dislocation of the lens as a result of weakness of the suspensory ligament. Cardiovascular complications (ascending aortic aneurysm formation, aortic dissection and aortic valve incompetence) are responsible for a greatly reduced lifespan.

Ehlers–Danlos syndrome

Inherited defects of collagen lead to fragility and hyperelasticity of skin with easy bruising, 'paper-thin' scars and hypermobility of joints. The wall of the aorta and gut are weak and may rarely rupture with catastrophic results.

Neurofibromatosis

Neurofibromatosis is an autosomal dominant disease with distinctive clinical features.

Type 1 (von Recklinghausen's disease) with the abnormal gene on chromosome 17. Clinical features include multiple cutaneous neurofibromas, multiple café-au-lait spots (light-brown macules of varying size), axillary freckling, scoliosis, and an increased incidence of a variety of neural tumours, e.g. meningioma, eighth nerve tumours, gliomas.

Type 2 with the abnormal gene on chromosome 22. Typically bilateral acoustic neuromas and other neural tumours.

DICTIONARY OF TERMS: DERMATOLOGY

ANNULAR LESIONS: lesions occurring in rings
ATROPHY: thinning of the skin
BULLA: a large vesicle
CRUST: dried exudate on the skin

ECCHYMOSES: bruises > 3 mm in diameter

ERYTHEMA: redness

ERYTHRODERMA: widespread redness of the skin with scaling

EXCORIATION: linear marks caused by scratching

MACULE: a flat circumscribed area of discoloration

MACULOPAPULE: a raised and discoloured circumscribed lesion

NODULE: a circumscribed large palpable mass > 1 cm in diameter

PAPULE: a circumscribed raised palpable area

PETECHIAE: bruises < 3 mm in diameter

PLAQUE: a disc-shaped lesion; can result from coalescence of papules

PURPURA: extravasation of blood into the skin; does not blanche on pressure

PUSTULE: a pus-filled blister

SCALES: dried flakes of dead skin

TELANGIECTASIA: a visible, small, dilated vessel on the skin

VESICLE: a small, visible, fluid-filled blister

WEAL: a transiently raised reddened area associated with scratching

FINAL MEDICINE EXAMINATION: DERMATOLOGY

1. What are the features and common causes of erythema nodosum? How would you investigate a patient with this condition?
2. Write short notes on the management of psoriasis.

ANSWERS

1. This is by far the most common question related to dermatology. The causes and clinical features of erythema nodosum are listed on page 517. Sarcoidosis and inflammatory bowel disease are the most common causes in the UK. A history of recent antibiotic ingestion, oral contraceptives or alteration in bowel habit should be sought. Basic investigations should include a full blood count, ESR and chest radiograph. Further investigations will depend on the history and associated clinical findings. In a patient who is otherwise well and with a single attack, further investigation may be unnecessary.
2. The management of psoriasis is outlined on page 515.

Index